Sports Biomechanics: Analyzing Human Movement

Sports Biomechanics: Analyzing Human Movement

Edited by Preston Hickey

SYRAWOOD
PUBLISHING HOUSE
New York

Published by Syrawood Publishing House,
750 Third Avenue, 9th Floor,
New York, NY 10017, USA
www.syrawoodpublishinghouse.com

Sports Biomechanics: Analyzing Human Movement
Edited by Preston Hickey

International Standard Book Number: 978-1-64740-254-9 (Hardback)

Cataloging-in-Publication Data

Sports biomechanics : analyzing human movement / edited by Preston Hickey.
p. cm.
Includes bibliographical references and index.
ISBN 978-1-64740-254-9
1. Human mechanics. 2. Sports--Physiological aspects. 3. Biomechanics. 4. Kinesiology.
5. Human physiology. I. Hickey, Preston.
QP303 .S66 2022
612.76--dc23

TABLE OF CONTENTS

PREFACE

The study of the function, structure and motion of the mechanical aspects of biological systems using methods of mechanics is known as biomechanics. Sports biomechanics seeks to employ the principles of biomechanics to analyze and assess human movement during sports. The primary functions of this field are minimizing the risk of sports related injuries and optimizing the performance of the players. Sports biomechanics analyzes body loading to ascertain the safest technique for performing a particular sport. Some of the tools used in this field are mathematical modeling, computer simulation and measurement. Sports biomechanics is an upcoming field of science that has undergone rapid development over the past few decades. The topics included in this book about this field are of utmost significance and bound to provide incredible insights to readers. Those in search of information to further their knowledge will be greatly assisted by this book.

After months of intensive research and writing, this book is the end result of all who devoted their time and efforts in the initiation and progress of this book. It will surely be a source of reference in enhancing the required knowledge of the new developments in the area. During the course of developing this book, certain measures such as accuracy, authenticity and research focused analytical studies were given preference in order to produce a comprehensive book in the area of study.

This book would not have been possible without the efforts of the authors and the publisher. I extend my sincere thanks to them. Secondly, I express my gratitude to my family and well-wishers. And most importantly, I thank my students for constantly expressing their willingness and curiosity in enhancing their knowledge in the field, which encourages me to take up further research projects for the advancement of the area.

Editor

1

ADDRESSING THE PHYSICAL ACTIVITY OF THE CHILDREN THAT DIFFERENTIATE THEM FROM THE ADULTS

Andrei DUMITRU

Faculty of Sciences

Department of Kinethic Therapy and Medical Assistance

University of Pitesti

Correspondence address: padrefortete@yahoo.com

Abstract: *The purpose* of this paper is to describe the measurement issues that complicate assessments of the physical activity specifically in children. Some of the issues are common to the challenges for any population but other factors stem from the unique developmental and behavioral aspects of children. Emphasis in this paper is on issues for pre-adolescent children since challenges in activity assessments are greater for younger children. While many issues remain for adolescents, they tend to become cognitively and behaviorally more similar to adults by the time they reach high school. By narrowing the focus on younger children we hope to address the substantive issues for assessments in young children in greater detail.

The goal is to health benefits through physical activity. The health benefits for adults are established through Public Health Departments. Similar links with children are not as well established since it takes time for unhealthy behaviors to influence chronic disease. Nevertheless, there has been tremendous interest in assessing and promoting physical activity among children. Much of this interest stems from the highly publicized increases in the prevalence of pediatric obesity. Studies have documented the important role that physical activity plays in weight control and significant tracking coefficients have been observed for obesity, coronary risk factors and physical activity/inactivity among youth.

The techniques for bringing on health are a numerous. They have been used to assess physical activity in a variety of populations (self-report, activity monitors, pedometers, heart rate monitors, doubly labeled water, and indirect calorimetry) and others that have been developed specifically for children (direct observation). Each of the measures has specific advantages and disadvantages that must be considered when selecting an instrument.

Key words: *self-reporting, activity monitors, observations, validity, movement patterns, kinetic program*

INTRODUCTION

The center to the understanding of some accurate assessment techniques of any population is a clear understanding of the nature of the individual or individuals being studied. Therefore, we will first describe the unique aspects of children's movement patterns and how these patterns influence the various measurement approaches used to assess physical activity. Next, we will review the current physical activity guidelines for children and clarify why it is important to use appropriate criteria when making determinations about the physical activity levels of children. Finally, we will review some of the more common physical assessment tools to determine the usefulness of each in studying children's physical activity [1].

Table 1. Characteristics That Differentiate Children From Adults in Physical Activity

Type	Characteristic	Implication
Biological	Need for high level of central nervous system arousal	•High volume of physical activity is typical •Low tolerance for total inactivity •Spontaneous activity is common
Cognitive Functioning	More concrete (less abstract) thought process	•Relatively short attention span on any given task •Less interest in continuous activity •Failure to see long term benefits of activity (e.g. health benefits)

	Less developed cognition	•Less accurate recall •Inability to accurately estimate time
Physiological	Limited tolerance for vigorous physical activity	•Activity typically intermittent in nature
	Weak relationship between fitness and physical activity	•Effort (active behavior) does not necessarily result in increases in fitness thus positive feedback for active behavior is lacking
Biomechanical	Poorer economy and efficiency of movement	•Quicker onset of fatigue, and need for frequent rest •Less interest in continuous activity
Psychological: (the "kid" factor)	More available free time	•More time to try new activities
	Natural curiosity and desire for pursuing new tasks	•Interest in exploring new activities

The Unique Nature of Children's Physical Activity Patterns

Several recent papers have provided insights as to the unique nature of children with respect to their propensity for physical activity. It was suggested a biological basis for the differences in activity patterns between children and adults. Children are inherently active primarily because it is physical movement that provides them with the necessary information required by the central nervous system for stimulation. Adults, on the other hand, achieve arousal of the central nervous system in a variety of non-locomotor activities such as reading, writing, artistic expression, problem solving, and vocational pursuits. The fact that children of nearly all animal species are more active than adult populations supports this idea, namely that children have an inherent biological need to be active.

An observational insight into the nature of children's activity habits will make us have a better understanding. Using a coding system calibrated against indirect calorimetry, it was recorded the intensity of children's activity every 3 s over a 12-hour period. Thus was allowed to characterize the "tempo" of physical activity in children, which was described as the natural variation in rate and intensity of activity events as well as the intervals between activity events. The median duration of low and moderate intensity activities were 6 s while the duration for high intensity activities were 3 s. Nearly all bouts of vigorous activity (95%) lasted less than 15 s and only 0.1% of the bouts were longer than a minute. No bout of high intensity activity longer than 10 minutes was recorded. The median duration between high intensity activities was 18 seconds, but ranged between 3 s and 21 min. Periods of rest were clearly long in proportion to periods of activity, but 95% of the 'rest' intervals were less than 4 min. and 15 s. This indicates that children do not remain inactive for extended periods of time. Collectively, these findings clearly document the highly transitory nature of children's physical activity. The authors suggest that short, intermittent bouts of vigorous physical activity (with frequent rest periods of longer duration) are typical of children and, in fact, may be necessary for normal growth and development [8].

Table 2. A Summary of Physical Activity Guidelines for Children

Guideline	Implications
Elementary school children should accumulate at least 30-60 minutes of age appropriate physical activity on all, or most days of the week.	•Children need longer periods of time in activity than adults (minimum standards). •Children are likely to accumulate activity in many intermittent activity bouts rather than single bouts of continuous activity.
An accumulation of more than 60 minutes and up to several hours per day of appropriate activities is encouraged for	•Sixty minutes (see guideline 1) is a minimum standard.

school aged children.	
Some of the child's activity each day should be in periods lasting 10 to 15 minutes or more and include moderate to vigorous activity. This activity will typically be intermittent in nature involving alternating moderate to vigorous activity with brief periods of rest and recovery.	•Some relatively long periods of time (at least 10-15 minutes) are necessary for children though activity need not be continuous or highly structured. •Both moderate and vigorous activity is necessary but is likely to be in intermittent spurts.
Extended periods of inactivity are discouraged for children.	•Activity sessions throughout the day are desirable and consistent with the developmental needs of children.
A variety of physical activities from the Physical Activity Pyramid are recommended.	•Children need variety to meet developmental needs and to retain interest in activity.

The guidelines of National Association for Sport and Physical Education on physical activity for children focus on the volume of activity and emphasize that intermittent activity is more likely to characterize their behavior than continuous activity. This document also highlights a number of other cognitive and behavioral differences between adults and children that should be considered when studying or promoting physical activity in children (see Table 1).

Each of the characteristics described in Table 1 also has implications for the assessment of physical activity. The fact that children have different patterns of activity (intermittent vs. continuous) necessitates that different intervals of assessment and/or outcome measures be used to assess their levels of activity. The less developed cognitive skills of children (characterized by concrete thinking) results in a lesser ability to effectively use self-report questionnaires. Biological differences in metabolism and biomechanical differences in efficiency and economy require different assumptions for measurement techniques that aim to estimate energy expended in physical activity. The implications of these various characteristics of children for each of the more common assessment techniques will be discussed later in this paper.

Unique Activity Guidelines for Children

Just as the unique characteristics of children should be considered when making decisions about the method of physical assessment so too should the unique expectations for children in activity to be considered .The need to assess physical activity in any population is based on the desire to determine the current activity status of that population and to determine if that population is meeting activity criteria that are appropriate for optimal health and development. For years, the activity guidelines for children were assumed to be similar to those recommended for adults. These guidelines generally indicated that activity must be of vigorous intensity for continuous periods of time (20+ minutes) to provide benefits. Some methods indicate (at 60% of heart rate reserve), a heart rate of 159 or 160 was calculated as a target for children. A consensus review of activity guidelines later indicated that heart rates of 139-140 were sufficient to define the threshold for activity in children. Both levels have been used in a number of studies to characterize children's activity levels, but the level of 140 has had more widespread usage.

Recently, there has been a shift toward the promotion of moderate-intensity physical activity for adults. This shift is based on the repeated observation that significant health benefits are obtained from modest levels of physical. The concept of accumulating intermittent activity is clearly consistent with children's normal movement patterns; however, most recommendations for 'lifestyle physical activity' are intended and designed for adults (e.g., incorporating stair climbing and yard work activities into one's daily routine). This model incorporates normal, intermittent free play as part of a child's natural activity and specifies how much activity children need on a regular basis (see Table 2). The recent physical activity guidelines for children are based conceptually and philosophically on this model. Similar guidelines for children have been developed in Europe [3]. These guidelines should be considered by those interested in the study of physical activity in children. Those interested in the study of physical activity in adolescents are referred to guidelines established by a recent international consensus group.

Table 3. Results of Selected Studies Characterizing Activity Levels in Children: A Comparison of Different Criteria and Measures.

Lead Author	Participants	Methods	Criterion	Results
		Heart Rate Monitoring Studies		
	163 boys and 107 girls ages 11-16	Continuous heart rate monitoring (12 hours)	• % of children with HR > 139 for 20 consecutive minutes • % of children with HR > 139 for 3, 5-minute bouts • Total number of minutes with HR > 139 (weekday)	• Girls: 12% active Boys: 23% active • Girls: 53% Boys: 70% • Girls: 32 minutes Boys: 45 minutes
	65 girls and 67 boys ages 10-11	Continuous heart rate monitoring (12 hours)	• % of children with HR > 139 for 20 consecutive minutes • % of children with HR > 139 for 3, 5-minute bouts • Total number of minutes with HR >139 (weekday)	• Girls: 34% active Boys: 39% • Girls: 85% Boys: 90% • Girls: 59 minutes Boys: 68 minutes
	43 girls and 86 boys ages 10-11	Continuous heart rate monitoring (12 hours/day over 3 days)	• % of children with HR > 139 for 20 consecutive minutes • % of children with HR > 139 for 3, 5-minute bouts • % of children with HR > 159 for 3, 5-minute bouts	• Girls: 37% Boys: 39.5% • Girls: 88% Boys: 92% • Girls: 70% Boys 79%
	18 girls and 22 boys ages 6-7	Continuous heart rate monitoring (12 hours)	• Total number of minutes with HR > 160 • Total number of minutes with HR > 140	• Girls: 9 minutes Boys: 21 minutes • Girls: 30 minutes Boys: 56 minutes
	76 girls and boys ages 6-17	Continuous heart rate monitoring (8-11 hours)	• % of children with HR > 60% of age predicted max for 20 minutes • Total number of minutes with HR > 60% of age predicted max ~ 155 bpm	• Total: 7% active • Total: 15 minutes
		Direct Observation Studies		
	14 girls and 10 boys ages 8-12	Direct observation on two days (12 hours)[1]	• % of children active for 20 consecutive minutes • % of children active for 14 minutes with only 1 stop or break • Total number of minutes of activity *(reported for those who were "active")*	• 8-13% of children • 58-63% of children • 61-71 total minutes of activity
	27 girls and 29 boys	Direct observation[2]	• % of children active for 20 consecutive minutes	• 14% of children active

		• % of children active for 10 consecutive minutes • Total minutes of activity	• 46% of children active • 88.5 minutes
Self-Report Instruments			
49 girls ages 8-11	Self-report of previous year	• Average minutes per day in moderate activity ≥ 4 METs	• 96.7 minutes
336 5th grade children	Two activity assessments 1. 24 hr recall 2. 16-item survey	• Number of minutes of moderate physical activity ≥ 6 METs computed with two measures	• Minutes per day for treatment and control groups 1. 72-82 minutes 2. 89-99 minutes
45 children (25 girls and 20 boys) in grades 6-8	Computerized activity recall	• Number of minutes of physical activity (no specification of intensity)	• Girls: 85 minutes Boys: 67 minutes
995 boys and girls ages 9-15	Self-Report of previous day (SAPAC)	• Number of minutes of physical activity	• Total: 168 minutes
National sample of 5th and 6th grade	Parent report of child's activity[3]	• % of children performing regular activity • Number of minutes of physical activity	• Girls: 49% Boys: 56% Total: 102-120 minutes
2410 3rd grade children	Activity Interview with a log	• Number of minutes of moderate to vigorous activity a day	• Girls: 83 minutes Boys: 97 minutes

[1]Activity defined as continuous slow or fast trunk movements
[2]Activity defined as being commensurate with a heart rate of 140 bpm
[3]Activity defined as "exercise involving large muscle groups in dynamic movement for periods of 20 minutes or longer 3 or more times a week."

Characterizing Activity Levels in Children

If the assessment of physical activity patterns of children is the goal, the standard used to define "being active" becomes highly relevant. Failure to use appropriate standards can lead to significant misinterpretations of both individual and group assessments of physical activity. Interpretations of studies on activity levels in children also can vary widely depending on what type of assessment is used. Some examples illustrate the importance of these issues for characterizing activity levels in children [4].

Prior to the development of specific physical activity standards for children, many studies were conducted to evaluate the habitual activity levels of children. To provide objective information about activity patterns, a number of studies used heart rate monitors or direct observation techniques. While varying slightly across the studies, the criteria in nearly all studies emphasized sustained aerobic activity for at least 10 minutes in duration. The percentage of children defined as "physically active" ranged from 8 to 39% depending on gender and nationality of the sample (see Table 3) leading most authors to conclude that children do not perform enough activity to obtain significant health benefits.

A different interpretation from these studies is possible when the data are examined using more current activity guidelines. In the two original studies, the majority of children (53-70% of 11-16-year-olds and 85-90% of 10-11-year-olds) had at least three 5-minute bouts of activity during the day. The total minutes spent at heart rates > 40 bpm ranged from 31-68 minutes. Using the criteria of minutes > 50% max heart rate (~ 149 bpm), other studies have reported means ranging from 29 minutes to 70-80 minutes. These mean levels of activity generally indicate that children perform a reasonable volume of activity during the course of the day.

Table 4. Methods of Assessment and the Characteristics of Physical Activity That Can Be Assessed.

Method of	Units of Measurement	Type of Output	Output Measure

Measurement			
Questionnaire	Time segments (often 10, 15, 30 min segments	1. Frequency of PA 2. Intensity of PA 3. Duration of PA 4. EE of PA	1. # of bouts > criterion level 2. Number or % of bouts 3. # minutes > criterion level 4. Estimates based on METS
Heart Rate	Beats per minute	1. Frequency of PA 2. Intensity of PA 3. Duration of PA 4. EE of PA	1. # of bouts > criterion level 2. Average HR per day or interval 3. # minutes > criterion level 4. Estimates from calibration equations.
Motion Sensors	Movement counts	1. Frequency of PA 2. Intensity of PA 3. Duration of PA 4. EE of PA	1. # of bouts > criterion level 2. Average counts per day or interval 3. # minutes > criterion level 4. Estimates from calibration equations
Direct Observation	Activity rating	1. Frequency of PA 2. Intensity of PA 3. Duration of PA 4. EE of PA	1. # of bouts > criterion level 2. Number or % of bouts 3. # minutes > criterion level 4. Estimates based on METS
Pedometers	Step counts	1. Frequency of PA 2. Intensity of PA 3. Duration of PA 4. EE of PA	1. NA 2. NA 3. Number of steps taken 4. NA
Indirect Calorimetry	O_2 consumption	1. Frequency of PA 2. Intensity of PA 3. Duration of PA 4. EE of PA	1. # of bouts > criterion level 2. Average VO_2 level 3. Monitored time above threshold 4. Total energy expenditure

Similar differences in interpretation are evident in the studies employing direct observation techniques. Some reported that only 8-13% of children were active continuously for 20 minutes, but 58-63% were considered active when less stringent criteria (14 minutes with one stop) were used. Other studies found only 14% of children to be active for 20 consecutive minutes but 46% had at least one sustained bout for over 10 minutes. These discrepancies also suggest that children are more likely to perform more intermittent activity. If bouts of activity are used as a criterion measure, the duration to define a bout of activity should be no greater than 10 minutes [5].

A number of studies have also used self-report instruments to characterize activity levels in the population, both for intervention and surveillance purposes. Many studies reported that average minutes of activity per day are summarized to provide a comparison to the other studies using heart rate and direct observation (see Table 3). The mean minutes of activity in these studies ranged from 67 to 168 min. per day. Because the activity levels reported in these (and other) studies are consistently higher than those reported with other instruments, the general consensus is that there is a consistent overestimation of activity using self-report instruments. This tendency was described in a comprehensive review of different surveillance instruments. It has also been noted that other studies compare self-reports to other objective measures.

While some degree of overestimation from self-report forms may be attributed to an exaggerated perception of time and effort, a certain amount can also be attributed to the sporadic nature of children's activity patterns and the nature of children themselves. Children may indicate that they were active while playing a sport or game but may have only been moving for a portion of the time. This is a more typical pattern of activity for children and their concrete thought processes causing them to view even short bouts of activity as significant. It is difficult to speculate on the degree of overestimation in children and it is also not clear if it is a consistent trend for all children. Specific efforts in some studies have been made to avoid this type of overestimation; however, it is not clear how they influenced the results.

Collectively, these comparisons reveal that the results of activity monitoring studies can vary greatly depending on how activity is measured and interpreted. This variability makes difficult to make any firm conclusions about activity levels in children. Generalizing information about activity levels from group data is also complicated by the large inter-individual variability in activity habits among children. Using the studies reviewed in Table 3, the coefficients of variation (SD / mean) were generally found to range from 50%-93% for the various studies employing self-report measures (these values were not calculated for the heart rate and observation studies due to small sample sizes). Activity patterns from children also tend to be positively skewed. Thus, the mean values for an assessment may be biased by a few children performing a lot of physical activity or a large number performing very little. To provide a more comprehensive view of activity patterns, investigators are encouraged to report the median as well as the inter-quartile ranges in their data, in addition to traditional descriptive statistics. A number of specific measurement issues influencing each of the assessments will be described in more detail in the subsequent section [6].

Measurement Issues for Assessing Physical Activity in Children

As conventionally defined, the term 'physical activity' refers to "any bodily movement produced by skeletal muscles resulting in energy expenditure". In actual practice, the specific operational definition of physical activity depends on how it is measured and scored. The variables of frequency, intensity, and duration are commonly used to characterize activity patterns; another variable of interest is energy expenditure that is a summary variable that incorporates all of the other indicators. Table 4 lists the various methods and highlights the units of measurement and the conversions required for calculation of these components.

The frequency of physical activity participation is typically reported as number of bouts per day or week or the percentage of children being active on a given day. Obtaining these values requires an appropriate criterion to define what constitutes "regular activity" and what counts as a 'bout' of activity. As previously described, criteria that are based on more structured, adult-patterns of activity (3 or more bouts of continuous activity for 10 or 20 minutes) are not appropriate for children. A better criterion to define frequency would emphasize the accumulation of intermittent activity throughout the day. Depending on the approach used, an appropriate criterion for children may be the percentage that reports 2-3 bouts of short, intermittent activity totaling 30-60 minutes on at least 5 days a week. Because of the large intra-individual variability in activity, conclusions about typical activity patterns should not be drawn from 1 or 2 isolated days of measurement.

The intensity of physical activity is often used to categorize physical activity but is not commonly used as an outcome measure. Several studies have reported mean heart rates or mean activity counts during the day or portion. While this may be useful for statistical comparisons, the values themselves are difficult to interpret. Because the majority of a child's day is spent in resting or light activities, mean values would be low and would not provide meaningful information about their true activity level. If mean levels were reported for a group, the large intra-individual variability in activity patterns in children would make interpretations of the data even more difficult [7].

The duration of activity is generally reported in minutes or percentage of time spent being active. Alternately, the amount of activity may be calculated in conjunction with intensity categories. For example, it is common to see breakdowns of the number of minutes spent in different activity categories (light, moderate, or vigorous). With observational measures and self-report instruments, the distinctions among activity levels are established a-priori according to a specific coding strategy or established categories on a questionnaire. For heart rate and motion sensing devices, cut points must be established by comparing the activity values against data from other measures (e.g., heart rate).

Obtaining energy expenditure estimates from physical activity requires information about the metabolic costs of the activities that are performed. For observation and self-report measures, estimates are typically made using multiples of resting metabolic rate (METS). Because the MET values for various activities are not well established for children, the estimates using these calculations may not be highly accurate. For heart rate and motion sensors, a calibration equation is needed to convert the raw unit of measurement into energy expenditure values. These equations are typically developed under lab situations using structured activities and may not generalize to field-based activities. Thus, these estimations must also be interpreted with caution.

It is apparent from Table 4 that a number of different approaches can be used to obtain a similar outcome measure. The ease and accuracy of assessing these different components varies among each of the instruments. The advantages, disadvantages, and specific measurement issues for assessing children's activity behaviors will be described below.

Self-Report Instruments

Self-report instruments provide a convenient way to assess activity patterns on large populations. While they have been commonly used for a variety of research purposes, there is a widespread concern about the accuracy of self-report data from children. Most validation studies with children have reported only moderate correlations between various self-report forms and other objective criteria. The lack of strong correspondence and the described tendency for overestimation have led to the consensus that children can not provide accurate self-report information about their activity patterns. Efforts have been made to describe the cognitive and methodological issues plaguing self-report instruments, but little is known about the specific cognitive skills required for children (or adults) to accurately complete self-reports.

While a number of different approaches have been tested, the consensus from several reviews is that previous-day recall instruments offer the most promise for use with children. A number of different instruments are now available for this type of assessment. A limitation of this format is that data must be obtained on multiple days in order to take into account the normal intra-individual variability in activity patterns. Because these instruments typically rely on a checklist of activities and coded intervals of time these instruments may be more susceptible to overestimation than other more general measures of activity. To avoid this type of error, some investigators recommend recording the number of "activity blocks" recorded by the participant rather than the time. Others have converted the data into an activity index that incorporates intensity and duration [2].

If the intent is to characterize general activity habits, alternative formats, that do not require estimates of time or amounts of activity, may be used. The Physical Activity Questionnaire for Children, for example, uses a series of questions about general activity patterns to calculate an overall activity score. While the score does not allow for estimations of frequency, intensity, or duration, it may be useful in discriminating between active and inactive children.

While self-report instruments have inherent limitations, there is considerable room for improvement in the way they are validated, scored, and interpreted. The increased use of computerized instruments offers promise to assist with recall and coding of activity. A computerized activity assessment is now available with the software versions. The use of electronic beepers may also be useful to prompt recall of activity in children. Regardless of what format is used, results will likely be improved if more attention is given to the setting for the assessment and the training needed for children to accurately complete the assessment. A description and copy of a number of different self-report instruments for children have recently been published to facilitate their use by both researchers and teachers.

Heart Rate Monitors

Heart rate monitors provide an objective indicator of the physiological effect of physical activity. They have been found to provide a valid measure of heart rate in children, and heart rate has been shown to be linearly related to energy expenditure during physical activity. However, the numerous other factors that influence heart rate under resting conditions contribute with considerable error when heart rate monitors are used for extended periods of monitoring. In a recent study, it was found that heart rate indicators were highly correlated with a direct observation measure under active conditions in physical education (r = .79), but weakly correlated under inactive conditions in the classroom (r = .49). While this type of error would bias measures of mean heart rate, they would not affect estimates of total minutes of activity (e.g., minutes > 140 bpm). Still, there are a number of difficulties inherent in using heart rate monitors for field-based research. Problems with 60-cycle interference and lost data from signal interruptions make data collection and data processing challenging. Delayed heart rate responses and the influence of other factors can add considerable error to heart rate recordings.

A promising application of heart rate monitoring techniques is for estimations of energy expenditure and for studies on obesity and weight control. Another promising option is the potential use of heart rate along with a motion sensing devices given by the predictions on energy expenditure, by using certain techniques, that show that these predictions can be improved, both to children and adults.

Activity monitors

Activity monitors provide an objective indicator of total body movement. Because most contemporary monitors feature time sampling capability, they can be used to assess the frequency, intensity, duration, and energy expenditure of physical activity. Numerous studies have examined the reliability and validity of these devices in children, and in lab. Similar to studies with adults, the general consensus is that they provide valid measures of physical activity but more questionable estimates of energy expenditure.

A well-described limitation of activity monitors is the inability to assess upper body activities such as throwing, catching, carrying, or lifting. Recent studies have documented that activity monitors significantly underestimate energy expenditure of common lifestyle activities in adults. While similar studies have not been conducted specifically in children, it is likely that activity monitors would also underestimate the energy expenditure estimates of children's intermittent activities. The use of 3-dimensional devices would appear to offer advantages over 1-dimensional devices but the results have been equivocal. Field-based calibration equations may improve the predictive accuracy of monitors. By reporting raw movement counts or using a different outcome variable (e.g., minutes of activity), the errors associated with energy expenditure estimations would be avoided.

One of the most common approaches for field-based research is to use "cut points" to determine the amount of time spent in different intensity categories. While this is a useful approach, it is important to recognize that cut points will underestimate activity levels in children if they are established based on the number of counts recorded during a continuous bout of activity. Because most accelerometry - based devices use an integrative procedure to summarize movement counts, the value at the end of the minute reflects the total counts within that time. Thus, short periods of vigorous activity may be obscured by alternating periods of rest when the total value for the minute is computed. Activity values for these minutes could be interpreted as "inactive" time periods if the cut points are based on how many counts would accrue during continuous activity. To avoid this potential error, the cut points must consider the intermittent nature of children's physical activity behavior. From this perspective, direct observation techniques using momentary time sampling procedures may provide the best criterion measure since they can address changes in activity levels within a minute. Another option is to process activity monitor data using time intervals less than 1 minute [9].

While there are limitations, activity monitors are one of the most useful tools to assess physical activity over extended periods of time. The cost and administrative time may be too high for large-scale studies, but they can be useful for smaller intervention studies, cross sectional comparisons, or validation of other assessment techniques.

Pedometers

Pedometers provide an objective indicator of step counts, a marker of total volume or duration of activity. They possess similar benefits and weaknesses to motion sensors but with less accuracy and precision. Because pedometers do not have time sampling capabilities, they cannot provide detail on frequency or intensity of physical activity. Energy expenditure estimates would likely be inaccurate due to the many assumptions needed to calculate this from step counts. Still, in terms of practicality, pedometers may offer the best solution for a low cost, objective monitoring tool. Recently, similar correlations with fitness and fatness measures were reported between pedometers and monitors. A recent study in adults suggested that 10,000 steps is a reasonable daily target for adults but similar studies are needed to determine guidelines for children.

Direct Observation

Direct observation techniques evaluate the behavioral aspects of physical activity and are well suited to studies on children. The merits of various instruments and coding strategies have been previously described. While considerable time and effort is required to conduct direct observation studies, the detail provided can be highly useful for characterizing children's activity. Direct observation techniques provide one of the best criterion measures to validate other assessment tools. For further information, readers should consult the specific protocols published with each instrument.

Summary

This paper is reviewing the nature of children's physical activity patterns and how the unique nature of children can impact the assessment of physical activity. To accurately assess children's activity patterns, an instrument must be sensitive enough to detect, code, or record sporadic and intermittent activity. Care also must be used to select criterion measures that reflect appropriate physical activity guidelines for children.

A number of different measurement approaches have been described for assessing children's activity, but no specific method can be identified as the best option for all studies. Selection of an appropriate instrument depends on the specific research question being addressed as well as the relative importance of accuracy and practicality. For example, accurate measures of energy expenditure using indirect calorimetry, or heart rate calibration equations may be needed for certain clinical studies, but the cost and inconvenience would make them impractical for field-based assessments on larger samples.

The "accuracy-practicality" compromise presents more challenging predicaments with children than for adults. In adults, a number of self-report instruments have been found useful for large epidemiological studies or interventions where less precision is needed. Because of developmental differences, especially in ability to think abstractly and perform detailed recall, children are less likely to make accurate self-report assessment than adults. Though self-report methods are still likely to be a principal source of information for many studies, other approaches (or the use of combined measures) may be needed to better characterize children's activity levels.

While objective instruments (e.g., direct observation or activity monitoring) require more time and resources than self-report, they are options available to simplify data collection. One approach may be to focus assessments on key times or places that allow children to be active. The time after school, for example, appears to be a critical period that defines their propensity for physical activity. Monitoring of entire groups for discrete periods of time (e.g., recess or physical education) may also be useful to understand variability in activity patterns since children would all be exposed to the same stimulus or opportunity to be active.

Proxy measures may also be useful in studying activity in children. For example, several studies have demonstrated that time spent outside is strongly predictive indicator of activity in children. Involvement in community sports programs may also be a useful proxy measure as sports programs have been found to account for approximately 55-65% of children's moderate to vigorous activity.

Another option for improving assessments in children is to employ multiple measures of physical activity. A number of studies have reported differences in levels of activity when activity monitors were compared with self-report data. The method of measurement has also been shown to influence the results of studies on the determinants of physical activity in children. While we do not currently know which measure is most accurate, reporting the results with different instruments provides a more complete description of children's activity and permit a triangulation of outcomes.

In summary, there remains no single way of obtaining a highly accurate account of physical activity or energy expenditure in children. The nature of children's movement patterns, the various types of activities engaged in, and the inherent limitations of each assessment tool limit the ultimate accuracy of these measurements. Future research should continue to characterize children's movement patterns so that better assessment techniques can be developed. There is a strong rationale that supports continued efforts to improve assessment techniques for epidemiological research. It is pointed out that relatively weak measures were probably sufficient to demonstrate general health benefits of physical activity, but that more sophisticated techniques are needed to answer the more complex research questions currently facing the field assessments. This is especially true for research with children since links with specific health outcomes are difficult to establish and variability in cognition and maturation complicate other outcomes. A reviewing of physical activity interventions in children also highlighted the importance of valid and reliable measures to assess change in physical activity behaviors over time. To advance research in pediatric exercise science it is important to continue work to improve current physical activity assessment techniques.

References

[1]. Welk, G.J., & Wood, K. (2000). Physical activity assessments in physical education: A practical review of instruments and their use in the curriculum. *Journal of Physical Education, Recreation and Dance*, vol. 71(1), 30-40

[2]. Zamora, Elena (2002): *Anatomie funcţională. Aparatul locomotor* vol.2. Cluj-Napoca: Ed. ALC Media Group, pp. 189-193

[3]. Şerbescu, Carmen (2011) *Kinetoterapia deficienţelor fizice* – note de curs, pp. 97-99

[4]. Hager, R. (1999). The *effect of television on children's opportunities for physical activity*. Unpublished doctoral dissertation, pp. 178-184

[5]. Epuran M., Marolicaru M., (2000), - *Metodologia cercetării în educaţie fizică şi sport*, Editura Risoprint, Cluj-Napoca, pp. 213-215

[6]. Epuran, M, Holdevici Irina, Tonita, Florentina, (2001), *Psihologia sportului de performanţă. Teorie şi practică*, Editura FEST, Bucureşti, pp. 80-92

[7]. Sbenghe, T., (2002), *Kinetologie. Ştiinţa mişcării*. Bucureşti, Ed. Medicală, pp. 188-193

[8]. Zamora, Elena (2000): *Anatomie funcţională. Aparatul locomotor vol.1*. Cluj-Napoca, Ed. Risoprint,, pp. 154-163

[9]. Rusu, I., Pascan, I., Grosu, E., Cucu, B.,(1998), *Gimnastica,* Editura G.M.I., Cluj-Napoca, pp. 172-177

2

EFFICIENCY OF PHYSICAL THERAPY AFTER ARTHROPLASTY OF THE HIP JOINT IN THE ELDERLY

Anca JIANU

Universitatea Spiru Haret, Sos. Berceni, Nr. 24, Sector 4, Bucureşti

Abstract: Background. Osteoarthritis is a condition common in people over the age of 50-60 years, a consequence to progressive destruction of articular cartilage of the hip joint , which determines stiffen evolving hip, accompanied by severe pain. We believe that the increased frequency of disease in elderly people, but also the middle-aged argue the necessity of applying kinetic means after hip prosthesis to these subjects.

Aims. Applying an early physical therapy program in subjects with osteoarthritis, upon which intervened surgically total hip arthroplasty leads to functional recovery of the hip-femoral joint and increase their quality of life.

Methods. This study, based on the method of the experiment, was performed on a number of 44 subjects diagnosed with osteoarthritis in the advanced stage.

Results. Analysis of the results reveals improve clinical and functional status of patients.

Conclusions. In subjects over 65 years, clinical parameters values followed during postoperative physical therapy program highlighted the efficiency of the recovery methods applied in order to regain normal functionality of the hip.

Key word: osteoarthritis, total arthroplasty, physiotherapy

Introduction

Osteoarthritis of the hip is the most disabling of arthritis, is a condition relatively common [1], especially in people aged 50-60 years.

Symptoms of the disease lies in the significant decrease in hip mobility and muscle tone, which is why patients realise difficult to perform daily activities such as boots, resting on a chair, walking, climbing or descending stairs [2].

All forms of osteoarthritis requires in each case, a different approach in the treatment of physical therapy [3]. In terms of an enhanced form of the condition is required initially surgery as total hip arthroplasty [4], after application of kinesiology. Total hip arthroplasty is a medical procedure effective in treating hip joint degeneration [5, 6].

A number of specialized studies mention the importance of total hip arthroplasty in hip pain relief and affected the functional independence of patients [7].

Although hip arthroplasty is used successfully in the treatment of coxarthrosis, literature data indicate the presence of postoperative complications in about 15% of patients, complications that arise as a weak pain and physical functions [8].

Vilardo, L. Shah, M. [9] support the possibility that postoperative become acute pain and to persist longer than 2 months after the intervention, under exclusion of other causes pain generators.

In this context should apply the benefits of physical therapy on his hip functionality and quality of life.

Hypotheses

Placing pre and postoperative physical therapy program appropriate to the age, associated pathology and exercise tolerance elderly contribute to reducing the negative consequences caused by surgery and increased functional independence of patients

Material and methods

Research protocol

a) *Period of the research*

This study was conducted from January 2014 - December 2014 and was based on the experimental method and the theoretical and practical method of documenting.

b) *Subjects*

The study was conducted on a sample of 44 subjects, aged 64-75 years.

All subjects were diagnosed with osteoarthritis in advanced stage and were selected from patients of Orthopaedics and Traumatology Hospital *Foişorul de Foc* in Bucharest .

To establish the role of physical therapy before and after surgery were established and recorded followed parameters to analysis and interpretation of results and the physical therapy program has been in patients of this study.

We note that all subjects have given their consent to participate in the study.

c) *Applied tests*

The subjects were evaluated in two test moments: initial (T_I) before hip arthroplasty and kinetic software application, and final (T_F), 4 weeks thereafter. The data collected were placed in tables and graphs.

For monitoring and quantifying the results, the following parameters were evaluated:

• Parameter postoperative pain revealed by Visual Analog Scales, a horizontal line of 10 cm with keywords on each end that the patient indicates a point that we believe is subjective perception of pain, anxiety and stress before surgery and joint replacement of the hip [10] ;

• Parameter joint amplitude at the hip-femoral joint on flexion and abduction on goniometer measured using [11];

• Parameter muscular hip of stabilizers: quadriceps, middle and big gluteal, psoas iliac, according to international standards measured through muscle testing scale of 0-5 [12, 13];

• Parameter thigh hypotrophy determined by measuring of thigh perimeter with metric tape at the crease subfesier, the patient beeing in standing with legs slightly apart and your body weight equally distributed on both feet [14];

• Parameter subjective assessment of quality of life Scale

• Parameter represented by gait.

d) Studied moments

Physical therapy applied pre- and postoperative (between times T_I and T_F) targeted the following general objectives.

Preoperative physical therapy program objectives [15] were represented by:

• Maintaining strength muscle,

• Maintaining joint mobility,

• Breath education,

• Enabling the general circulation,

• Balancing mental patient.

The means for achieving the targets were isometric exercises for the buttocks and quadriceps muscle contraction lasting 6 seconds and pause 12 seconds, and isotonic exercises for the leg muscles affected to the healthy upper limb ,individualized dose (10-20 reps with pause 5 or 10 repetitions).

The general objectives of postoperative physical therapy [16] were:

• Pain relief,

• Fighting muscle contractures,

• Improving muscle strength of the lower limb joints stabilizers,

• Improved knee and hip joint mobility with respect to specific restrictions,

• Walking reeducation.

The means used to attain these objectives were: posture operated leg in abduction of 20° using triunghiulare Muller pillow, correcting the tendency of external rotation with a splint or a scroll type lateral Brown, breathing exercises accompanied by movements of the limbs upper and inhale and exhale exercises against resistance (exhales through the tube immersed in a jar of water) in the first five days and, not least, learned exercises before surgery.

They performed leg exercises supine healthy and exercises with leg operated as follows:

• Phase I (48 hours) consisted of isometric contractions of the quadriceps (10 repetitions), exercises in all planes at the ankle (20-30 reps),

• Stage II (4-5 days) represented earlier exercises, to which was added without gravity hip abduction (20 repetitions) activo-passive flexion of the hip with the knee extended (10 repetitions), balancing in set (40 repetitions), walking frame loading of the hip prosthesis and respect normal step,

• Phase III (6-7 days) was the previous stage exercises, hip abduction of decubitus cushion between your knees heterolateral of isometric prone buttocks, knees flexed, from sitting to standing with support lifting the healthy leg frame (2x6 repetitions),

• Phase IV (days 8-9) with exercises increase muscle strength in the legs,

• Phase V was (10-11 days) is addressed with the involvement of tolerance to walk with crutches or (with progressively increasing load and increased flexion and extension); 4-6 weeks after surgery with a crutch or a cane going to facilitate recovery,

• Phase IV (days 8-9) with exercises increase muscle strength in the legs,

• Phase V was (10-11 days) is addressed with the involvement of tolerance to walk with crutches or (with progressively increasing load and increased flexion and extension); 4-6 weeks after surgery with a crutch or a cane going to facilitate recovery

In applying individualized physical therapy programs have kept in mind the following methods:

• Maintain abduct the hip with a pillow between your legs, the patient was in lateral decubitus ventral

• Use assistive devices to prevent flexion greater than 90 °, and sat operated leg will stay extended

• Avoid crossing one's legs or rotation inwards and outwards peaks feet.

e) The statistical methods used

The software used for statistical analysis was used Microsoft Excel 2013.

Statistical indicators followed were arithmetic averages and the difference between the initial and final values of the parameters evaluated.

Results

Following evaluations made were noted as follows:

• The data showed a higher number of female subjects, the percentage is 68, 8%.

• Monitoring of postoperative pain as "*acute response to surgery*" [17] highlighted the good evolution of this parameter in the experimental group at 4 weeks postoperatively, according to Table. 1.

Table no.1. The pain intensity in the two tests:

The pain intensity in the two tests	Initială Tests(T_I)	Final tests (T_F)
Absence of pain	2	15
Mild pain	5	21
Moderate pain	28	6
Violent pain	9	2

• Parametrul Parameter joint mobility on flexion and hip abduction increased articular mobility

Table no. 2. Evolution of mobility on hip flexion

	Before physical therapy	After physical therapy
Flexion with the extended knee over 90^0	9	3
Flexion with the extended knee over 90^0	5	4
Flexion with the flexed knee over 90^0	4	6
Flexion with the flexed knee below 90^0	15	19
Passive flexion limited	11	12

Subjects in the experimental group were increases in flexion between 20°-35°, and the movement of 15°-25° abduction.

After rehabilitation complex treatment is successfully improving active extension with the knee flexed at values above 150° in 25 cases, while 19 cases were executed passive extension around 15-20 degrees or slightly above it.

Preoperatively 32 patients (72.72%) had abnormal gait (limping), and after application of postoperative physical therapy only 12 patients had abnormal gait .

Resumtion of gait and its training requires values lower limb muscle strength grade five.

The scale of subjective assessment of quality of life had initial value of 4.69 to the average score of the 44 subjects their condition well, and finally 7.8.

Discussions

Speciality literature mentions the benefit of preoperative physical therapy for individuals affected hip arthroplasty, respectively of the postoperative aimed at improving muscle tone [18]. Jack, Ș., C. [19] believes that the preoperative physical therapy intervention on physical functionality, and similar studies converge on the same physical improvement in performance.

The study by Trăilă, L., A. [20] attest to the prevalence of coxarthrosis and hip arthroplasty in individuals females.

Postoperative pain relief confirms that pre- and postoperative physical therapy program well led, individualized reduces postoperative complications.

Similar studies notes following the intervention, reducing postoperative pain in approximately 84% of patients, while 76% reported improvements in functional recovery of physiological [21].

The decrease decompensation allowed algetic active physical therapy techniques are applied to recover stability and mobility of hip surgery.

Movements of the abduction, adduction, internal rotation, external rotation so the knee extended and flexed with him were affected in most patients and their evolution after physical therapy is less significant.

The results correspond to data obtained from the literature that the exercise properly dosed and applied in accordance with methodical guidelines for the application of physical therapy in elderly increase quality of live.

Conclusions

1. The people most affected by osteoarthritis are female.
2. A well dosed kinetic program, individualized reflected in minimizing complications of hip joint replacement.
3. Postoperative pain decreases in most patients within one month.
4. Preoperative physical therapy has a major role on the functional capacity of the elderly, but this, along with postoperative physical therapy contributes effectively to achieve the state of balance and physical and mental health.
5. Evolution experiment followed parameters in subjects us to say that physical therapy program developed and achieved its goal.
6. Physical treatment advanced coxarthrosis lead to improved stability and specific joint mobility, and to increase exercise capacity and quality of life of the elderly.

Acknowledgments

The authors would like to thank all participants in this experimental study.

References

[1].Ciocoi-Pop, D., R., (2008). *Metode de evaluare şi explorare în kinetoterapie-bolile reumatice*. Cluj-Napoca: Editura Risoprint, p. 82.

[2]. Lin, S., Y., Davey, R., C., Cochrane, T., (2012). *Community rehabilitation for older adults withosteoarthritis falls risk and physical function in older adults with lower-extremity osteoarthritis*. Arch Phys Med Rehabil; 93(1), p. 27-34.

[3]. Moraru, G., Pâncotan, V., (2008). *Evaluare şi recuperare kinetică în reumatologie*, Editura Universităţii din Oradea, p. 211.

[4]. Quintana, J., M., Arostegui, I., Escobar, A., Azkarate, J., Goenaga, I., Lafuente, I., (2008). *Prevalence of knee and hip osteoarthritis and the appropriateness of joint replacement in an older population*. Arch Int Med, 168, p. 1576-1584.

[5]. Knutsson, S., Engberg, I., B., (2011). *An evaluation of patients' quality of life before, 6 weeks and 6 months after total hip replacement surgery*. J Adv Nurs ; 30 (6), p. 1349-1359.

[6]. Smith, T., O., Blake, V., Hing, C., B., (2011). *Minimally invasive versus conventional exposure for total hip arthroplasty: a systematic review and meta-analysis of clinical and radiological outcomes*. International Orthop; 35(2), p. 173-184.

[7]. MacWilliam, C., H., Ulcickas, Y., M, Verner, J., McCarthy, B., D., Ward, R., E., (1996). *Patient related risk factors which predict poor outcome after total hip replacement*. Health Services Research; 31, p. 623-638.

[8]. Rosenberger, P., H., Ickovics, J., R., Epel, E., S., D'Entremont, D., Jokl, P.. (2004). *Physical recovery in arthroscopic knee surgery: unique contributions of coping behaviors to clinical outcomes and stress reactivity*. Psychology & Health, Vol. 19, p.307-320.

[9]. Vilardo, L., Shah, M., (2011). *Techniques in Regional Anesthesia. Pain Management*; 15(3), p. 110-115.

[10]. Filip, N., Ciulei, R., Pocol, P., Georgescu, A., (2012), *Medical, demographic and psychological predictors of functional status and postoperative pain in patients with hip arthroplasty* în Palestrica Mileniului III - Civilizaţie şi Sport, 13 (3), p. 234 -240.

[11]. Cordun, M. (2011). *Bioenergetică şi Ergometrie în Sport*. Editura CD Press Bucureşti, p. 281.

[12]. Chiriac, M.,(2000). *Testarea manuală a forţei musculare*, Editura Universităţii din Oradea, p. 128-152.

[13]. Sidenco, E., L., (2003). *Coloana vertebrală şi membrul inferior. Evaluare mioarticulară în kinetoterapie şi în medicina sportivă.* Editura Fundaţiei *România de Mâine* Bucureşti, p. 20-72.

[14]. Cordun, M., (2009). *Kinantropometrie*. Editura CD Press Bucureşti, p. 36-67.
[15]. Pascalău, N., Cioară, F., (2011). *Actualităţi în managementul coxartrozei*. Editura Universităţii din Oradea.
[16]. Moţet, D., (2010). *Enciclopedia de kinetoterapie, vol. II*, Editura Semne Bucureşti, p. 671-695.
[17]. Khan, R., S., Ahmed, K., Blakeway, E., (2011). *Catastrophizing: a predictive factor for postoperative pain*. American Journal Surgery, 201(1), p. 122-131.
[18]. Dauty, M., Genty, M., Ribinik, P., (2007). *Physical training in rehabilitation programs before and after total hip and knee arthroplasty*. Ann Readapt Med Phys, 50(6), p. 462-468.
[19]. Jack, S., West, M., Grocott, MP., (2011), *Perioperative exercise training inelderly subjects*. Best Pract Res Clin Anaesthesiol, 25(3), p. 461-472.
[20]. Trăilă, L., A., (2015). *Present considerations in the kinetic treatment of coxarthrosis* în Journal of Sport and Kinetic Movement, Editura Universităţii din Craiova, 1(26), p. 241-245.
[21]. Filip, N., Ciulei, R., Pocol, P., Georgescu, A., (2012), *Pre and post surgery changes in the quality of life of patients receiving total hip arthroplasty* în Palestrica Mileniului III - Civilizaţie şi Sport, 13 (3), p. 188 -193.

3

CONTROL TESTS FOR THE SELECTION OF TALENTS IN ATHLETICS

Alina Elena ALBINĂ, Constantin ALBINĂ

The University of Craiova, the Faculty of Physical Education and Sports, Romania

Abstract: Introduction. An essential problem is the need for an organized scientifically system, to permit that based on some objective criteria and the said forecast, to select among large groups of children and young people the most endowed, which after a suitable training to achieve the model of the performer.

Methods

The initial selection of children in athletics is considered as integer part of the research plan aiming the vast selection process in athletics. After the choice of the research theme, at the indications of the department of athletics we have established the plan of work, the hypothesis, the purpose and tasks of research, taking into account also the volume of data collected on the basis of these considerations we set the research methods so that all activity to be conducted with greater efficiency.

We made a selection of children with athletic predisposition, identifying and engaging the best in the athletic department in the School Sports Club of Craiova "Petrache Trişcu".

Result

Comparing the results of boys and girls of 11 and 12 years old, we notice that there is a continuous increase in all parameters, both morphological and motor.

Conclusion

For an efficient selection and accurate predictive assessment of future evolution of the one selected, it must that the base tests remain the speed test on 50 m; start running from standing position, long jump off place; throwing ball dating; running of resistance to 600 m to 800 m up to 11 years old and for girls of 12 years old 800 m, and boys of 12 years old 1000 m and detention on the vertical.

Keywords*:* selection, talents, control tests, athletes.

Introduction

Selection act is not an isolated act and do not represent in any way an end in itself because once completed, it provide a training process that leads to another moment of selection [1].

So the selection is a process conducted until reaching the upper limits of performance [2].

This is why the selection and training concepts have been brought together in a phrase that suggests a complex process linked and directed towards a certain specialization of children and junior [3].

The selection leads to an early specialization expressing the concern for directing the child to a sports test or branch from an early age [4].

According to N. Alexe (1983) „The selection process is an organized and repeated, of detection of innate availabilities in child, junior, using a complex system of criteria (medical, biological, psycho-sociological and motor), for the practice and his later specialization into a discipline or sports test" [5].

The same author says that, the advantages of the selection are:

- Ensures high performance achievement
- Substantially reduces training time
- Helps increase rapidly the elements detected by selection
- Helping to increase sports longevity
- Favours applying effort in compliance with the particularities of modern training concept
- Avoids an unnecessary amount of work and material investments which can not be capitalized
- Detects limited athletes
- Facilitate the recruitment of young elements
- Forming beliefs for work perspective
- Increases the possibilities of affirming international.

Talent is a college education or a group of capabilities with some specificity, above the average of a group of subjects to which they relate[6].

The purpose of the work

The purpose of this paper is to observe how the primary selection is carried out in athletics and based on findings from the harvested data to bring a modest contribution, the present system of selection

Methods

We made a selection of children of 11 to 12 years old, with athletic predisposition, identifying and engaging the best athletic department in the School Sports Club of Craiova "Petrache Trişcu".

Primary selection is based on international test of physical ability known as „Standard Fitness

Test" adopted by the International Federation of Physical Education.

The test contained eight testing.

For a uniform assessment of the results was set a system of scaling of the performance for each age, separately for boys and girls, each getting a performance equivalent in points. We chose six of these tests that are more important in our view:

1. Running of speed - 50 m
2. Long jump off place
3. Throwing the ball dating
4. Lifting the trunk from lying to sitting
5. Running of resistance
6. Detention on the vertical

I did a comparison of the test results of children and minimum standards for grade 5 of the S.U.V.A.D.

Results

The survey data were collected and grouped by sex and age resulting (tables T1-T4) with primary data that we've attached the paper.

We insisted on the average, amplitude and coefficient of variability because it optimal characterizes both tendency and dispersion of data strings.

Table 1 The results of the control samples Girls 11 years

Tests Ind. statistics	The waist (cm)	Weight (kg)	50 m (sec)	Long jump off place (cm)	Throwing the ball dating (m)	Sit-up 30" (nr.)	600 m (min. and sec.)	Detention on the vertical (cm)
N	20	20	20	20	20	20	20	20
X	139.1	31.9	8"54	165.6	21.2	22.9	2'32"	31.2
Xmin	135	29	7"42	138	14	18	2'02"	26
Xmax	148	36	9"40	198	29	29	2'55"	39
W	13	7	1"98	60	15	11	0'53"	13
S	3.2	1.7	0.69	16.3	4.6	3.3	0.13	4.67
Cv	2.32%	5.3%	8.07%	9.8%	21.6%	14.4%	5.6%	14.9%

Note:N - total number of cases
X - average
X min - the lowest value of the results
X max - the largest value of the results
W - the amplitude distribution
S - standard deviation
Cv - the coefficient of variability

Tabel 2 The results of the control samples Boys 11 years

Tests Ind. statistics	The waist (cm)	Weight (kg)	50 m (sec)	Long jump off place (cm)	Throwing the ball dating (m)	Sit-up 30" (nr.)	600 m (min. and sec.)	Detention on the vertical (cm)
N	21	21	21	21	21	21	21	21
X	133.3	31.6	8"15	174.4	29.6	24.1	2'05"	33.2
Xmin	137	27	7"20	160	26	18	1'58"	27
Xmax	154	42	9"03	200	37.5	29	2'40"	43
W	17	15	1"83	40	11.5	11	0'82"	16
S	12.5	3.7	0"64	11.3	3	3.4	0.29	5.1
Cv	9.3%	11.7%	7.8%	6.4%	10.7%	14.45	14.15	15.3%

Note:N - total number of cases
X - average
X min - the lowest value of the results
X max - the largest value of the results
W - the amplitude distribution
S - standard deviation
Cv - the coefficient of variability

The arithmetic average of data samples "Standard Fitness Test" compared to the minimum scales of rules for obtaining Note 5 S.U.V.A.D. have higher values in all control samples.

Table 3 The results of the control samples Girls 12 years

Tests Ind. statistics	The waist (cm)	Weight (kg)	50 m (sec)	Long jump off place (cm)	Throwing the ball dating (m)	Sit-up 30" (nr.)	600 m (min. and sec.)	Detention on the vertical (cm)
N	21	21	21	21	21	21	21	21
X	151.5	38.1	7.6	176.8	24.6	23.2	2'99"	33.4
Xmin	142	30	6"90	155	18	19	2'30"	27
Xmax	162	50	8"52	210	33.5	30	4'04"	40
W	20	20	1.62	55	15.5	11	1'34"	13
S	6.06	5.5	0.51	16.6	3.7	3.7	0.58	4.3
Cv	4%	14.6%	6.71%	9.3%	15%	15.9%	19.39%	12.8%

Note:N - total number of cases
X - average
X min - the lowest value of the results
X max - the largest value of the results
W - the amplitude distribution
S - standard deviation
Cv - the coefficient of variability

Table 4 The results of the control samples Boys 12 years

Tests Ind. statistics	The waist (cm)	Weight (kg)	50 m (sec)	Long jump off place (cm)	Throwing the ball dating (m)	Sit-up 30" (nr.)	600 m (min. and sec.)	Detention on the vertical (cm)
N	16	16	16	16	16	16	16	16
X	152.3	36.1	7"60	187.6	33.6	25.5	4'01"	37.9
Xmin	110	27	7"00	168	24	20	3'28"	29
Xmax	165	42	8"48	220	42.5	31	4'49"	43
W	25	15	1"48	52	18.5	11	1'21"	14
S	7.8	4.8	0.50	19.4	5.4	3.28	0.46	4.12
Cv	5.2%	13.2%	6.57%	10.3%	17.10%	12.8%	11.2%	10.2%

Note:N - total number of cases
X - average
X min - the lowest value of the results
X max - the largest value of the results
W - the amplitude distribution
S - standard deviation
Cv - the coefficient of variability

Reporting at the rules for primary selection of the 5 multilateral physical training tests only 30'' sit-ups is the only sample that exceeded the score of 60 points out of all 5 tests and the average score of 50 points over the "Fitness Standard Test" exceeded the scale by only 50 m running with start from standing position and long jump off place.

Conclusions

Only on the basis of objective criteria and a realistic prognosis can select from large masses of children and youth the most gifted, which after an appropriate training to accomplish without a model
In appreciation of multilateral physical training at the 6 testing tested there is a continuous improvement of performance in the studied period, but with few exceptions, even if the growth is in rhythms or different values.
For an efficient selection and accurate predictive assessment of future evolution of the one selected, it must that the base tests remain the speed test on 50 m; start running from standing position, long jump off place; throwing the ball dating; running of resistance to 600 m to 800 m up to 11 years old and for girls of 12 years old 800 m, and boys of 12 years old 1000 m and detention on the vertical.

Acknowledgement
All authors have equal contribution.

References:

[1] Alexandrescu D., Tatu T., Ardelean T., (1983) *Atletism*, Bucureşti, Didactică şi Pedagogică, p.227.

[2] Cârstea Gh., (1993) *Metodica Educaţiei Fizice şi Sportului*, Universul, Bucureşti, p.30.

[3] Paraschiv, V. (1984) *Studiul privind eficienţa criteriilor de selecţie în selecţiile de copii şi juniori ale cluburilor sportive,* Bucureşti, Sport-Turism, p.80.

[4] Gaisi G., (1977) *Bazele teoretice ale depistării talentelor în sport ţinând cont de criteriile antropometrice şi fiziologice*, Bucureşti, Sportul la copii şi juniori, vol. XX-XII, p.35.

[5] Alexe N., (1993) *Antrenamentul sportiv modern*, Bucureşti, Editis, p.43.

[6] Kupoinov R., (1977) *Capacitatea şi talentul,* Bucureşti, Sportul la copii şi juniori, vol. XX-XII, p. 35

4

DETERMINATION OF THE VOLLEYBALL PLAYERS' PROBLEM SOLVING SKILLS IN TERMS OF SOME VARIABLES

Sefa Sahan BIROL, Elif USTUN, Veysel TEMEL

Karamanoglu Mehmetbey University, Physical Education and Sports High School, Karaman.

ABSTRACT: Purpose: Done with the aim of revealing whether problem solving skills differ in terms of different variables or not.

Methods: Research group consisted of 50 male and 59 female players who played at youth volleyball league in Konya city center. In this study, "Problem Solving Skills Inventory" developed by Heppner and Petersen (1982) and the adaptation work of this scale to Turkish was conducted by Şahin, Şahin and Heppner (1993)was used as data collection tool. The unique Kolmogorov Smirnov Test was used in order to determine whether measures were suitable for normal dispersion or not. T-test and One Way Anova (one way variance analysis) were used on analyzing and interpreting of data since it was a normal dispersion for impetuous approach, from sub dimensions of the problem solving skills, and tukey test was used in order to determine the differences between groups and meaningfulness was determined as P>0,05 and also, Kruskal Wallis-H test and Mann Whitney-U test were used on analyzing and evaluating the data for Total Point skills and considering, avoidant, Evaluator, self-confidence and planned approaches, from sub dimensions of the Problem Solving Skills.

Findings: Problem solving total point average of the athletes participated in the research with (Mean=95,1651), impetuous approach point average with (Mean=31,0183), considering approach point average with (Mean=13,6514), avoidant approach point average with (Mean=11,6697), Evaluator approach point average with (Mean=9,0000),Self-confidence approach point average with (Mean=19,4128) and planed approach point average with (Mean=10,4128), from sub dimensions of the Problem Solving Skills, were low.

Results: Meaningful difference was found in terms of personal characteristic on problem solving total and sub dimensions of the problem solving skills of participants 'team which they play at', 'gender', 'education' and "sport beginning age' and 'family member number' variables whereas meaningful difference was not found on "parents education", "parents occupation", "family income" and "place in which they spend most of their life" variables.

Key Words: Problem Solving, Athletes, Volleyball, University

INTRODUCTION

Life could consider as a process of problem solving. From birth to death human-being encounters with lots of problems regardless its quality and quantity. Solving this problems and methods of solving problems become effective on adaptation to life and life balance. On Eric Ericson's theory about psychosocial development states that "Problems make people mature; individuals who have reached successful identity status, are the people who have confronted and solved problems in their lives." According to Ericson, what really matters is to consider problems as a development opportunity [4].

Individuals may react in different ways to problems. Among these reactions; there are different ways such as; to find a good solution to problem, in other words to decide; to ignore problem; to anticipate the problem disappear; to wait someone to find a solution; to postpone deciding and to put problem on someone's shoulders. While anticipated reactions to problems could vary depending on the situation and individual, 'finding a good solution to problem' namely solving the problem is thought to be the healthiest reaction in most cases [15].

Thus, solving a problem which is a complex mental activity composed of auperior cognitive abilities and activities; visuality, connotation, abstraction, comprehension, reasoning, analysis, synthesis, generalisation is a complex combination of abilities with the components such as cognitive, behavioral and attitudinal [2].

According to [1] evaluation in problem solving process occurs after the action is taken and this is arranged for changing the real result . If this process does not occur, individuals could insist on an indecisive performance, instead of discovering rational solutions for their problems. Briefly, success on problem solving depends on the true definition of problem at first. In addition to true definition of problem, one should acquire adequate knowledge and formulate multiple behaviours that possibly puzzle out the problem and start with option assumed as a way to best solution. Available options are applied and if it works after evaluation this option is continued to conduct, otherwise another option is applied.

The problem is the difference between his current situation and his desired situation. This difference means a problem as a result of various obstacle to individuals who aim to reach their goals. According to this description, the same situation could a problem for an individual while it is not for another person. The reason of considering this as a problem is the following grounds:

- Innovation or excentricity ("I don't know what to do.")
- Hardship ("This is too complicated.")
- Paradoxical targets ("I don't know which one to choose.")
- Deficiency of ability ("I can't do it, because I don't know how to do.")
- Deficiency of source ("I don't have enough time to deal with it.")
- Uncertainty ("What's going on?)
- Emotional Distress ("I prefer not to do anything, because I am afraid of failure after I try.") [17].

Individuals face with small or big problems in different ways, in certain terms of their lives. Reactions to problems depend on individual. People endeavour solving same problem with different approach and some may achive, some may fail. Problems' area is not only limited to mathematics. Life needs solutions for a set of problems. Problem emerges when individual is hindered from reaching his target [6].

One of the fields of problems that individual encounters in his life is the interpersonal problems. "Interpersonal problem is defined as at least one of the interacting parties is aware of the difference between current interaction style and ideal style and as a consequence he feels the tension, attempts to supress however inhibits from doing it. Solving interpersonal problem could be expressed as cognitive and behavioral process that include attemps for supressing the tension arising from this interpersonal problem, and awarness of difference between current situation and desired situation in interpersonal relations [18].

[3] suggests that problem solving process is affected by factors such as creative Considering, intelligence, emotions, will and taking actions, needs, targets, values, abilities, habits (past experiences) and attitudes[3]. These factors form as a result of personal perception, past experiences and given meaning to them. Hence, it could affect what individual perceives about problem and how he solves it. Generally, first perception would not be the plain truth in problem case. Problem solving process, is affected by personal perception. Factors are affected by problem solving abilities are given below:

- Self-confidence
- Age
- Social learning and take someone as a model
- Individual differences
- Socio-economic level
- Sense of responsibility
- Knowledge about personal problems
- Emotions
- Past and life experiences
- Interaction
- Personality [14]

It turns out that people who can not solve their problems effectively are more anxious and insecure than people who have ability to solve their problems effectively [12,13,17]. Besides, effectless problem solving stimulates stress and psychological disharmony [9].

In a case of a problem and a case to overcome, individual uses all his sources, goes through previously obtained datas with the aim of obtaining some opinions and hints to solve problem. Success in problem solving is subject to problem solving ability [1].

Problem solving ability is a virtual lifetime ability and it includes all cases from basic to complex in lifetime. Problems in one's life, sometimes can be solved with easy actions, sometimes with concentrated Considering and sometimes with one's abilities [10]. It is also valid for people who are interested in sport. Athlete should decide his location and move regarding to his opponent's location and move and also his teammate's location and move on field, in hall, in boxing ring, on mat [14].

METHOD

This chapter involves information about the model of research, the research group, the collection of data, data collection tools and the operations which were conducted in the process of analysis of the data.

The Model of Research

Research is a descriptive work. Descriptive statistics, a collection of numerical values of a variable are statistical operations that allow description and presentation [5].

The Research Group

The research group involves 109 athletes of whom consists 50 male and 59 female players in Youth League of the city center of Konya.

The Collection of Data

First of all, current information related to the aim of the research are given systematically with scanning the literature. Therefore, a theoretical framework on the subject was created. Secondly, the Problem Solving Inventory (PSI) which was developed by [11], (Problem Solving Inventory, Form-A (PSA-A) was applied over the participants surveyed through random sampling.

The Data Collection Tools

Data collection tools that required achieving the defined objectives related to the research are listed below in order:

The Personal Information Form

Information form which consists 11 questions, were prepared by the researcher to collect information about personal characteristics of 109 players who played in the Youth League of the city center of Konya and in order to create independent variables about the subject of the research.

Problem Solving Inventory (PSI)

Problem solving inventory (PSI) was developed with the purpose of to determine the dimensions of the problem-solving methods right along with the competence to solve the people's problems as well as how he was perceived by taking into consideration some problem-solving steps such as "general orientation" "description of the problem,"alternative production", "decision-making" and "evaluation" which are resulting from various researches by [11,20]. The translation studies within the framework of the Turkish version studies of the scale was finished by [8,22, 21] orderly; and validity and reliability studies as finished by Taylan (1990), Şahin, Şahin and P.P. Heppner (1993) and Çam (1995). As a result of the analysis of factor that is conducted by Şahin and Heppner (1993), it is indicated that the scale is formed by 6 factors such as 1. Impetuous Approach: 13, 14, 15, 17, 21, 25, 26, 30 and 32. items, $\alpha = 0.78$, 2. Considering Approach: 18, 20, 31, 33 or 35 items, $\alpha = 0.76$, 3. Avoidant Approach: 1, 2, 3 and 4 items, $\alpha = 0.74$, 4. Evaluator Approach: 6, 7 and 8. items, $\alpha = 0.69$, 5. Self-assured Approach: 5, 11, 23, 24, 27, 28 and 34 items, $\alpha = 0.64$, Planned Approach: 10, 12, 16 and 19 items, $\alpha = 0{:}59$. The answers given is evaluated with scores ranging from 1 to 6. In scoring, 9, 22 and 29. items are kept off the scoring. Scoring is done through 32 items. 1, 2, 3, 4, 11, 13, 14, 15, 17, 21, 25, 26, 30 and 34. items are scored revers scored inversely. The range of points that are taken from inventory is between 32-192. The highness of the total score from the scale indicates problem-solving skills of individuals as inadequate. In decrease in the total score on the scale, the perception of individual's problem-solving skills is considered to be positive. While the scale aims to measure problem-solving skills of physical education and sports teachers. The reliability coefficient of internal consistency (Cronbach alpha) was found as 0.72.

Data Analysis

While the solution and interpretation of data, with the usage of Kruskal-Wallis H and Mann-Whitney U test, significance was estimated as $P<0{,}05$. In the evaluation and the calculation of the data, SPSS 21 (Statistical package for social sciences) packaged program was used.

FINDINGS

Table 1. Sub-Dimensions Of Participants in General Problem Solving and The Results of The Total Score's Average and Standard Deviation Values

	N	Mean	Ss	Min	Max	The lowest and the highest score that can be obtained from the scale
Impetuous Approach	109	31,0183	5,25460	22,00	49,00	9-54
Considering Approach	109	13,6514	5,10515	5,00	29,00	5-30
Avoidant Approach	109	11,6697	5,30209	5,00	24,00	4-24
Evaluator Approach	109	9,0000	2,71143	3,00	16,00	3-18
Self-assured Approach	109	19,4128	5,56479	9,00	34,00	7-42
Planned Approach	109	10,4128	4,12358	4,00	22,00	4-24
Total Point	109	95,1651	20,36178	60,00	162,00	32-192

In Table 1, it is indicated that, the point average of problem-solving (Avg. = 95.1651), the point average of impetuous approach which is the sub-dimension of problem-solving skills (Avg. = 31.0183), the point average of considering approach (Avg. = 13.6514), the point average of avoidant approach (Avg. = 11.6697), the point average of evaluator approach (Avg. = 9.00000), the point average of self-assured approach (Avg. = 19.4128), and the point average of planned approach (Avg. = 10.4128) are low.

Table 2. The Total and Sub-Dimension Results of Mann Whitney U Test According to The Participants Genders Related to Problem-Solving

		N	Mean Rank	Rank Sum	U	Z	P
Impetuous Approach	Female	50	43,44	2172,00	897,000	-3,528	,000
	Male	59	64,80	3823,00			
Considering Approach	Female	50	46,66	2333,00	1058,000	-2,548	,011
	Male	59	62,07	3662,00			
Avoidant Approach	Female	50	43,13	2156,50	881,500	-3,655	,000
	Male	59	65,06	3838,50			
Evaluator Approach	Female	50	56,67	2833,50	1391,500	-,517	,030
	Male	59	53,58	3161,50			
Self-assured Approach	Female	50	42,15	2107,50	832,500	-3,927	,000
	Male	59	65,89	3887,50			
Planned Approach	Male	50	45,49	2274,50	999,500	-2,948	,003
	Female	59	63,06	3720,50			
Total Point	Male	50	40,70	2035,00	760,000	-4,354	,000
	Female	59	67,12	3960,00			

In Table 2, it was examined the total and sub-dimension results with Mann Whitney U test according to the participants genders related to problem-solving. In the study results, impetuous Approach (U: 897.000 P <0.05) considering approach (U: 1058.000 P <0.05) avoidant approach (U: 881.500 P <0.05) evaluator approach (U: 897.000 P <0.05) self-assured approach (U: 832.500 P <0.05) planned approach (U: 999.500 P <0.05) total point (U: 760,000 P <0.05) differences between sub-dimensions was founded substantive.

Table 3. According to The Team Variables of Participants, Kruskall-Wallis Test Results for The Total and Sub-Dimensions in Problem Solving

		N	Mean Rank	Sd	X^2	P	Meaningful Differences
Impetuous Approach	Güneş Spor (female)	13	40,19	6	8,716	,190	-----
	Konya Fener (female)	14	41,57				
	Selçuklu belediye (female)	14	36,71				
	Gençlik spor (female)	13	45,35				
	Konya spor (male)	12	60,54				
	Konya büyükşehir (male)	14	53,11				
	Gençlik spor (male)	14	56,21				
Considering Approach	Güneş spor (female)	13	45,23	6	6,588	,361	-----
	Konya fener (female)	14	48,07				
	Selçuklu belediye (female)	14	34,07				
	Gençlik spor (female)	13	46,27				
	Konya spor (male)	12	51,38				
	Konya büyükşehir (male)	14	48,21				
	Gençlik spor (male)	14	59,57				
Avoidant Approach	Güneş spor (female)	13	28,15	6	16,687	,011*	7-1
	Konya fener (female)	14	48,61				
	Selçuklu belediye (female)	14	35,43				
	Gençlik spor (female)	13	51,42				
	Konya spor (male)	12	49,08				
	Konya büyükşehir (male)	14	54,14				
	Gençlik spor (male)	14	64,79				
Evaluator Approach	Güneş spor (female)	13	56,58	6	3,434	,753	-----
	Konya fener (female)	14	43,79				
	Selçuklu belediye (female)	14	51,82				
	Gençlik spor (female)	13	50,38				
	Konya spor (male)	12	41,96				
	Konya büyükşehir (male)	14	42,18				
	Gençlik spor (male)	14	45,86				
Self-assured Approach	Güneş spor (female)	13	32,92	6	20,138	,003*	7-3
	Konya fener (female)	14	49,14				
	Selçuklu belediye (female)	14	26,07				
	Gençlik spor (female)	13	55,88				
	Konya spor (male)	12	52,88				
	Konya büyükşehir (male)	14	51,36				
	Gençlik spor (male)	14	64,57				
Planned	Güneş spor (female)	13	32,31	6	12,709	,048*	7-1

Approach	Konya fener (female)	14	46,89				
	Selçuklu belediye (female)	14	33,96				
	Gençlik spor (female)	13	55,65				
	Konya spor (male)	12	52,75				
	Konya büyükşehir (male)	14	52,25				
	Gençlik spor (male)	14	58,93				
Total Point	Güneş spor (female)	13	34,77	6	16,616	,011*	7-3
	Konya fener (female)	14	45,54				
	Selçuklu belediye (female)	14	29,11				
	Gençlik spor (female)	13	51,77				
	Konya spor (male)	12	54,38				
	Konya büyükşehir (male)	14	52,32				
	Gençlik spor (male)	14	65,00				

*p<0,05

The sub-dimension of problem-solving for volleyball player and total score according to team variables and whether it became different or not were examimed with the Kurskal Walis test in Table 3. In the study result, there isn't any signifiant division among the sub-dimension of Impetuous, Considering and evaluator approach, however, significant division was found according to avoidant approach (X2 =16,687 P<0.05), self-assured approach (X2 =20,138 P<0.05), planned approach (X2 =12, 709 P<0.05) and total point approach (X2 =16,616 P<0.05).

Table 4. The Result of Kruskal-Wallis Test Telated To The Factor For Participant's Starting Gym According to Problem-Solving Tatl and Sub-Dimensions.

		N	Mean Rank	Sd	X^2	P	Meaningful Differences
Impetuous Approach	5-7	11	37,64	2	5,959	,051	-----
	8-10	31	49,95				
	11-13	67	60,19				
Considering Approach	5-7	11	33,50	2	6,174	,046	3-1
	8-10	31	54,24				
	11-13	67	58,88				
Avoidant Approach	5-7	11	25,05	2	13,366	,001	3-1
	8-10	31	51,65				
	11-13	67	61,47				
Evaluator Approach	5-7	11	64,23	2	1,307	,520	3-1
	8-10	31	56,15				
	11-13	67	52,96				
Self-assured Approach	5-7	11	24,45	2	13,970	,001	3-1
	8-10	31	51,15				
	11-13	67	61,80				
Planned Approach	5-7	11	36,55	2	6,274	,043	3-1
	8-10	31	50,66				
	11-13	67	60,04				
Total Point	5-7	11	24,86	2	14,524	,001	3-1
	8-10	31	49,77				
	11-13	67	62,37				

*p<0,05

The sub-dimension of problem-solving for volleyball player and total score according to their gym start and whether it became different or not related to their factor were examimed with the Kurskal Walis test in Table 4. In the study result, there isn't any signifiant division among the sub-dimension of Impetuous approach, however, significant division was found according to considering approach (X^2 =6,174 P<0.05), avoidant approach (X^2 =13,366 P<0.05), evaluator approach (X^2 =1,307 P<0.05), self-assured approach (X^2 =13,970 P<0.05), planned approach (X^2 =6,274 P<0.05) and total point approach (X^2 =14,524 P<0.05).

Table 5. The Result of Kruskal-Wallis Test Related to The Factor for Participant's Education Status According to Problem-Solving Total and Sub-Dimensions.

		N	Mean Rank	Sd	X^2	P	Meaningful Differences
Impetuous Approach	High school	48	64,60	2	12,459	,002*	2-3
	University	11	65,64				
	Other	50	43,44				
Considering Approach	High school	48	62,15	2	6,492	,039*	3-1
	University	11	61,73				
	Other	50	46,66				
Avoidant Approach	High school	48	61,36	2	16,964	,000*	2-3
	University	11	81,18				
	Other	50	43,13				
Evaluator Approach	High school	48	52,66	2	,498	,779	-----
	University	11	57,64				
	Other	50	56,67				
Self-assured Approach	High school	48	66,28	2	15,457	,000*	3-1
	University	11	64,18				
	Other	50	42,15				
Planned Approach	High school	48	64,36	2	9,149	,010*	3-1
	University	11	57,36				
	Other	50	45,49				
Total Point	High school	48	65,63	2	19,534	,000*	2-3
	University	11	73,64				
	Other	50	40,70				

The sub-dimension of problem-solving for volleyball player and total score according to their eduation status and whether it became different or not related to this factor were examimed with the Kurskal Walis test in Table 5. In the study result, there isn't any signifiant division among the sub-dimension of Evaluator approach, however, significant division was found according to considering approach (X^2 =6,492 P<0.05), avoidant approach (X^2 =16,964P<0.05), impetuous approach (X^2 =12,459 P<0.05), self-assured approach (X^2 =15,457 P<0.05), planned approach (X^2 =9,149 P<0.05) and total point approach (X^2 =19,534 P<0.05)

Table 6. The Result of Kruskal-Wallis Test Related to The Factor For Number Of Participant's Family Member According to Problem-Solving Total and Sub-Dimensions.

		N	Mean rank	Sd	X^2	P	Meaningful Differences
Impetuous Approach	3	14	53,86	3	8,836	,032*	3-2
	4	34	43,10				
	5	37	58,58				
	6	24	67,00				

Considering Approach	3	14	50,14	3	1,254	,740	-----
	4	34	52,22				
	5	37	56,15				
	6	24	60,00				
Avoidant Approach	3	14	52,32	3	3,584	,310	-----
	4	34	48,43				
	5	37	56,35				
	6	24	63,79				
Evaluator Approach	3	14	60,54	3	2,945	,400	-----
	4	34	55,87				
	5	37	48,42				
	6	24	60,69				
Self-assured Approach	3	14	47,79	3	3,206	,361	-----
	4	34	50,90				
	5	37	55,81				
	6	24	63,77				
Planned Approach	3	14	40,93	3	5,058	,168	-----
	4	34	55,15				
	5	37	54,18				
	6	24	64,27				
Total Point	3	14	51,82	3	5,010	,171	-----
	4	34	47,38				
	5	37	56,16				
	6	24	65,85				

*p<0,05

The sub-dimension of problem-solving for volleyball player and total score according to their number of family member and whether it became different or not related to this factor were examimed with the Kurskal Walis test in Table 6. In the study result, there isn't any signifiant division among the sub-dimension of evaluator approach, considering approach, avoidant approach, self-assured approach, planned approach and total score factor however, significant division was found according to impetuous approach (X^2 =8,836 P<0.05).

THE DISCUSSION OF RESULTS

It was indicated that mean total score of problem-solving, the point average of the sub-dimensions of problem-solving skill as, Impetuous, Considering avoidant, Evaluator, self-assured and planned approach are low. According to gender factor, Impetuous, Considering, avoidant, Evaluator, self-assured, planned approach in total score has been identified as significant in all sub-dimensions. It was thought that in overcoming the problems faced by women and men, the perception of the problem, acceptance and have different perceptions to reach a solution. These results are in line with the work that has done by [24].

According to the factor of the team which they play volleyball; the ratio of volleyball player in Gençlik Spor Erkek team is higher than the volleyball players who play in Güneş Spor Kız team in the level of sub-dimension of avoidant approach. At a level of the sub-dimension of the self-assured approach, it was indicated that the ratio of the volleyball male players in Gençlik Spor is higher than the female players in Selçuklu Belediye Kız. At a level of the sub-dimension of the planned approach, it was determined that the ratio of volleyball player in Gençlik Spor Erkek team is higher than the volleyball players who play in Güneş Spor Kız team. And at a level of the sub-dimension of the total score, the ratio of volleyball player in Gençlik Spor Erkek team is higher than the volleyball players who play in Selçuklu Belediye Kız team. The reason of male player's attitude, such as self-confidence that is showed in the case of a problem and to be assured as well as ignoring the problems they face while coping with a problem, the behavior of not being aware of the problem might differ according to their position within the team and gender.

According to the starting age of volleyball factors, it is shown that in the sub-dimension of Considering approach, avoidant approach, Evaluator approach, self-assured approach, planned approach and total score, the rate for starting sport between the ages 11-13 is higher that the age group of 5-7. It can be said that the ones that have older age are more adequate according to event detection, monitoring, and evaluation. The finding from the study of [23] are showing similarities.

According to the factor of education status, while the rate of Impetuous approach, avoidant approach and total score who has chosen the selection of "other" is higher than who has chosen the selection of "university", self-assured and planned approach at the level of the ratio of the other options, educational level as other is higher than the option "high shool". By taking into consideration, the thing that is expected from education is the necessity of Considering versatile in the problem-solving for individuals, we can express that the level of education could affect the size of approaches against problems. The finding from the study of [19] are showing similarities.

According to the factor of the number of family members, while the rate of Impetuous approach with a number of 5 members is higher than with a number of 4 members. We can say that, according to the family size, the problem-solving skills are different, the solving process might be late in case of a large number of family members, and because of that, in the face of the problems encountered, the attitude of moving towards without taking into account different factors is displayed.

References

[1]. **Ağır, M. (2007).** Üniversite Öğrencilerinin Bilişsel Çarpıtma Düzeyleri İle Problem Çözme Becerileri ve Umutsuzluk Düzeyleri Arasındaki İlişki, Yayımlanmamış Doktora Tezi, İstanbul Üniversitesi Sosyal Bilimler Enstitüsü, İstanbul.

[2]. **Aksan N. (2006).** Üniversite Öğrencilerinin Epistemolojik inançları ile Problem Çözme Becerileri Arasındaki ilişki. Yayınlanmamış Yüksek Lisans Tezi. Çanakkale On Sekiz Mart Üniversitesi, Sosyal Bilimler Enstitüsü, Eğitim Bilimleri Anabilim Dalı, Çanakkale.

[3]. **Bingham A. (2004).** Çocuklarda Problem Çözme Yeteneklerinin Geliştirilmesi. (Çeviri A.F. Oğuzhan) İstanbul. Türkiye Cumhuriyeti Milli Eğitim Bakanlığı Yayınları.;6.

[4]. **Burger M.J., (2006).** "Kişilik", Kaknüs Yayınları, 1. Basım, İstanbul.

[5]. **Büyüköztürk, Ş. (2010)** Sosyal bilimler için veri analizi el kitabı. Ankara: Pegem Akademi Yayınları.

[6]. **Cüceloğlu D. (2004).** İnsan ve Davranış. İstanbul. Remzi Kitapevi.

[7]. **Çam, S., (1995)** Öğretmen Adaylarının Ego Durumları ile Problem Çözme Becerisi Algısı İlişkisinin İncelenmesi. Psikolojik Danışma ve Rehberlik Dergisi. 6(2), 37-42.

[8]. **Ferah, D., (2000)** Kara Harp Okulu Öğrencilerinin Problem Çözme Becerilerini Algılamalarının ve Problem Çözme Yaklaşım Biçimlerinin Cinsiyet, Sınıf, Akademik Basarı ve Liderlik Yapma Açısından İncelenmesi. Yayınlanmamış Yüksek Lisans Tezi. Hacettepe Üniversitesi, Sosyal Bilimler Enstitüsü, Eğitim Bilimleri Anabilim Dalı, Ankara.

[9]. **Güçlü, N. (2003).** Lise Müdürlerinin Problem Çözme Becerileri. Milli Eğitim80.Yıl Özel Sayısı. Sayı: 160, 272-300

[10]. **Gülşen, D. (2008).** Farklı Lig Düzeyinde Oynayan Futbolcuların Oynadıkları Mevkilere, Öğrenim Durumu ve Spor Yaşlarına Göre Problem Çözme Becerilerinin İncelenmesi,, Yayımlanmamış Yüksek Lisans Tezi, Adana

[11]. **Heppner PP., Petersen CH. (1982)** "The development and a implications of a personal problem solving inventory", Journal of Counseling Psychology, 29(1), 66–75.

[12]. **Heppner PP, Baumgardner AH, Jackson J. (1985).** Depression and Attributional Style: Are They Related? Cognitive Therapy and Research; 9: 105–113

[13]. **Izgar H. (2008).** Headteachers Leadership Behavior and Problem Solving Skills: A Comperative Study. Social Behavior and Personality [serial online] [12.02.2012] 36(4) Availible from: http://apps.ısıknowledg.com.

[14]. **Karabulut, E.O. (2009).** Beden Eğitimi ve Spor Öğretmenliği Bölümü Öğrencilerinin Problem Çözme Becerileri ile Kişilik Özelliklerinin Bazı Değişkenler Bakımından Belirlenmesi ve Karşılaştırılması (Ahi Evran Üniversitesi ve Gazi Üniversitesi Örneği), Yayımlanmamış Doktora Tezi, Gazi Üniversitesi, Ankara.

[15]. **Korkut, F. (2002).** Lise Öğrencilerinin Problem Çözme Becerileri. Hacettepe

Üniversitesi Eğitim Fakültesi Dergisi, 22: 177-184.

[16]. **Nezu AM. (1985).** Differences in Psychological Distress Between Effective and İneffective Problem Solvers. Journal of Counselling Psychology; 42: 42–48.

[17]. **Nezu AM, D' Zurilla TJ. (2007).** Solving Life's Problems: A5 Step Guide To Enhanced Well-Being, New York. Springer Publishing Company. 4.

[18]. **Öğülmüş S. (2006).** Kişilerarası Sorun Çözme Becerileri ve Eğitimi. Ankara. Nobel Yayınları, 9

[19]. **Saracaloğlu A.S., Serin O., Bozkurt N. (2001).** Dokuz Eylül Üniversitesi Eğitim Bilimleri Enstitüsü Öğrencilerinin Problem Çözme Becerileri İle Başarıları Arasındaki İlişki, M.Ü. Atatürk Eğitim Fakültesi Eğitim Bilimleri Dergisi, 14, 132.

[20]. **Savaşır, İ., ve Şahin, N. H. (1997)** Bilişsel-Davranışçı Terapilerde Değerlendirme: Sık Kullanılan Ölçekler, Ankara: Türk Psikologlar Derneği Yayınları, No: 9.

[21]. **Şahin N., Şahin NH., Heppner PP. (1993)** "Psychometric propoties of the Problem Solving Inventory in a group of Turkish university students", Cogn Ther Res, 17: 379-396.

[22]. **Taylan, S. (1990)** Heppner'in Problem Çözme Envanteri'nin Uyarlama, Güvenirlik ve Geçerlik Çalışmaları, Yayınlanmamış Yüksek Lisans Tezi, Ankara Üniversitesi, Sosyal Bilimler Enstitüsü, Ankara.

[23]. **Temel V., Ayan V. (2015).** Beden Eğitimi ve Spor Öğretmenlerinin Problem Çözme Becerileri, KMÜ Sosyal ve Ekonomik Araştırmalar Dergisi 17 (29), 75.

[24]. **Yıldırım A., Hacıhasanoğlu R., Karakurt P., Türkleş S. (2011).** Lise Öğrencilerinin Problem Çözme Becerileri Ve Etkileyen Faktörler, Uluslararası İnsan Bilimleri Dergisi, 8(1), 905.

5

DEVELOPMENT STRATEGIES FOR A NATIONAL SPORTS ORGANIZATION: METHODOLOGY AND APPLICATIONS

Prof. PhD H.C. Adrian DRAGNEA
University of Târgovişte

Abstract: In the field of sports, development strategies (by level) include: the social mission of sport, the vision of accomplishing the mission, the values that must result from activities carried out over long periods of time (more than 12 years).
In Romania, there have been developed strategies at the national level by field of activity, such as the economic, cultural, educational, sporting and financial ones, as well as at the region, county and local levels.
Designing a strategy involves completing an acknowledged methodology specifically applied to a field, depending on its traits and dimensions.
The disharmony existing between the statements of leaders and current realities, the lack of knowledge of the basic concepts and their contents, and consequently the sports-specific categories, the appointment of leaders based on political criteria and the sponsors unprepared specifically represent handicaps which are difficult to overcome when developing strategies in the field
Key words: Development strategies, national sports, organization

1. Introduction

Strategos (Greek), meaning the leader, the commander of an army or a general, is a term that has changed its content in the time of Pericles (450 BC), when it started denoting leadership (in administrative, oratorical, power-related terms). Throughout the years, the term has evolved. Thus, according to Napoleon Bonaparte, strategy is the art of application, and according to Clausewitz, strategy is the art of using military forces to achieve the goals set by policy. Nowadays, strategy is perceived intentionally and is concretized in programs, plans and methods aiming at the future of a country, the social area, institutions, sports federations, sports clubs, firms and the operations involved to reach the objectives. It is also perceived as the sum of objectives set by leaders, which must be reached within a given time.
In the field of sports, development strategies (by level) include: the social mission of sport, the vision of accomplishing the mission, the values that must result from activities carried out over long periods of time (more than 12 years).
In Romania, there have been developed strategies at the national level by field of activity, such as the economic, cultural, educational, sporting and financial ones, as well as at the region, county and local levels.
All these have become necessary and possible in an increasingly globalized external environment integrating the social, economic, cultural and other areas. The internal environment seeks forms of understanding according to the dominant ideology, animated by policies with different scopes.
National sports organizations are concerned, in a broad sense, with their prospective development, optimization of the activity, construction of the own future over a long period of time. Strategy development is laborious, because sport has become a cultural, educational, economic and managerial field with increasingly complex social functions.
The durations of strategies in sport are relatively easy to establish if one takes into account the 4-year periodicity of the Olympics. In sport, there are conventionally used the following periods: the near (4 years), medium (8 years) and large (12 years or more) ones.

2. Material and method

Designing a strategy involves completing an acknowledged methodology specifically applied to a field, depending on its traits and dimensions.
The strategies of organizations, particularly of national sports federations and sports clubs, include the following phases:

- Defining the mission of the organization
- Purpose of the activity or its strategic target/targets delimited and described as clearly as possible
- Explicit vision of the way of action for achieving the mission, based on data resulting from:

o An analysis of the external environment in which the organization performs
o An analysis of the internal environment of the organization
• Strategic targets by subsystem (globally)
• Strategic objectives by subsystem (sport for all, performance sport, adapted sport) or department (technical, economic, financial, human resources)
• Activities for achieving the objectives
• Factors with responsibilities (duties)
• Performance indicators
• Human resources
• Strategy implementation (phases, stages, roles)
• Assessing the performance indicators (objectives, activities) and the achievement of strategic targets

3. Results

3.1. The objectives of a federation are to grow and develop activity in the sport it administers, and they are established according to policies, as shown in Figure 1:

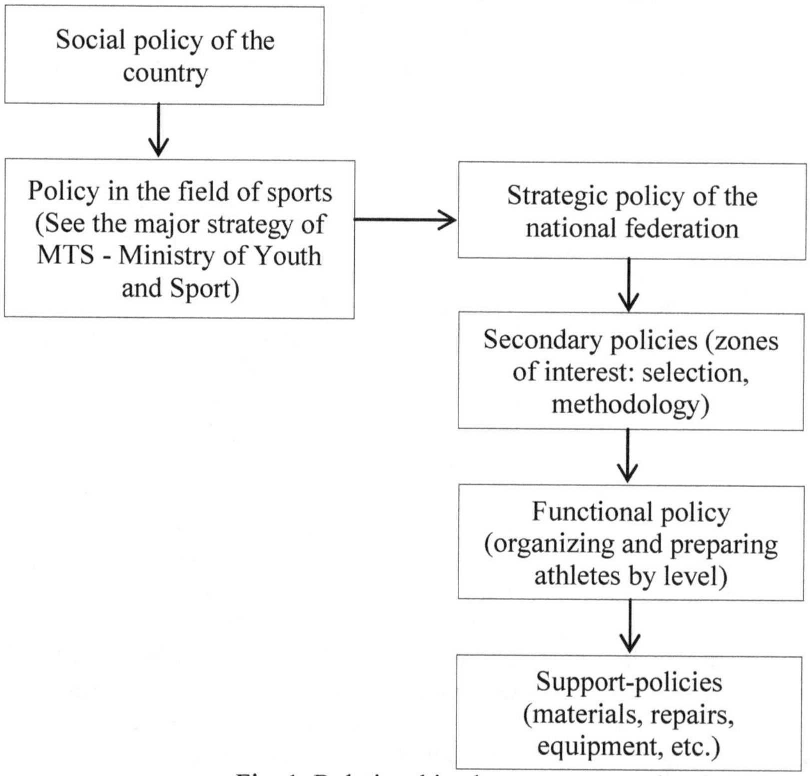

Fig. 1. Relationships between sports development policies

3.2. Explicit vision resulting from:
• An analysis of the external environment:
- Political factor: the strategy of Romanian sport is developed in the European context, in compliance with and by applying the legislation drawn up to increase the social role of sport, as seen in Figure 2.
- Sociocultural factor:
o Performance sport – Athletes Without Frontiers (AWF)
o Sport as a cultural and human development factor:
▪ Mutations and development directions
▪ Emergence of new sports
▪ Training reconceptualization and restructuring. Directions of action in performance development
- Economic factor
- Technological factor
• An analysis of the internal environment:
- National policy on sport is concretized in a series of laws and normative acts, among which the most important are:

o Law of Physical Education and Sport no. 69/2000, with subsequent amendments
o Law of National Education no. 1/2011, with subsequent amendments
o Normative acts and government emergency ordinances on the organization of sport, the fight against doping, financing, human resources, the professionalism status, etc.

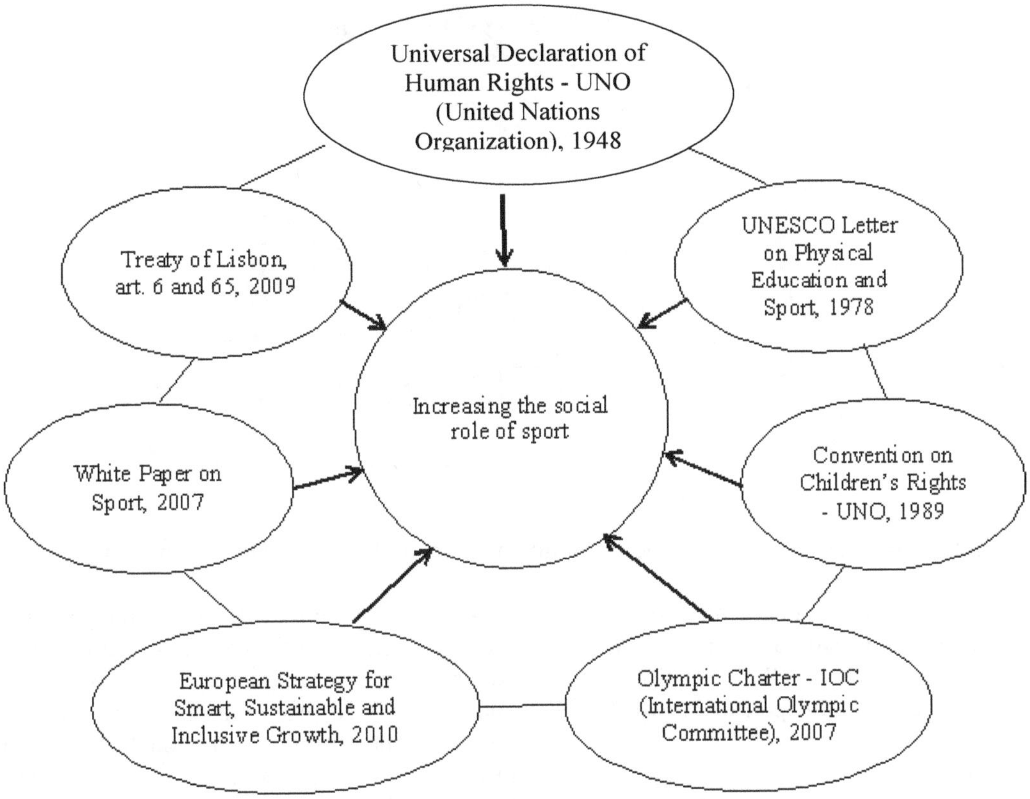

Fig. 2. International political context in which the Romanian sport is developing

The defining notes of Romanian sport and implicitly of subjacent organizations are shown in Figure 3.

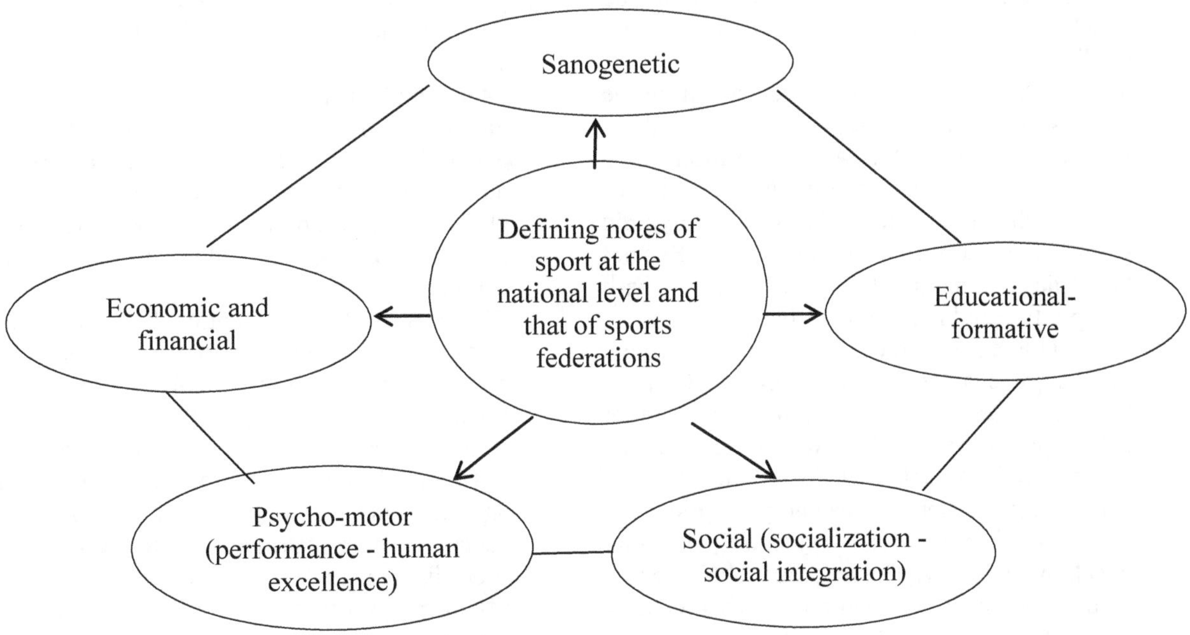

Fig. 3. Dimensions of sport

3.3. SWOT analysis has emphasized several aspects:

3.3.1. As regards sport for all (European Commission, Eurobarometer Sport and Physical Activity, March 2014), it is noted that, among the 28 European countries, the percentage of Romanian population not involved in the practice of sport reaches 60% (Figure 4).

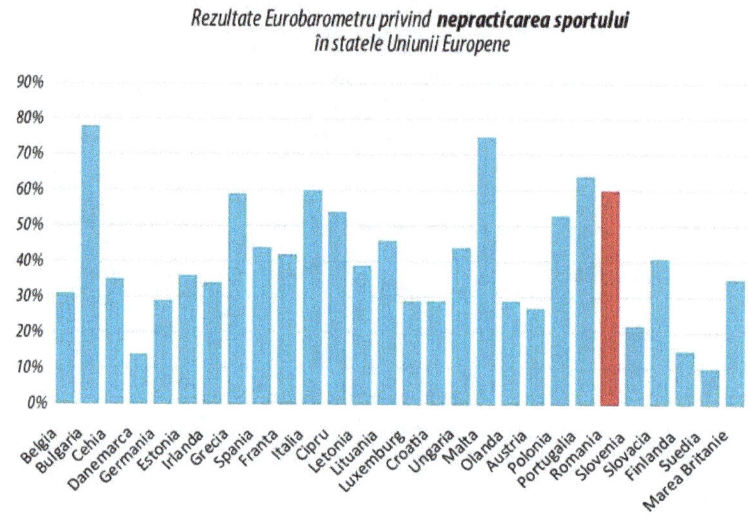

Fig. 4. Eurobarometer results on the non-practice of sport in the European Union countries

3.3.2. Performance sport is characterized, at the national level (total federations), by the following data provided by INS (National Institute of Statistics) for the period between 1924 and 2012:

- 96 Olympic medals
- 976 medals at the World Championships and European Championships
- a drastic decrease in the number of registered athletes
- a decrease in the number of employed coaches, especially those with higher qualification

3.3.3. Adapted sport is organized based on the models of good practice provided by three institutions: Sport for All Federation (also concerned with the integration of sport for people with disabilities), National Paralympic Committee (performance level) and Special Olympics Romania (sport for all - with competitive and non-competitive forms).

3.3.4. Human resources. On 14 July 2016, the number of coaches in the records of CNPFA (National Center for the Training and Further Development of Coaches) was 41020, for the 66 federations acknowledged and for all categories: Master, 1st category; Senior, 2nd category; 3rd category; 4th category; assistant coach, 5th category. The records include people in the documents of the center, whether they are in the country, abroad, employed or not engaged in the profession.

Weaknesses: poor qualification (many people); non-involvement of specialists from higher education in awarding categories; unaccredited and not updated programs; lack of correlation between the training of coaches and the provisions of Law no. 1/2011; inexistence of an occupational standard for coaches; conflicts of interest between the institutions involved; inexistence of a Sectoral Committee for Sport; lack of professional associations, etc.

3.3.5. International resources. Scientific research and methodological assistance

The specificity of research is interdisciplinarity.

Factors involved: INCS (National Institute for Sport Research); few research centers for human performance within the faculties for physical education and sport; INMS (National Institute of Sports Medicine); scientific conferences.

Weaknesses: low international visibility; low transfer of knowledge to applications; low number of experts involved; precarious financing, etc.

3.3.6. Material resources - infrastructure. In 2013, in Romania, there were 417 sports organizations, among which: 276 clubs, central administration structures; 48 subordinated to MTS; 220 subordinated to MENCS (Ministry of National Education and Scientific Research); 141 structures/clubs subordinated to local administration; 69

structures of joint-stock companies; 3843 private structures/clubs.

3.4. Strategic targets and objectives

Strategic targets derive from the mission and generate the strategic objectives by subsystem:

- Examples of strategic targets and objectives for a subsystem
  - Increasing active and systematic participation of the population of all ages in sports activities to promote health, education, social integration and cohesion

- Increasing the number of participants and facilitating access to sports programs
- Enhancing the level of information and education about sports and other physical activities

- Examples of strategic targets and objectives for a sports club
  - Contributing to the improvement of general health status of the population registered at the club
  - Promoting annually 1 or 2 athletes from each section of the club to national sports teams

- Increasing the number of participants in sports competitions for all organized by the club
- Enlarging the selection base and making up 2 or 3 groups of children and juniors in each section

Each subsystem or organization ends with the performance indicators expressed in an objective way. For instance, increasing annually by 10% the number of participants in the competitions organized by the club

- Example regarding scientific research
  - Development of scientific research at the club level by assigning tasks to the own specialists

- Preparing information documents for the population about the sports actions organized and the assistance provided
- Improving the selection system and highlighting the dynamics of skills by age

The same methodology is applied for:

- Material resources - infrastructure
- Human resources
- Financial resources

3.5. Strategy implementation

- Factors involved
- Activities by factor
- Strategy restructuring depending on future evolutions of the external and internal environments

3.6. Forms of assessment

- Periodic balance sheet (annually or biannually)
- Auditing
- Synthesis reports

4. Discussions and conclusions

1. Developing long-term strategies in the field of sports, in general, or of sports branches, in particular, is necessary in order to guide the development, specify the performances achieved by organizations, formulate and implement decisions, systematically control the actions undertaken.
2. Strategies are characterized rather by generalities, they reflecting the external environment patterns, fully harmonized ideologically and politically.
3. The goals of the activity must reflect the conceptual structure of the assumed social mission, of policies, by teleological judgment, giving meaning to the involved parties.
4. Strategies, regardless of the type of sports organization and its level, are developed in the context of new communicational strategies.
5. The structure of any medium- or long-term strategy must comply with the scientific methodology of strategic management: mission, vision, values, purpose and/or strategic targets, objectives, activities, factors involved, performance indicators, implementation and forms of assessment.
6. Strategy proposals for the Romanian sports development in the past 20 years were developed in an artisanal, autodidactic way by people incompletely prepared, in the context of the conflicts of interest between departments, largely focusing on the financial aspects and those related to the material base. The professionalism of human resources was the task of departments associated to sports.
7. The disharmony existing between the statements of leaders and current realities, the lack of knowledge of the basic concepts and their contents, and consequently the sports-specific categories, the appointment of leaders based on political criteria and the sponsors unprepared specifically represent handicaps which are difficult to overcome when developing strategies in the field.

References

[1]. Bloyce, D., & Smith, A. (2010). *Sport Policy and Development: An Introduction.* London & New York: Routledge.

[2]. Council of the European Union (2013). *The Health-Enhancing Physical Activity.*

[3]. De Bosscher, V. (2007). *Sport Policy Factors Leading to International Sporting Success*. Brussels: VUB Press.

[4]. Dragnea, A. (coord.) (2002). *Teoria educaţiei fizice şi sportului*. Bucureşti: FEST.

[5]. Dragnea, A., & Teodorescu, S. (2002). *Teoria sportului*. Bucureşti: FEST.

[6]. European Commission (2010). *Europe 2020. A European Strategy for Smart, Sustainable and Inclusive Growth.*

[7]. European Commission (March, 2014). *Eurobarometer - Sport and Physical Activity.*

[8]. Green, M., & Houlihan, B. (2005). *Elite Sport Development: Policy Learning and Political Priorities*. London & New York: Routledge.

[9]. Houlihan, B. (1997). *Sport, Policy and Politics: A Comparative Analysis*. London: Routledge.

[10]. Institutul Naţional de Sănătate Publică (2013). *Raportul Naţional de Sănătate a Copiilor şi Tinerilor*. Bucureşti.

[11]. International Olympic Committee (2007). *Olympic Charter*.

[12]. Naneş, M. (2001). *Strategii de firmă*. Bucureşti: Sylvi.

[13]. Societatea Română pentru Educaţie Fizică şi Sport (2004). *Strategia de dezvoltare a educaţiei fizice şi sportului în România*. Bucureşti.

[14]. *Strategia de dezvoltare teritorială a României. România policentrică 2035 - coeziune şi competitivitate teritorială, dezvoltare de şanse egale pentru oameni.*

[15]. World Health Organization (2004). *Global Strategy on Diet, Physical Activity and Health.*

[16]. Strategii elaborate de salariaţii MTS pentru anii 2008, 2009, ... 2013, 2014, 2015 (propuneri nefinalizate).

(Note: Because the strategies submitted to authorities do not include the sources of inspiration, except for explicit official data on some situations, states and other exigencies, we present only the documents that have been used in this paper.)

6

ATTRACTIVE WAYS TO IMPROVE THE FENCERS LOWER LIMB STRENGTH THROUGH MOVEMENT GAMES

Cătălin FORȚAN, Gabriel MANGRA, Camelia VLĂSCEANU, Cătălin POPESCU

University of Craiova

Abstract: The physical preparation in fencing occupies an important place in the athletes' training, the basic positions requiring a permanent contraction of the lower limbs. The paper aims to highlight the role which the non-specific means of the physical training has on the development of the force in the lower limbs.

Method. Thus, a group of 18 athletes (aged 11-12) have participated in a training program in which nonspecific means were introduced in the physical training, especially in gymnastics and movement games. The subjects were tested pre and post intervention, aiming at the development of explosive strength of the legs.

Results. The recorded data showed significant progress concerning the detent (11.13%), the lower limb strength recorded statistically significant differences after applying the new means.

Keywords: fencing, strength, unspecific means,

Introduction

The force is regarded as one of the most important capabilities that greatly influences the manifestation of all the motor components. It is expressed in the body through its ability to achieve efforts based on the muscle contraction with the defeat of a resistance. [1,2]

Fencers should train lower-body power emphasizing horizontal displacement, noting that this seems to offset any advantage one would expect fencers of a taller stature to have.[3] To meet the demands of the discipline, one uses appropriate programs of strength and conditioning, program in which strength, power, and power-endurance qualities (including economy of movement) can be enhanced.[4]

Cosma et al, sustained that lack of unspecific physical training can lead to the situation when athletes have satisfactory results only to a certain stage of training and at the seniorship abruptly fall because they can't handle different movement situation[5]. The fencers' training consists of combining physical, technical, tactical and moral-volitional training; such a training strengthens the multilateral, physical and moral health, it develops the strength of the functional systems of the body and influences the achievement of the the best sport results.

Therefore, this paper aims to validate the working programs, with the purpose of optimization of the beginner fencers' training by applying the means of physical training based on non-specific gymnastic exercises and movement games.

Methods

A group of 18 beginner fencers participated in training for 6 months, which had in their structure non-specific fencing means to develop the strength in the lower limbs. The subjects have been practicing fencing for 1 year and are assigned to the beginner group. The means used were mainly motion games that have contained many jumps, but there were also means specific to gymnastics. The subjects were tested before and after implementing the work programs, the tests were the following:

LONG JUMP FROM STANDSTILL. The test is common to both sexes. It allows a single swinging of the arms for take-off. There are given two attempts and recorded the best jump. It is measured the distance from the tiptoe (starting position) to the heel (landing position). The jumping surface must be smooth and non-slippery. One jumps barefoot or wearing tennis shoes. The results are recorded in centimeters and converted into points according to the tables.

VERTICAL DETENT. This test evaluates the ability of the explosive force of the lower limbs. The performer sits with a shoulder to the wall at a distance of one foot. They wet their middle finger of the hand from the wall, execute a slight take-off bending the knees and depart trying to leave, with the wet finger, a trace on the wall as high as possible. Then, they sit against the wall with the relaxed arm up and leave another trace behind under the first one. It is measured in cm. the distance between the two traces. After two attempts, it is recorded the best result.

VERTICAL DETENT - 50cm. This test measures the jump height after landing from a height of 50cm. More than in the previous test, in this muscle effort there are involved the contractile fibers and the elastic ones of the lower body. It is aimed at the testing of the participation in the effort of the slow fibers (red) which enable a high oxygen raport, and although they cannot develop great strength, they are resistant to fatigue, and the fast fibers (white) with high level of concentration, but short-lived.

The trainee, with the shoulder to the wall, after having moistened the middle finger, starts from a right position after a platform situated at a height of 50cm and after landing in a square of 30cm performs a rapid depreciation followed by a high jump, vertically, leaving a trace, landing again in the same square. Then, he sits back against the wall with his arm raised in an unforced position, leaving another trace after the first one. It is measured the distance in centimeters between the two signs, checking the best result in two attempts.

MOVING 10M WITH ONE STEP FORWARD It is measured the forward speed of the fencers; considering the optimal distance to check only the speed of execution, without the involvement of other motric qualities. The athlete in the guard position with the front toe at the starting line, must undergo, at the highest speed, the 10m route with a step forward, without turning the movement into running or into added step forward. The timing is started at the beginning of the movement, and the result is recorded in seconds and tenths of seconds. There is recorded the best result in two attempts.

MOVING 10M. WITH ONE STEP BACKWARDS. It is measured the speed of the fencers. The athlete sits in the guard position, with his foot back (left foot for the right-handed, right foot for the left-handed) at the starting line, having to complete, steps back, a distance of 10m. without turning the movement into running or into added step back; there is minuted the time at the lifting of the back foot and the reaching of the same leg of the line situated at 10m and it is recorded in seconds and tenths of seconds ; from two attempts whichever is the best result is recorded.

Results

Following the initial and final testing, the subjects recorded the following data (Table No. 1 and Table No. 2)

Table no.1 Initial and final testing on explosive strength

Nr.	Name	VERTICAL DETENT T1	VERTICAL DETENT T2	VERTICAL DETENT 50cm T1	VERTICAL DETENT 50cm T2	Standing long jump T1	Standing long jump T2
1.	B.I.	40	42	41	43	195	200
2.	B.E.	41	42	39	41	198	204
3.	A.I.	39	41	39	40	180	185
4.	H.I.	38	39	37	38	184	187
5.	S.S.	36	39	36	39	175	180
6.	D.C.	37	40	40	43	180	182
7.	R.A.	32	35	31	36	170	174
8.	D.A.	33	36	34	37	184	189
9.	I.N.	30	34	30	34	173	179
10.	F.F	37	38	39	42	178	180
11.	C.I.	36	39	36	38	180	183
12.	B.C.	41	42	43	46	179	191
13.	S.I.	40	41	41	44	175	178

14.	S.M.	42	44	43	45	208	212
15.	L.A.	38	40	37	40	186	190
16.	B.O.	39	40	41	13	200	205
17.	V.D.	36	37	36	38	189	191
18.	A.S	37	39	38	40	178	180
Mean		35.39	39.33	37.78	40.39	180.78	188.33
Average		8.93	2.61	8.98	7.17	18.27	10.64
p		0.02		0.03		0.01	
Dif.		3.94		2.61		7.55	
Dif%		11.13		6.90		4.2%	

Table no.2 Initial and final testing after specific evaluation

Nr.	**Name**	**10m. p.int.**	**10m forward T2**	**10m. p.in**	**10 m backward T2**
1.	B.I.	3”60	3”52	4”28	4”01
2.	B.E.	3”79	3”70	4”25	4”13
3.	A.I.	3”80	3”74	4”32	4”03
4.	H.I.	3”72	3”60	4”80	4”54
5.	S.S.	4”00	3”55	4”84	4”62
6.	D.C.	3”66	3”33	4”25	4”01
7.	R.A.	4”22	4”05	4”47	4”14
8.	D.A.	3”68	3”32	4”06	3”85
9.	I.N.	3”56	3”29	4”06	3”90
10.	F.F	3”46	3”32	3”58	3”32
11.	C.I.	4”00	3”87	4”12	4”02
12.	B.C.	3”52	3”48	4”00	3”89
13.	S.I.	3”47	3”32	4”10	4”02
14.	S.M.	3”41	3”35	3”56	3”41
15.	L.A.	3”15	3”03	3”66	3”48
16.	B.O.	3”03	2”95	3”27	3”15
17.	V.D.	3”34	3”25	4”29	4”20
18.	A.S	3”87	3”62	4”48	4”21
Mean		3.63	3.46	4.13	3.94
Average		0.30	0.28	0.41	0.39
p		0,02		0,02	
Dif.		0,17		0,19	
Dif%		4,68		4,60	

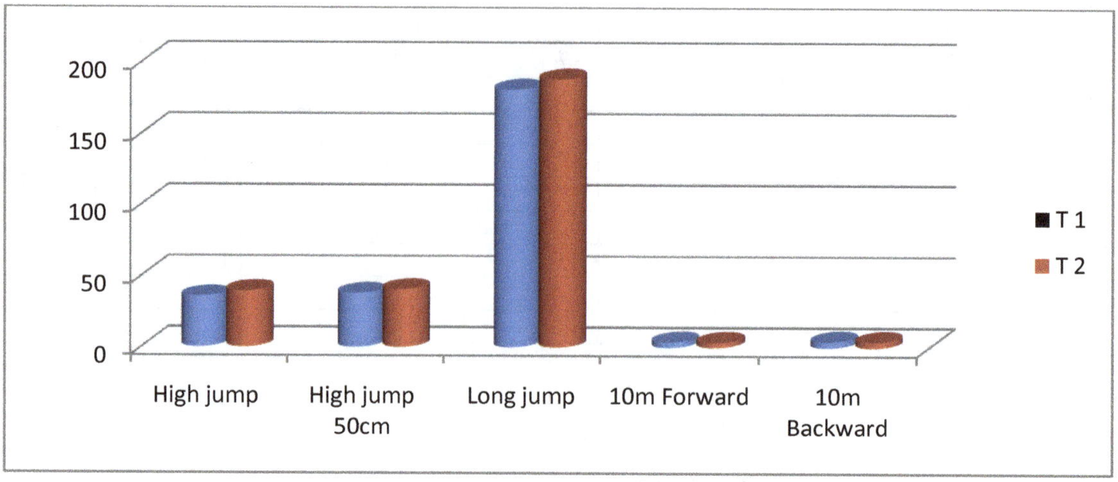

Chart no. 1 Initial and final testing

In the detent test, there was recorded in the initial testing an average of 35.39 (± 8.93cm) and in the final one, after applying the work program, the average rose to 39.33 (± 2.61cm) (chart no.1), registering the progress of 11.13%.

In the detent test -50cm, there was recorded in the initial testing an average of 37.7 (± 8.98cm), and in the final testing, the subjects had an average of 40.39 (± 7.17cm) the progress being 6.90%.

The long jump test recorded in the initial testing an average of 180.78 (± 18.27cm), in the final testing, the subjects had an average of 188.33 (± 10.64cm), the progress being 4.2%.

The specific tests, the movement 10m with one step forward and step backward registered significant progress (4.68% and 4.60%). Thus, the accumulations within the motric tests were found also in the specific tests, thus the explosive force positively influenced movement on the fencers'board.

Conclutions

The current trends in sports performance show that the specialists in the field are always looking for new means or improving existing ones, in order to increase the sports performance, which were introduced since the junior stage. The means applied in our progress have proven their effectiveness, the lower limb strength is improved, the difference of the initial and final averages was statistically significant at a threshold of $p < 0.05$. Besides the fact that the means were effective, we could see an increase in competition within the training, the exercises being extremely attractive to the athletes.

References:

[1] Rață, G. Rață, (2006), *Aptitudinile în activitatea motrică*, editura EduSoft, Bacău, p.183

[2] Dragnea A, (1996), *Antrenamentul sportiv,* Editura Didactică şi Pedagogică, R.A., Bucureşti, p.85

[3] Turner, A., Bishop C., Chavda S., Edwards M., Brazier J., Kilduff LP., (2016), *Physical characteristics underpinning lunging and change of direction speed in fencing, Journal of Strength and conditioning research*, vol.30, Issue 8, pp.2235-2241

[4] Turner A., Miller S., Steward P., Cree J., Ingram R., Dimitriou L., Moody J., Killduf , *Strength and Conditioning for Fencing.* Available from: https://www.researchgate.net/publication/235790920_Strength_*and_Conditioning_for_Fencing* [accessed Oct 17, 2016].

[5] Cosma A., Orțănescu D., Cosma G., (2014), The role of gymnastics elements in training junior volleyball players, *Procedia Social and Behavioral Science* 117 (2014) pp. 427-430

7

EXERCISES AND MOVEMENT GAMES FOR CORRECT POSTURE EDUCATION IN YOUNG PUPILS

Constantin ALBINĂ, Alina Elena ALBINĂ

The University of Craiova, Faculty of Physical Education and Sports, Romania

Abstract: Introduction. The strengthening and consolidation of the body, the improvement of movement skills and basic motor skills development are primordial components of the tasks system of physical education at young school age.

Methods

The experiment that I conducted took place at the Middle School No.39 with Classes I-VIII Craiova, Dolj County, during October 2015 - April 2016.

For a more extensive knowledge of the students subject of the research, we turned to a series of tests, regarding the somatic side, making anthropometric measurements, and also some traction tests.

We used a set of exercises, games and relay race utility applications for forming a correct posture in young pupils.

Results

After the initial and final evaluations, we found significant differences in favour of the experiment group, through the continuous use of exercises, games and relays race utility applications.

Conclusions

The tests carried out during the experiment, and the results of the experiment group confirm the effectiveness of the methods and procedures used, leading to very good results in control tests used.

Keywords*:* methods, young pupils, exercises, correct posture.

Introduction

The process of physical education is an active process which involves direct pedagogical initiative and child responsibility; it represents the efficient method of education, consolidation, compensation and fortification and is considered an integral part of the educational process [1].

The level and the effectiveness of the teaching-learning process of the motor skills, condition the accomplishment of the other components of training, respectively the harmonious physical development, the positive development of motor skills, the ability to act in an organized manner, both individually and collectively, the ability to generalize the application expressed by the participation in dynamic games play, relays race, applicative pathways, competitions [2].

The acquisition, enhancement and improvement of basic motor skills, of utility and specific to some sport branches, occupy a central position, reflected by both the objectives and the content of the physical education curriculum, in all classes [3].

The purpose of the work

Consists in selecting exercises and games applications utility appropriate capacity development coordination to students, from a middle school.

Methods

The research lasted for one school year (2015-2016) and included students from two fifth grade classes, from a middle school in Craiova.

In the class experiment were mainly used exercises, movement games and relay races of utility applications during physical education classes and sports, and the other pupils class (control group), which worked following the school curriculum for fifth grade. [4, 5, 6, 7, 8]

We used different exercises for balance training:

- On an area of 20 cm wide, drawn on the ground is executed: walking in balance, with the back straight, head up, eyes forward, arms outstretched to the side; the leg executing the walk is stretched, stepping on the ground with the toe;
- Reducing the support area or the execution conditions (walking on tiptoe, standing on one leg, etc.);
- Return at 360 degrees at the middle of the trail;
- Handling of objects (scarves, clubs, circles).

Relay race utility applications used for balance training:

- Walking in balance on the gym bench to the end, descent, running to a fixed point, return, walk in balance to the end with relay race to the next continuing the action;

- Walking in balance on the gym bench to the end, raising a knee to the chest, return, walk in balance until the end of the bench, with relay race to the next pupil continuing the action.

We used different exercises to train crawling:

- Starting position - support on the knee. Moves forward at a distance of 1/2 step, one knee and opposite arm, followed by the forward movement of the two other limbs;
- Lying on the face, support on the hands, arms outstretched, forward motion on the palms, the body remains stretched and tiptoes supported on the ground.

We used different exercises to train climbing:

- Face at the fixed ladder, feet resting on the last lath, arms bent, hands gripped to the lath at the chest level. The left foot is lifted on the first lath, is pushed on it to lift the body, while simultaneously lifting the opposite arm on the next lath. Continue the climbing action;
- Climbs up to the middle of the ladder, after moving left or right side, with arm and leg on the same side, and then follows the other arm and leg approach. You can also switch from one ladder to another.

Relay race utility applications used in climbing:

1. Running, climbing on the fixed ladder, descent, running and handing over to the next continuing the relay race action.
2. Running, climbing the sailor ladder to the top, descent, running and handing over to the next continuing the relay race action.
3. Running, climbing up to the top of the rope, descent, running and handing over to the next continuing the relay race action.

Through exercises and games we used in the experiment group, over this period, we monitored the general physical development and the training of basic motor skills.

Results

Somatic indices hereby confirm the fact that when the physical education teaching is carried out as planned, while fully respecting the curriculum, the growth in height and weight is within normal proportionality parameters.

The obtained results reveal that during lessons were continuously monitored the executions of children, correcting whenever needed, explaining the stages of implementation, the basic moments and how to make their connection, so that the global implementation to offer an unitary picture (tables 1,2,3,4).

Table 1 The results of the control tests (initial testing and final testing) Experiment group

No. crt.	Subjects Girls	Shuttle 3x5m (sec)		Long jump/ On the spot (cm)		Applied relay race (sec)	
		T.I.	T.F.	T.I.	T.F.	T.I.	T.F.
1	A.D	15,4	15,1	92	98	38	21
2	B.C.	15,9	15,5	88	94	43	24
3	B.V.	16,0	15,7	96	103	48	25
4	C.A.	15,2	14,9	76	82	39	22
5	C.M.	15,7	15,2	102	108	38	23
6	P.V.	16,2	15,5	98	105	37	20
7	R.G.	15,3	14,7	106	113	34	18
8	T.E.	15,6	15,0	103	109	35	19
X		15,66	15,20	95,12	101,5	39	21,5
S		0,33	0,32	9,10	9,31	4,24	2,29
Cv		0,02	0,02	0,10	0,09	0,11	0,11

Note: X - average S - standard deviation Cv - the coefficient of variability

Table 2 The results of the control tests (initial testing and final testing) Control group

No. crt.	Subjects Girls	Shuttle 3x5m (sec)		Long jump/ On the spot (cm)		Applied relay race (sec)	
		T.I.	T.F.	T.I.	T.F.	T.I.	T.F.
1	B.G.	15,5	15,4	78	83	46	36
2	B.F.	16,0	15,9	102	107	35	29
3	C.d.	16,3	16,0	80	86	42	28
4	C.F.	15,7	15,7	92	96	40	26

5	G.I.	15,9	15,7	98	101	36	24
6	I.E.	16,2	16,1	104	107	32	25
7	P.V.	15,8	15,6	104	108	30	20
8	Ş.A.	16,1	15,9	106	110	32	23
X		15,94	15,79	95,50	99,75	36,62	26,37
S		0,25	0,21	10,38	9,77	5,22	4,50
Cv		0,02	0,01	0,11	0,10	0,14	0,17

Note: X - average S - standard deviation Cv - the coefficient of variability

Table 3 The results of the control tests (initial testing and final testing)
Experiment group

No crt.	Subjects Boys	Shuttle 3x5m (sec)		Long jump/ On the spot (cm)		Applied relay race (sec)	
		T.I.	T.F.	T.I.	T.F.	T.I.	T.F.
1	A.I.	14,3	14,0	88	94	40	27
2	B.C.	14,8	14,2	84	91	42	29
3	B.V.	14,5	14,1	85	92	38	24
4	C.M.	14,1	13,8	103	112	28	20
5	C.A.	14,9	14,5	98	108	39	27
6	I.I.	14,2	14,1	104	113	30	19
7	P.A.	14,7	14,3	110	122	25	17
8	P.I.	14,6	14,0	92	108	37	22
X		14,51	14,13	95,50	105,00	34,87	23,12
S		0,27	0,20	9,06	10,64	5,88	4,04
Cv		0,02	0,01	0,09	0,10	0,17	0,17

Note: X - average S - standard deviation Cv - the coefficient of variability

Table 4 The results of the control tests (initial testing and final testing)
Control group

No. crt.	Subjects Boys	Shuttle 3x5m (sec)		Long jump/ On the spot (cm)		Applied relay race (sec)	
		T.I.	T.F.	T.I.	T.F.	T.I.	T.F.
1	A.I.	14,3	14,2	92	95	37	28
2	B.M.	15,0	15,3	108	112	32	26
3	B.G.	14,8	14,6	84	88	29	23
4	B.I.	14,6	15,0	76	80	41	29
5	C.A.	15,2	15,0	88	91	39	30
6	C.B.	14,5	14,3	98	102	33	27
7	C.F.	14,4	14,0	104	108	30	22
8	G.F.	15,1	15,0	106	112	28	19
x		14,74	14,68	94,50	98,50	33,62	25,50
σ		0,32	0,44	10,71	11,11	4,53	3,57
Cv		0,02	0,03	0,11	0,11	0,13	0,14

Note: X - average S - standard deviation Cv - the coefficient of variability

Using permanently exercises, within physical education lessons, games of movement, as they became attractive, capturing the attention of children, asking them a high physical effort, an effective participation, and thus helping to increase the results of the entire group.

Conclusion

1. Based on the findings both in terms motor and somatic parameters, we concluded that the bio-motor development both in the control group and the experiment, correspond to the level of training, but at the same time to the peculiarities of age and sex, confirming the validity of the experiment.

2. The forms of generalization-application (dynamic games, relay races, trails, complex exercises, competitions, contests) that have particular impact on children on motor and

mental plan and are loved by them, cannot be executed without requiring them to master motor skills.

3. Engaging the whole body in motion, the skills require the complex manifestation and permanent of the kinaesthetic sense, muscles and tendons transmitting "information" on the contraction and requesting level, generating spontaneous adaptations.

4. Learning motor skills applied and their application in complex forms attract an extensive physical participation of the child leading to the education of some traits and qualities that can turn into lifelong stable characteristics.

Acknowledgement

All authors have equal contribution.

References:

[1] Cârstea, Gh., (1993) *Teoria şi metodica educaţiei fizice şi sportului*, Bucureşti, Universul, p.23.

[2] Mitra, Gh., Mogoş, Al.,(1980) *Metodica educaţiei fizice şcolare*, Bucureşti, Sport Turism, p.175.

[3] Barta A., Dragomir P.,(1995) *Deprinderi motrice la preşcolari*, Bucureşti, Integral, p. 76.

[4] Barcan Ţibuliuc, E., (1976) *Exerciţii şi jocuri pentru preşcolari*, Bucureşti, Sport-Turism, p.163.

[5] Bucur. C.I., (1979) *Jocuri dinamice pentru clasele I-IV,* Timişoara, Centrul Metodologic de studii şi documentare, p.36 .

[6] Corneşeanu, T., (1970) *Exerciţii şi jocuri aplicative pentru şcolari*, Bucureşti, Stadion, p. 89.

[7] Niculescu, Al., Cruli, N., (1976) *Exerciţii şi jocuri în şcoală*, Bucureşti, Sport Turism,p. 45.

[8] Teodorescu,D,T., (1994) *Exerciţii de educaţie fizică şi ştafete pentru clasele I-IV*, Craiova, GHE. Cîrţu Alexandru, p.70.

8

DEVELOPMENT OF MOTOR QUALITIES THROUGH MEANS SPECIFIC TO FOOTBALL IN MIDDLE SCHOOLS

Aurora UNGUREANU - DOBRE[1], Doru STOICA [1], Roxana DUMITRU[1], Gheorghe VERGU[2]

University of Craiova, Faculty of Physical Education and Sports, Brestei Street, No. 156
"Matei Basarab" National College of Informatics, Râmnicu Vâlcea, Henri Coanda Street, No. 21

Abstract : This paper represents the applied research for the elaboration of the Grade I Paper of professor V.G., at "Matei Basarab" National College of Informatics from Râmnicu Vâlcea. The issued hypothesis, that was verified, aimed to develop the motor qualities through technical methods specific to football, at the level of the representative school team, but also the efficiency and attractivity in comparison to the traditional means. The subjects of the research were students from 6th - 8th grades, members of the representative team of the abovementioned school. The applied control trials were: Speed 5x10m – for acceleration speed; Jumps over the gymnastics bench - for the strength of the lower limbs; dribbling among cones - for skill, and Short Marathon - for resistance. After applying the technical methods from football for the development of the motor qualities of the representative team of the school, that were the aim of the control trials, and after analysing the results from the control trials, from the initial testing until the final testing, progress was made concerning all control trials. We concluded that the hypothesis was confirmed, the applied means were efficient and attractive in comparison to the traditional ones.

Key words: representative team, speed, coordination, resistance, strength.

Introduction

The football game is characterized by the alternation of the maximal, submaximal and medium efforts with active or passive, sometimes unequal and incomplete, pauses, as well as by physical, spontaneous and unforeseen actions like duration and intensity.

Agility, coordination and speed are important components of a football player`s performance needed to play football, and then these can be developed through taking part in playing football systematically and regularly. [1]

To date speed, agility, coordination, dribbling and kicking theoretically and practically found to be the issue which numerous studies suggested, a paramount difference has been observed in the physical capacity of the team compared with the past. Numerous research studies has brought sufficient evidence that in the game situation, agility, coordination and speed are the components of the dribbling and kicking performance of football players. [2]

Apparently, speed, coordination, agility, dribbling and kicking are becoming more and more imperative in football game situations. It is not surprising, the intensity of the game, the attacking movements, the breaks from out of defense and changes in the tempo of the game require greater and nonstop endurance on the part of the players. [3]

A vast number of publications revealed that agility, coordination, speed, dribbling and accuracy pass has been the fundamental components of a successful football player`s performance. [4]

One of the most overlooked aspects in the game of soccer is the importance of the overall physical conditioning. It has been my experience that many soccer coaches understand the benefits of strength training, but view it as secondary to skill training or simply misunderstand its importance in the game. Contrary to popular belief, strength training has a positive effect on an athlete's speed and explosive power. In addition, strength training helps to reduce injuries and aids in a faster recovery should the unfortunate occur. [5]

The main aim of fitness training in football is to target the physiological mechanisms causing fatigue and thereby limiting physical football performance. A higher fatigue resistance will allow the players to utilize their technical and tactical capacity throughout a game and especially during the critical game periods. [6]

In middle schools, the activity with the representative football team can start simultaneously with the school year, adding, of course, in its composition, other students, after a selection from the middle school classes, considering that the students from the previous 8th grade have gone to high school.

A lesson carried out with the student of the representative team is similar to a training class at junior level, it being planned 3 times per week or every day, if possible, especially around the time of competitions.

Teaching soccer on a reduced field, at middle school, was conducted using the analytical method, every technique being isolated taught for acquisition, respecting the teaching methodology of this discipline.

After the learning stage, we will pass to the binding of the learned procedures into technical and tactical structures which will be consolidated through repetition. Subsequently, the leaned and consolidated technical processes, and technical and tactical actions will be applied in the bilateral game with simplified rules which will lead to their perfecting. Thus, the student, will must resolve some game phases using the available motor luggage and especially overcoming the opponent, who, during the game, is active and with unforeseen actions.

The integral game can't be practiced without the students having the minimum theoretical knowledge in addition to the specific motor skills.

As a conclusion, the isolated learning of the technical processes will be for a short period, insisting on their consolidation during the technical and tactical structures and activities of the game, and through practicing the bilateral game.

In the present research we tried to determine whether the use of the technical processes from football, which have reached the consolidation stage, will be effective for the development of motor qualities at the students of the representative school team.

Material and methods

The hypothesis from which we started the research was: is the development of the motor qualities using the technical methods specific to football, at the level of the representative boys team of the school, more effective and more attractive than using traditional means.

The experiment was performed at the representative team of "Matei Basarab" National College of Informatics from Râmnicu Vâlcea, boys from the 6th to 8th grades, during the two semesters.

We have worked with the students of the representative school team, after the planning documents drafted, involving their participation in sport competitions provided for the middle schools.

The applied control trials at the initial and final testing were: Control trial 1 - Speed 5x10m - from acceleration speed; Control trial 2 - Jumps over gymnastics bench - force of the lower limbs; Control trial 3 - Dribbling between cones (skill), and Control trial 4 - Short Marathon (resistance).

Working with the students of the representative school team in the training lesson followed the traditional means, treating the speed or skill theme at the beginning of the fundamental part (never both in the same lesson), and the force and/or resistance theme at the end of the fundamental part. These were permanently coupled with football themes.

The motor qualities themes were covered using the game and emulation means, the means being the technical methods specific to the football game, reached in the consolidation stage, and the methodical succession of the discipline teaching was respected for the football themes.

Next we exempify/mention a few the actuation means (Ungureanu A. 2009) specific to football for motor qualities targeted to develop in the present experiment: "The pitches into a semicircle", "The pitches into a circle", "Following it on the front", "The man and the ball", "Emulations for force". [7]

Results

Table no.1 - The Table of the control trial results of the initial testing (T_I) and final testing (T_F)

No.	The students ' initials	Class	Control Trial 1		Control Trial 2		Control Trial 3		Control Trial 4		Control Trial 5	
			T_I	T_F	T_I	T_F	T_I	T_F	T_I	T_F	T_I	T_F
1	A.O.	VIII A	14.40	14.03	35	42	11.42	11.21	89	83	1.37	1.23
2	C.S.	VIII A	13.87	13.10	36	38	12.41	12.04	38	47	1.40	1.22
3	P.L.	VIII A	14.05	13.80	32	37	13.04	12.84	81	92	1.41	1.20

4	S.A.	VIII A	13.25	13.07	31	34	12.85	12.70	56	58	1.38	1.23
5	F.L.	VIII B	13.66	13.23	41	43	11.85	11.25	187	212	1.31	1.24
6	D.R.	VIII C	13.93	13.60	34	38	13.04	12.53	57	84	1.38	1.22
7	D.A.	VIII C	12.93	12.85	44	45	10.44	10.24	158	184	1.35	1.23
8	D.Ş.	VIII C	13. 23	13.03	30	38	13.89	12.74	55	65	1.38	1.24
9	O.A.	VIII C	14. 24	13.70	31	42	11.94	11.25	46	54	1.38	1.30
10	T.R.	VIII C	14.84	14.17	35	39	13.50	12.90	42	50	1.43	1.35
11	G.R.	VIII D	14.42	13.95	34	40	12.14	12.05	88	76	1.44	1.36
12	P.B.	VIII D	14.12	14.00	32	36	11.87	11.07	75	81	1.41	1.33
13	I.Ş.	VIII E	13.88	13.65	36	38	13.94	12.91	47	51	1.38	1.30
14	P.D.	VIII E	13. 23	13.13	33	35	12.91	12.24	45	57	1.30	1.24
15	P.M.	VIII E	14.34	14.10	33	37	10.40	10.22	108	113	1.35	1.27
16	P.E.	VII A	13.57	13.11	42	44	10.82	10.64	123	119	1.36	1.30
17	S..C.	VII E	13. 95	13.21	38	40	11.91	11.77	51	64	1.37	1.30
18	T.A.	VII E	14.57	14.11	30	35	12.21	11.65	84	91	1.45	1.37
19	R.L.	VII C	13.81	13.52	40	43	10.97	10.41	103	125	1.39	1.32
20	P.E.	VII C	13.75	13.40	36	35	11.96	11.42	175	205	1.42	1.40
21	T.V.	VII D	13.21	13.10	41	42	13.40	12.90	43	57	1.39	1.38
22	T.A.	VI B	13.84	13.70	34	32	10.11	10.15	39	28	1.41	1.39

Legend:
T_i - Initial testing
T_f - Final testing

Discussions

Table no. 2 - The Table of the differences and progress between the initial and final testing at all control trial

The control trial	Speed 5x10m	Force - - Jumps over gimnasticsbeanch in 30″	Skill - Dribling between cones on 10 m	Skill - Kepping the ball in the air using both legs	Resistence - Short Marthon
D	0.42	3.41	0.45	9.36	0.10
D%	2.99 %	10.24 %	3.59 %	12.43 %	6.95 %

Legend: D-difference; D% -difference in % (the progress)

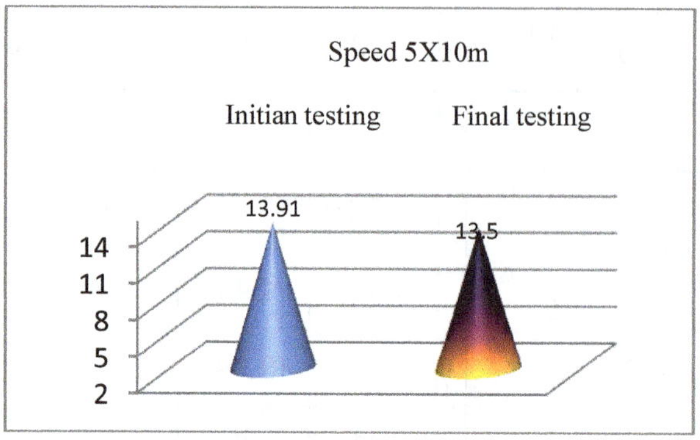

Graphic no. 1. Average of the initial testing (13,91) and of the final testing (13,5) of the control trial Speed 5x10m

1. At the control trial Speed 5x10m for the testing of the acceleration speed it **was** obtained an average of 13.91 seconds at the initial testing, and at the final testing of 13.50 seconds, recording an increase of 0.42 seconds and a progress of 2.99 % (graphic no 1.)

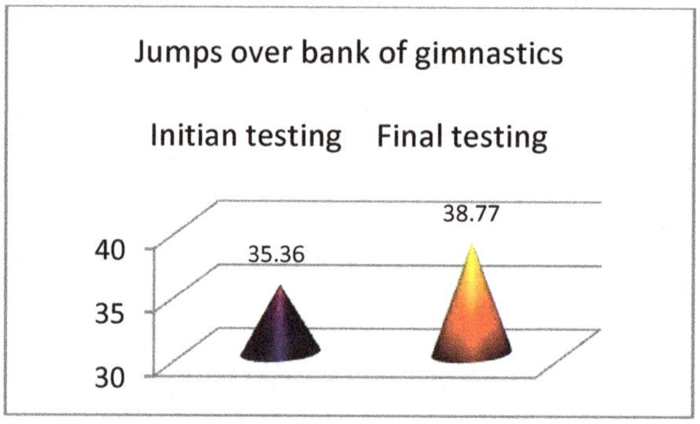

Graphic no. 2. Average of the initial testing (35,36) and of the final testing (38,77) of the control trial of Jumps over the gimnastics beanch for 30 seconds

2. For testing the **force** of the lower limbs, the control trial of Jumps over the gimnastics beanch for 30 seconds was applied, and the average at the initial testing was of 35.36 seconds and at the final testing of 38.77 second, recording an increase of 3.41 seconds corresponding to the progress of 10.24 % comparison withthe initial testing (graphic no. 2).

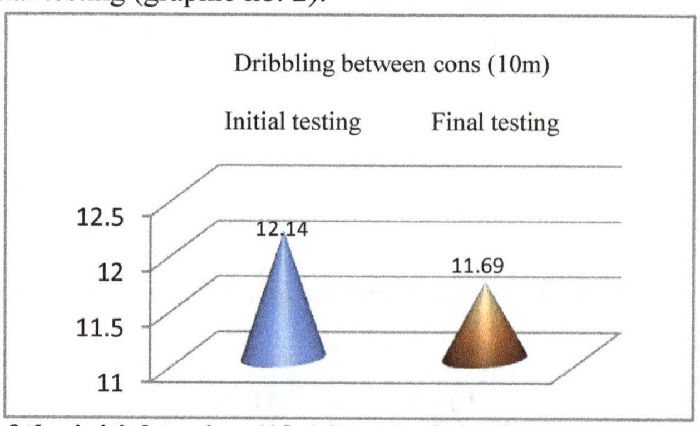

Graphic no. 3. Average of the initial testing (12,14) and of the final testing (11,69) of the control trial Driddling between cons (10 m)

3. The trial Dribbling between cones which focussed on **skill** wich, at the final testing records an increase of 0.45 seconds (the rate of the progress is of 3.59%) in comparison with the initial testing, the averages being of 12.14 seconds at the initial testing and of 11.69 seconds at the final testing (graphic no. 3.).

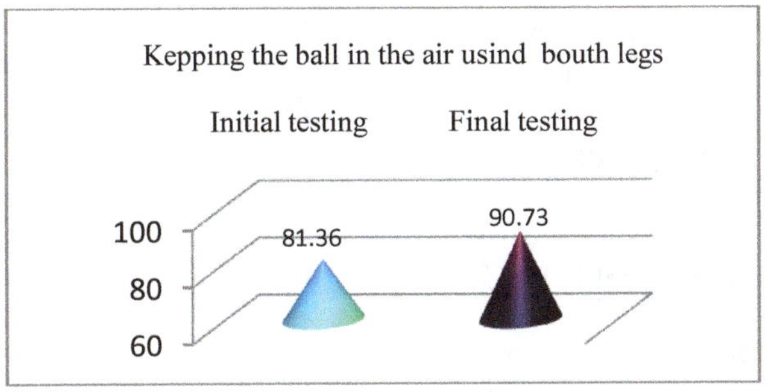

Graphic no. 4. Average of the initial testing (81,36) and of the final testing (90,73) of the control trial Kepping the ball in the air using both legs

4. The skill specific to football was tested also through the trial Kepping the ball in the air using both legs and at the final testing (90.73) it is recorded an increase of 1.15 (the progress rate is of 33.10%) in comparison with the initial testing (81.36) - (graphic no. 4.)

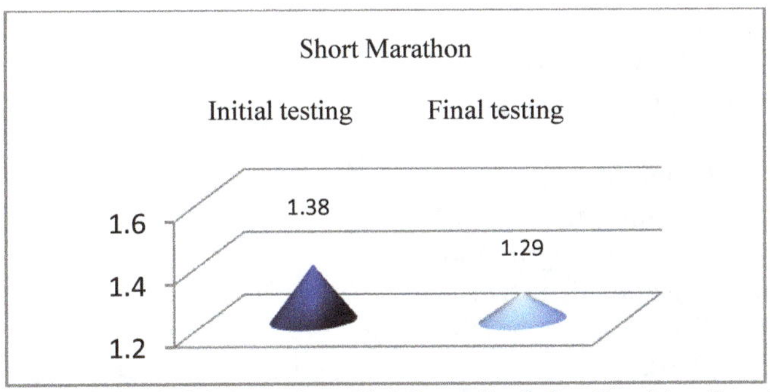

Graphic no. 5. Average of the initial testing (1,38) and of the final testing (1,29) of the control trial Short Marathon

5. The resistence in speed, specific to game phases on reduced field, was tested through the - Short Marathon obtaining an average of 1.38 seconds at the initial testing and of 1.29 seconds at the final testing and it was recorded an increase of 0.10 seconds (the progress rate is of 6.95 %) in comparison with the initial testing (graphic no. 5.).

Conclusions

1. From the initial testing to the final testing, the development indices of the motor qualities have improved, at all control trails, as:

✓ for the motor quality SPEED at the control trial *Speed 5x10 m,* the progress was of 2.99%;

✓ In the FORCE cases, the evolution the performances at Jumps over gimnastics beanch it was recorded a progress of 10.24;

✓ for the motor quality SKILL two control trials were applied and the evolution of the performances at Dribbling between cones it was recorded a progress of 3.59 %, and at the control trial - Kepping the ball in the air using both legs, it was marked an substantial increase of 33.10%;

✓ for the motor quality RESISTENCE at the control trial – The Short Marathon it was recorded a progress of 6.95%.

2. The differences and the progress between the averages from initial and final testing, are significative at all control trials, therefore we can say that using the tehnical methods specific to football, at this level, for development of the motor qualities (speed, force, resistence, skill) had expected efficiency, the hypotesis being confirmed.

References

[1]. Silassie, A.G., & Demena, T. (2016) - A study of agility, coordination and speed as related to dribbling and kicking performance of Jimma, Woliso and Sebeta town male football players. Journal of Physical Education Research, Volume 3, Issue I, pp 47-55.

[2]. John, F.G. (2014) - Agility training for athletic performance , http://www.performbetter.com/webapp/wcs/stores/servlet/PBOnePieceView?storeId=10151&catalogId=10751&pagename=347 - (Accessed 21 September, 2016).

[3]. Fahey, T.D., Roth, W.T., & Insel, P.M. (2003). Fit & well: core concepts and labs in physical fitness and wellness with online learning center bind-in card and daily fitness and nutrition journal (4th ed.), USA, McGraw-Hillcompanies, Inc, pp.31-32.

[4]. Neopolion, M, & Rani, U. (2014). Predict of football playing ability on selected skill related Variables & motor fitness variables of school level male football players. Indian Journal of Applied Research, *4*(5), 540-541.

[5]. Williams Sport Trainning (2012) - http://williamssport.com/lorem-ipsum-dolor/Reasons why - Speed, Strength and Power is important for the game of soccer - posted of January 26, 2012 by wstadmin (Accessed 21 September, 2016).

[6]. Mohr, M., & Iaia, F. M. (2014). Physiological basis of fatigue resistance training in competitive football. Sports Science, 27(126), 1-9, https://secure.footprint.net/gatorade/stg/gssiweb/pdf/SSE126_MohrIaia.pdf

[7]. Ungureanu A. (2009) - Predarea lecției de educație fizică prin jocuri de mișcare, Craiova, Editura Universitaria Craiova, pp: 205 - 245.

9

ISSUES ON LEARNING METHODOLOGY IN TENNIS RIGHT COUP IN CHILDREN

Claudiu Cristian TEUŞDEA

Faculty of Physical Education and Sport, Spiru Haret Spiru Haret University

Abstract: Kick right has evolved over time due to increases in velocity of the ball striking the upward trend, before the ball is hit on the downward trend, driving the opponent of placement median outside the sidelines of the field by opening angles and sending balls diagonally long before it is sent median, sending the ball diagonally short and the long line of positions of increasingly advanced followed the attack at the net before the ball being played at the bottom of the field, switching from using outlets fixed the changeable switch from using blows with the flat effect, changing the biomechanics of strokes.

Keywords: tennis, methodical kick right, kids, technique.

Introduction

In today's modern game, kick right is used by most players to put your opponent under pressure and win the point.

Initiation into tennis begins with learning the kick right.

Material and method

Tennis

Game that takes place between 2-4 players or players who send the ball over the net with rockets.

Technical

Sports Technique is a method or combination of methods, learned through the year in order to resolve as economically, rationally and with maximum efficacy with a task-based movement (in other words, a motor problem).[1]

Technique playing tennis is a set of motor skills specific form and content, consisting of hitting the ball with the racket on the spot and displacement achieved in order to practice in the most efficient game of tennis, in accordance with rules game official .[2]

Forehand

The kick is taken by right-handed right side of the body, and the left-handed left side of the body.

Consists in sending shot after ground contact ball over the net.

Kick right is a basic element in the game of tennis technique.[2]

Technical forehand include:

-fundamental position;

-outlet;

-preparation, impact and end the coup.

The techniques are composed of four basic points, ensuring their development:

- preparation mechanism;

-training mechanism for kicking the ball away;

-the mechanism of hitting the ball;

-completion mechanism of actions of hitting the ball. [3]

Kick right procedures are:

-stepping off place;-shift to ball;-spin (figure 1) [4];-cut (figure 2) [5];-flat (figure 3) [6].

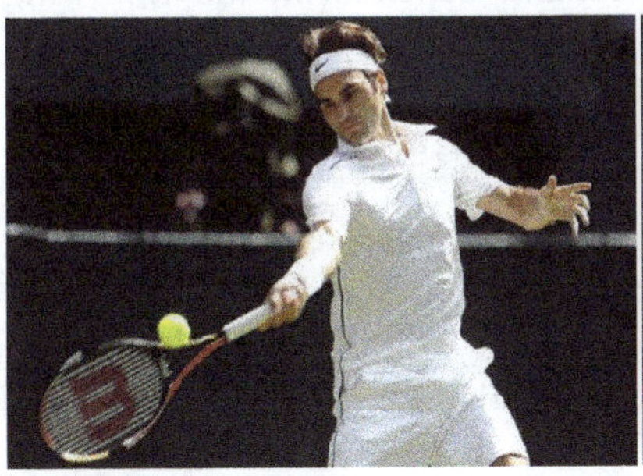

Fig.1 Spin right Kick [4]

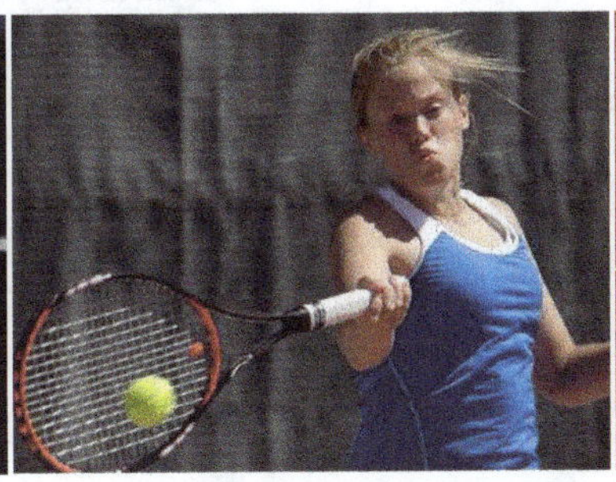

Fig.2 Cut right kick [5]

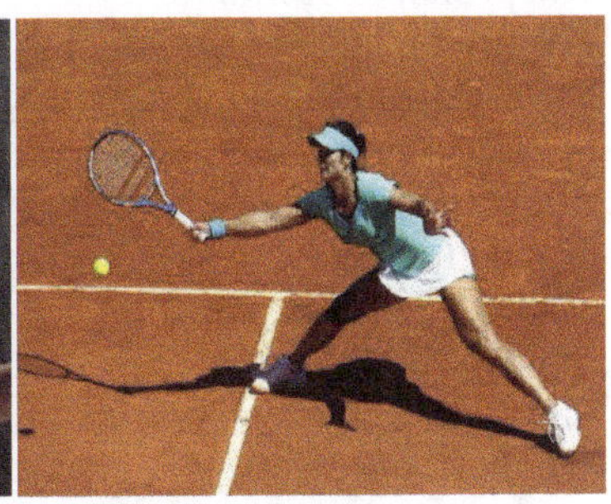

Fig.3 Flat right kick [6]

Children

In our days an increasing number of children are becoming more involved in recreational and competitive tennis.

From the age of 4-5 years old children can practice mini tennis, mini participate in training and competitions as required 10 Tennis imposed by the International Tennis Federation (ITF) from 2012.

Method

With the work we used the method of ascertaining study, bibliographic study method and the method of video movie about the coup learning techniques and methods right, taken from the "You Tube" processed by Freemake Video Downloader Defragmenter.

Learning Methodology

Theory of effective practice or active theory with practical finality. [7]

Methodology used in learning and perfecting technique and tactics of the game of tennis coach must solve the following tasks:

- creating an accurate representation of the item and the process taught;
- ensuring a proper execution of movements;
- formation of specific motor skills improvement;
- training - improvement of technical and tactical skills, accurate and effective.

Methodical orientation in teaching the game of tennis is based on a series of principles and methods that correspond to the principles and methods of instruction in physical education and sports training.

In tennis lesson may apply didactic principles (general and specific) and training methods.

General principles and teaching methods are:

- The principle of active and conscious participation.
- The principle of intuition.
- The principle of accessibility.
- Systematization and continuity principle.
- Modeling principle.
- The principle of sustainability.

Training methods:

- Method-verbal explanation.
- Intuitive method.
- The demonstration, observation.
- Method of practice - practice (analytical, global).

Specific sports training principles are:

- The principle of active and conscious participation.
- The principle of intuition.
- The principle of accessibility.
- Systematization principle.
- The principle of sustainability.
- Going concern.
- The principle that.
- The principle of specification.
- The principle of multilateralism. [8]

Learning forehand

Learning is a lasting change in behavior that occurs during interaction between organism and environment.[9]

Motor learning is specific to physical education and sport.

In motor learning elements exteroceptive, proprioceptive or are involved with different weights rational by nature of activity and actions that compose them. [9]

Synthesis bibliographic information specialist can draw the following types of motor learning presented below.

After driving skills approach:

- global learning (recommended by most experts for simple skills);
- partial or analytical learning (recommended for complex skills). [7]

The current trend, called "modern" in motor learning is to start with global learning and then move, if possible and appropriate, partial learning (for "polishing" technique).

By type of learning driving skills:

- intensive learning. when addressing one theme of driving skills in the same business;
- extensive learning, when addressing two or more themes driving skills in the same activity. [7].

Motor learning stages and their main objectives are:

- initiation stage primary properties;
- consolidation phase driving habit;
- improving the skill driving stage.

Learning forehand depends on the following factors:

Order learning: first blow.

Place execution: by age on the field red, orange and green.

Structure movement: analytical; overall.

Teacher actions: given the ball thrown and released.

Condition of practice: relieved, with coach; with a partner.

Structure motor : the place; walking, running.

Number of subjects: in groups, with partner, individually.

Effect ball: spin, flat, cut.

Direction coup: median; long line; long diagonal and short diagonal.

Learning the right kick is done in three steps:
1. Execution blow to a ball without rocket.
2. Imitating the right socket and rocket blow
3. Execution kick racquet and ball.

Right coup learning exercises propose the following structure for the three steps listed above:

1. Execution blow to a ball without rocket.

The objective of the exercise:
- learning hits the ball with the heel of the hand dexterous arm (figure 4,5);
- release arm ball adroitly learning (figure 6).

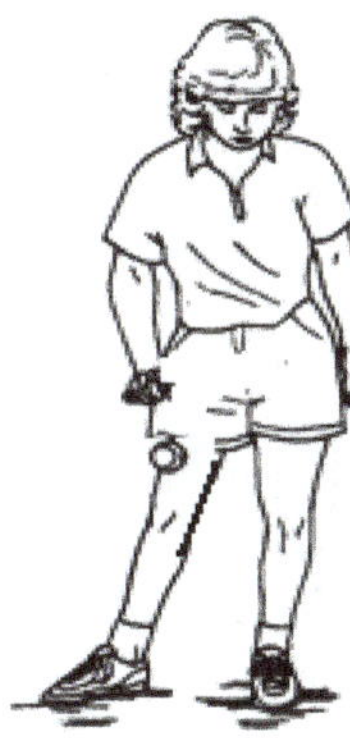

Figure 4.
Whipping the ball on the ground

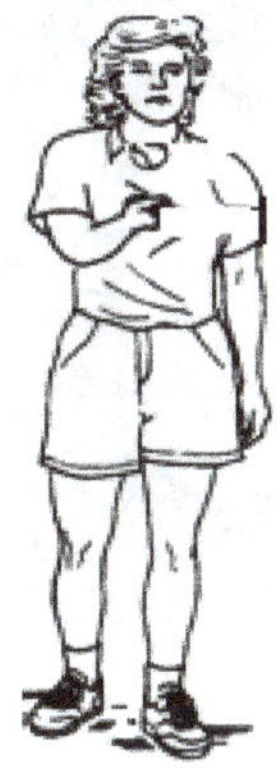

Figure 5.
Churning up the ball

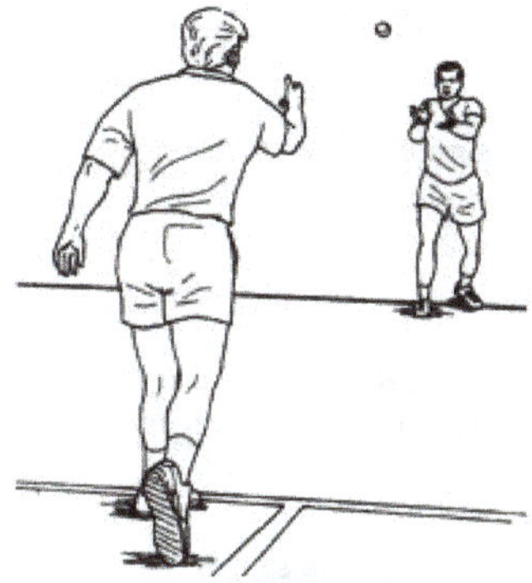

Figure 6.
Launch ball

2. Imitating the right socket and rocket blow

The objective of the exercise:
- learning to blow right socket (figure 7);
- learning the right technique coup place (figure 8)of running away (figure 9).

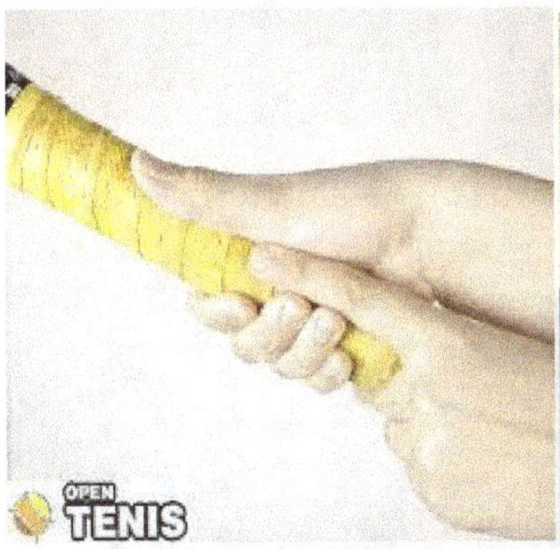

Figure7. Fixing right takeoff [10]

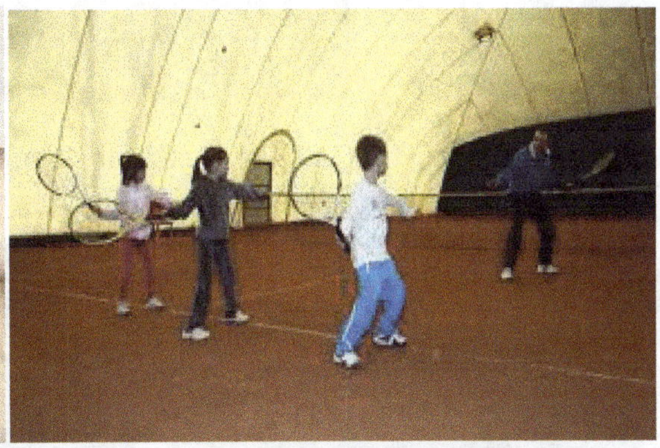

Figure 8. Imitating the right analytical coup [11]

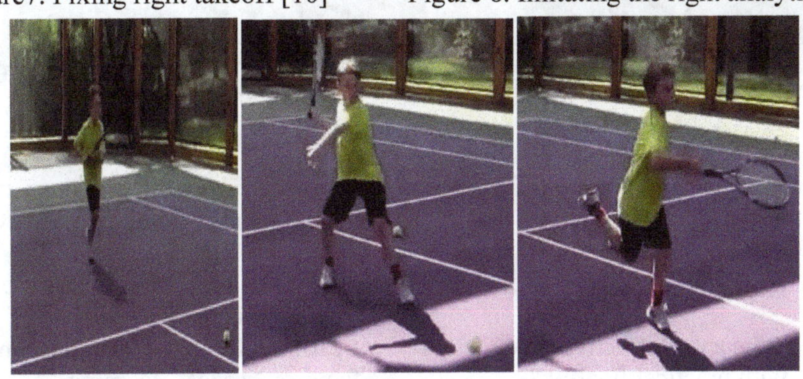

Figure 9. Kick right of running [12]

3. Execution kick racquet and ball.

The objective of the exercise:

- learning to blow right socket (figure 10,11);
- learning the right technique coup instead of running, analytical and globally (figure 12,13, 14, 15,16).

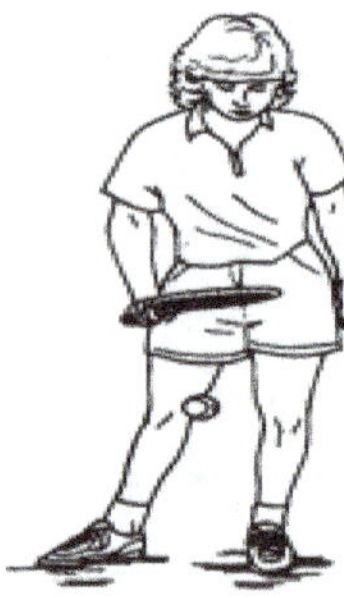

Figure 10. Striking the ball

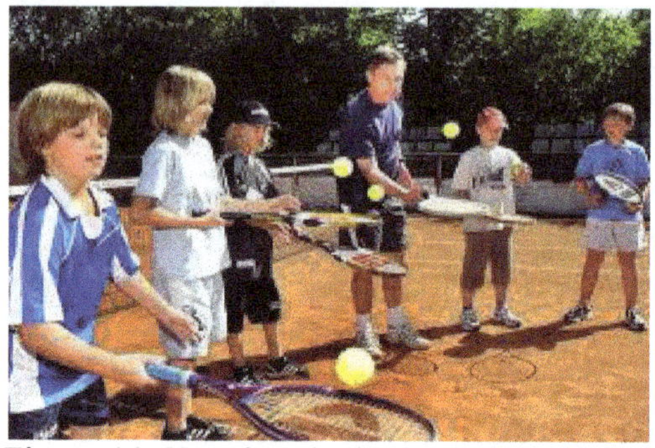

Figure 11. Keeping the ball on racket [13]

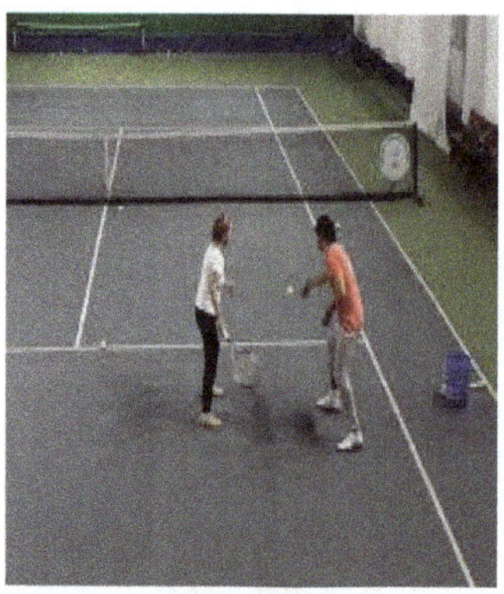

Figure 12. Kick ball provided [11]

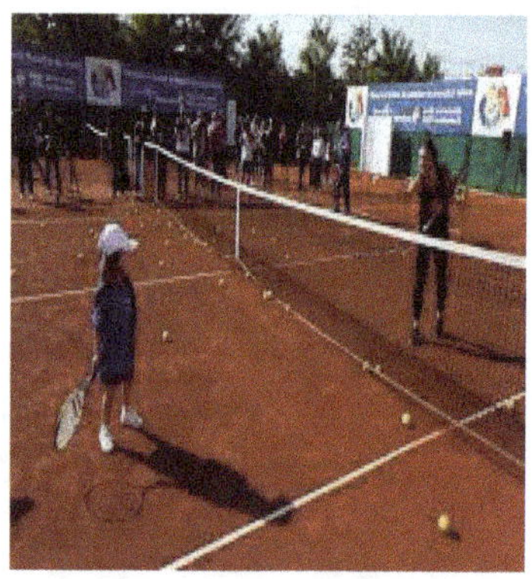

Figure 13. Kick ball thrown [14]

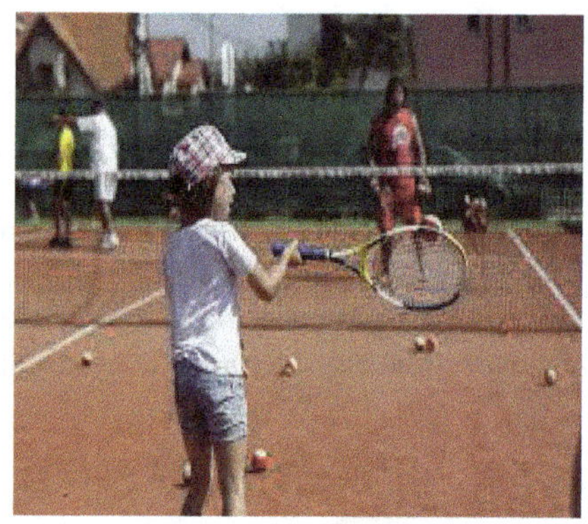

Figure 14. Kick ball launch [15]

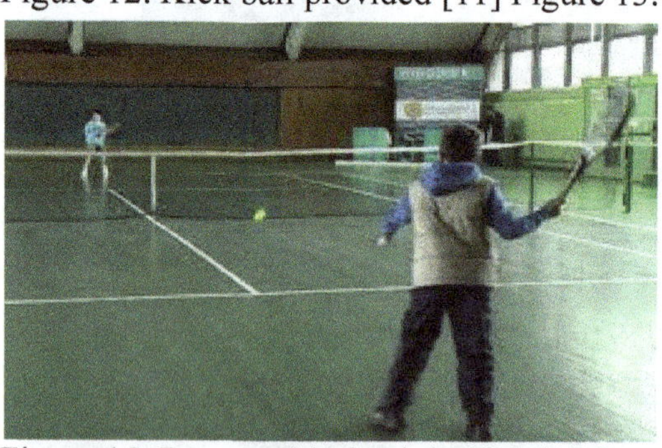

Figure 15. Passes with the right kick [16]

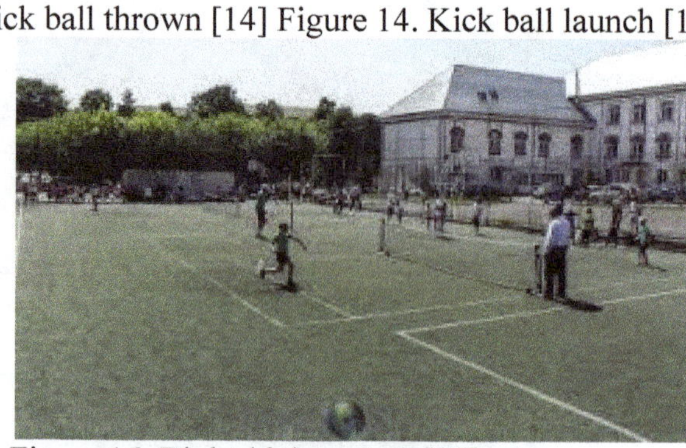

Figure 16. Right-kick contest [17]

Results and discussions

The literature on learning in tennis right coup in children is extensive.

Technical forehand include:-fundamental position, outlet, preparation, impact and end the coup.

Methodology is a "theory of effective practice" or "active theory with practical finality."

Learning is a lasting change in behavior that occurs during interaction between organism and environment.

Motor learning is specific to physical education and sport.

Learning forehand depends on the following factors: order learning, place execution, structure movement, teacher actions, condition

of practice, structure motor, number of subjects, effect ball, direction coup.
Learning the right kick is done in three steps: execution blow to a ball without rocket, imitating the right socket and rocket blow, execution kick racquet and ball.

Conclusion
The kick is made by right handed right side of the body, and the left-handed left side of the body.
Hit the right is done in three sequences linked unit.
In tennis lesson may apply didactic principles (general and specific) and training methods.
Learning the right kick to be achieved in stages through age-specific methods and means and it is conditional on a series of factors.
From the age of 4-5 years old children can practice mini tennis, mini participate in training and competitions as required 10 Tennis imposed by the International Tennis Federation (ITF) from 2012.

References
[1]. Baciu, M. (2008). *Antrenamentul în tenisul de câmp.* Cluj Napoca: Editura Napoca Star, pag. 5.
[2]. Gh. Moise, D. Moise, Ş. Doboşi (1995). *Tenis pentru începători* Cluj Napoca:Editura Garamond, pag.17, pag. 25.
[3]. Dan George Moise, Gheorghe Moise (1999) . *Tenis Modele de lecţii de antrenament pentru pregătirea tehnico-tactică de performanţă* Constanţa:Editura Leda Muntenia, pag.25, 26.
[4]. www.cursuritenis.info/blog/ forehand federer.jpg.
[5]. http://www.cursuritenis.info/blog/forehand slice.jpg.
[6]. http://www.tenis.info.ro/secretele-tenisului/825.html
[7]. Gheorghe, Cârstea. (2000). *Teoria şi Metodica Educaţiei Fizice şi Sportului* Bucureşti: Editura AN-DA, pag.8, pag 69.
[8]. Gheorghe, Daniel. (2005).*Teoria Antrenamentului Sportiv* Bucureşti: Editura Fundaţiei *România de Mâine*, pag.47
[9]. Gheorghe, Ioana. (2013). *Teoria Activităţilor Motrice, Curs în tehnologia IFR* Bucureşti: Editura Fundaţiei *România de Mâine*, pag.181.
[10]. http:// www.opentenis.ro
[11]. http://www.Sizzyreduceri.ro
[12]. http://youtu.be/pDXsLpUvdIA
[13]. http://www.bocaso-sport.ro
[14]. http://doartenis.ro
[15]. http://www berlinsport.ro.
[16]. http://www.protv.md.
[17]. http://www.cronicadefalticeni.ro

10

COORDINATION - AMBIDEXTROUS - IN SPORTS GAMES

Florentina Popescu[1], Porfireanu Maria-Cristiana[2]

Faculty of Physical Education and Sport Spiru Haret[1], Academy of Economic Studies[2]
flory_bk@yahoo.com

Abstract: Sports games have multiple meanings formative and educative. By content, form and effect, they show great advantages for learning, training and strengthening the habits and skills of basic motor, utility-applied and specific, as for the development of motor skills: conditional and coordination, processes and mental traits personality. Technique of a sports game is the driving movements executed by a player during practice and game respecting the rules. The technique involves defining the rational and economical movements of a particular type of specific sports game, made in order to obtain maximum efficiency in the difficult conditions of the game. The technique has its support as the main mode of manifesting superior driving ability. The level of technical training of a player depends largely on the initial conditional and coordination development capabilities and experience of its motor. Coordination capabilities are required for mastery of situations that require quick and rational action, it is important in the relationship game. Ambidextrous most commonly occurs as a result of education clumsy hand (any awkwardness that due to social factors have become right-handed). We know all that until recently awkwardly school students were forced to write with his right hand.
There are sports that involve a strong lateralization (throws, jumps) and others that require symmetrical movements, ambidextrous such as swimming, skiing, and running.
Keywords: coordination, ambidextrous, learning technique games

Introduction

Childhood is the age of growth and development, maturation and progressive fulfillment of personality. The largest increase capacity in children ante driving puberty occurs at age 5. Motor stimulant that age has an important role to improve the physical development of children. The correct dosage of effort must take into account the capacity of the child at this age, closely related to the degree of morphological development of the organism.

Cortical Plasticity in particular, facilitates the work of physical education teacher, who guides children in learning specific skills sports.

During this period, growth and development of morpho-functional schoolchildren are much faster and generally more uniform than up to that age.

At the age of 6-7 ends the differentiation of cortical neurons and peripheral and efferent and afferent fibers nucleizarea all.

„*The brain weighs approximately equal to that for adults, but from a functional perspective, its development is complete. There is a better development of the first signaling system; complex motor cortical area is only at 13-17 years"* [1].

Phylogenetic older segments of the somatic nervous system (spinal cord, bulb, bridge, midbrain, paleostriatul etc.) mature faster than new ones (neostriatul and neopallium).

From a functional perspective most striking is the lack of balance between fundamental cortical processes, pointing out a clear predominance of excitation. Of the various forms of inhibition, particularly inhibition of differentiation (one of the main forms of internal inhibition, conditioned) is underdeveloped. Predominance of cortical excitation is largely responsible for exaggerated cheerfulness, eternal restlessness, irritability, restlessness permanent pupil ante pubertal age. Poor development of inhibition (internal) determines conditional relative instability of concentration and difficulty maintaining attention longer.

Special plasticity of the central nervous system at this age is one of the biggest advantages that confers younger generation functional receptivity increased compared to adults including the driveability.

This plasticity increased brain early age children ensure receiving a relatively large number of information from the external environment and form directed the education process child may acquire a large amount of concepts and knowledge of the various fields of different sciences. Increased responsiveness and ability to initiate children by themselves do not ensure the acquisition of motor skills, but only through a systematic repetition. This difficulty results from the weak development of inhibition of differentiation mentioned earlier, that does not help, but rather hinders cortical fixation element again received. Sabău et al. *study shows in early age, the expression of the lateralization dominant, through gestures and motor acts, is not complete. The motor tasks that require ambidexterity expressed simultaneousness indicate similar manifestations in boys and girls at early age* [2].

Special plasticity of the central nervous system and motor skills default, they put a special mark on the handling side and feet side.

„Functional dominance over another part of the body , especially the hands, resulting in preferential use of it . So there are right-handed and left-handed. [3]. Delimited, the term refers to skills, manual dexterity. *„There is a disguised one of the dominant right hands in activities that are carried out symmetrically with both hands. It is considered that the right hand is skillful, while the left hand is stronger*"[3].

Laterality occurrence in older children a year, is dependent on a progressive brain hemispheres dominance over the other.

This dominance is expressed as:

- establishing a dominant guidelines to specific excitation sources;
- simultaneous inhibition correlated to other centers.

So dominance can translate by creating a hotbed of excitement, which can occur in different areas, while inhibition from other pathogens. The principle of dominance occurs on all floors central nervous system.

The working relationship indicates the predominance of one of the two cerebral hemispheres is called cerebral hemispheric dominance. It is usually dominant left hemisphere which is expressed in the right half of the body but can be dominant right hemisphere. Dominance translates into a more high-temporal organization of area parietooccipito hemisphere that as a result of management actions gnostic-praxico-phase finer and more accurate.

In everyday life we are accustomed to find that man uses symmetric elements of the body in the same way or with the same frequency.

All human motility, roughly, is asymmetrical: speech centers and motor centers are situated to the left. This asymmetry induces nervous, but apparently a motor asymmetry: most people are right-handed. Laterality is an expression of development asymmetric key feature of the processes involved in developing and growing tendency towards harmonization of organized inter psychophysiological correlate different structures and functions.

Asymmetry is the most educated. Child seems to be „symmetrical" at least in terms of the upper limbs: he grabbed with both hands. Over time, these movements are inhibited and coordinated driving under the influence of images created by imitating gestures and adult education directed permanent motor: eat and write with his right hand, left hand does not give etc. So we can say that at this age we can act with real results in education ambidextry of children.

Hand laterality, sometimes called „skill", reveals stronger especially when running complex and expressive movements like shooting the basketball, the shot on goal handball, volleyball to accommodate the service and throwing with the same hand in track and field.

In the work carried out with both hands, ruling that bears more complex work , doing other work on coordination of completion. *„The left hand generally carried out preparatory action, while the right hand complement the activities*" [3]. For example, in archery athlete stretchs rope with his right hand to launch the arrow, the right-hander takes pole vault pole with the right hand.

Grodin (1997) quated by Criotoru presents *„ice hockey by as interesting as the way of keeping the object (right or left on the butt end) depends on laterality, printing outlet and a certain style of play: based those who hold the power to stick with your dominant hand or finesse the puck leadership to others*" [3].

A good coordination is a prerequisite execution as faithful as possible to the model (program) motor fixed, it depends in turn on the accuracy of information from analyzers, whose integrity and level of training plays a decisive role here.

In coordination processes, some sectors of the action come are automatic, not subject to constant scrutiny of consciousness. This action only in the event of unforeseen changes, programmed sequence.

Coordination abilities differ from motor skills: *„while motor skills are acts motive concrete reinforced, partially automated capabilities of the coordinative represent conditions strengthened generality, that fundamental* *human performance in relation to a series of acts gesture*"[4].

From specialty materials, distinguish the general and special coordinative abilities. General coordination abilities arise, as a result of various actions polyvalent training gestural driving or sports. They manifest in different areas of everyday activity, but also in sports because gestural some problems can be solved creatively. Special coordinative capabilities grow more within sports being specialized skills.

Coordination capacity can be regarded as psychomotor which is based on the correlation between the central nervous system and skeletal muscles while performing an act or motor action.

Coordinative skills development *are particularly effective in increasing difficulties execution, as disturbing (strengthening or weakening) the information provided by analyzers*. Harre quoted by Manno, *proposes a whole range of means*"[5].

- Execution variation movement or engaging each partial phases of a driving sequence (technical sports, motor skill base) or running partially on each of them or modifying the pace.
- Changes in external conditions - it is about changing data and dimensions of the environment or installations: the height of a grid or a gate diameter ball sports games, ways of a way, etc.
- The combination of skills (technical) already automated. Acquired motor skills are executed simultaneously or chained form, that implies that they are perfectly mastered (phase coordination fine), otherwise error may occur intermittently or exercise and is impossible.
- Practicing with time control. Exercises known are executed at a rate as fast as possible or succeed the minimum and maximum ranges. Times are timed and communicated to the athlete.
- Variation information. Information received from sports can be enhanced or simplified either by changing the environment or making use of simple devices. An amplification of this information using video carriers, accelerometers platforms ergometer etc. increases the capacity of the athlete's control.
- Exercises performed on the substance of fatigue. Exercise used for it, must be mastered in order to avoid unpleasant consequences due to poor execution.

Establishing a finality requires immediate and prepare a program selection engine. This program should be developed as closely in relation to the proposed model, which corresponds to what the player has already repeated on several occasions to acquire a precise motive images and a sequence of movements corresponding to concrete implementation.

A too weak line between program and achieving its deficiencies may be due to the conditional nature (eg insufficient strength in the initial phase of technical execution or lack of resistance).

Motor memory, which records the movement program performed his transformations that occur through specific exercises similar fragments already registered movement is essential to learning.

Coordinative capacity building training process is oriented in two directions:

- development of overall coordination;
- development „skill" sport specific branches.

The training lessons envisages the following methodological guidance for the development and coordination abilities:

- training emphasis will be placed on mastering a large number of specific motor skills play sports;
- exercises must show a high degree of difficulty; as the player gets used to the exercise, will increase its difficulty increasing requirements for precision movement, full coordination of the movement and its components and spontaneity change the situation;
- providing pauses long enough to allow full recovery of exercise capacity;
- workload in a lesson must be low, instead will schedule a large number of training lessons with objectives of development of the various components of skill;
- the most favorable periods for skill development are childhood, puberty and adolescence, when the body has a greater plasticity than adults.

Ambidextrous human is the ability to use the same skill with the same ease both hands in everyday life.

Ambidextrous most commonly occurs as a result of educating our skillful hand (any awkwardness that due to social factors have become right-handed). We know all that until recently awkwardly school students were forced to write with his right hand which hinder the development of ambidextry.

There are sports that involve a strong lateralization (throws, jumps) and others that require symmetrical movements, ambidextrous such as swimming, skiing, running. Sports games are between these two categories. It is worth mentioning here that the regulation requires the use of rhythmic gymnastics official nondominant hand (fumble) in a proportion of 20 percent of all evidence submitted in the course of the contest.

In basketball, for example, it is looking for left-handers for the effectiveness of their action against right-handed but must not forget that most times the conditions of ambience (the playing field with the right and left), passes that can be sent and received either right or left, collective technical and tactical actions that can take place depending on the game situation (blockage to the player with the ball can be made on both sides) - all these are arguments for ambidextrous in sports. Therefore in sports training is needed to ensure functional symmetry.

Conclusions and discussion

Learning the art in games sportive depends on the level of development of capabilities of the coordinative and driving (coordination, ambidextrous, laterality).

Left-handed assault athletes in sport is increasingly higher. The subjects that excel are those of left-handers and individual direct confrontation, where opponents uncomfortable. Laterality unusual awkwardness sometimes becomes a determining factor in achieving success by targeting their unexpected offensive actions in sports games.

„In basketball the players choose to make a pass or shot with the weaker hand"[6].

According to Alparslan et al.'s results of a research, *„combining strength workouts with tennis technique and coordination training develops strength as much as hand-eye coordination within the children that are 6 years old and do regular tennis exercises*" [7].

Mosoi's research shows *„that athletes who feature left hand laterality or are ambidextrous have a higer level of neuromuscular control that athletes who distinguish themselves than right laterality*" [8].

According to Badau'study *„females have a superior general coordination than the males. This statement adds up to the results of other studies a"cording to which women have a better orientation in space as compared to men, as well as a better perception and space visualization*" [9].

References

[1] Negulescu, C. (1994). *Particularităţile morfo-funcţionale şi psiho-motrice ale juniorilor. Variaţii specifice juniorilor baschetbalişti*. Bucureşti: Editura ANEFS

[2] Sabău, E., Gheorghe, D., Popescu, F., Ioniţă, M., Alupoaie, M., Săndulache, Şt., Teuşdea, C. (2007). *Study on lateralization and ambidexterity in children of early childhood age – first grade*. In: Analele Universitatii Spiru Haret, Anul IV, nr. 4, 2007, pp. 9

[3] Croitoru, D. (1999). *Ambidextrie în jocurile sportive. Exemplificări şi aplicaţii în volei*. Bucureşti: Editura ANEFS, pp 38, 49

[4] Tudor, V. (1999). *Capacităţile condiţionale, coordonative şi intermediare, componente ale capacităţii motrice*. Bucureşti: Ed. Rai, pp 121

[5] Manno, R. (1996). *Les bases de l' Entrainement sportif*. Bucureşti: SDP, 371-374, pp. 144

[6]https://en.wikipedia.org/wiki/Ambidexterity accessed on 4th October 2016

[7] Alparslan, E., Çağlar, Ö., Asuman, Ş., Neşe, T. (2011). *Effect of Strength Training on Coordination in 6 Years Old Tennis Players*. In: Conference Proceedings Volume (1/2011) 4th Annual International Conference Physical Education Sport and Health 18 – 19 November, 2011 http://www.sportconference.ro/images/stories/58._Erman_Alparslan.pdf

[8] Mosoi, A.A., Gugu Gramatopol, C. (2012). *Neuromuscular control and Lateralization in the game of tennis*. In: The 5th International Conference Edu-World 2012. Education Facing Contemporary World Issues. Procedia–Social and Behavioral Sciences 76 (2013) pp. 553-558.

[9] Badau, D. (2013). *Identification of General Coordination Level According to Laterality in Handball*. In: Coaching, Trening and Testing, 2013, pp. 71 http://www.eqol.uns.ac.rs/3rd%20eqol/3%20coaching.pdf

11

AEROBICS – A WAY TO IMPROVE THE STUDETS PHYSICAL FITNESS

Germina COSMA, Dorina ORȚĂNESCU, Ligia RUSU, Roxana DUMITRU

University of Craiova, Faculty of Physical Education and Sport

Correspondence adresse: germinacosma@yahoo.com

Abstract. Introduction. Aerobics is an attractive discipline that can be practiced at any age successfully. The purpose of the study was to identify the effects of practicing aerobics programs for 12 weeks for a group of 19 students (female, aged 19 1.5 years) who attended the aerobics program twice a week.

Methods. Research subjects were evaluated before and after implementing the work programs both in anthropometric terms, and on muscle strength and flexibility. The aerobic gymnastics session lasted 50 minutes, the means being selected so as to target mainly the abdominal area and the legs.

Results. At the end of the experiment, there have been significant advances in terms of muscle strength and flexibility, the statistical effects of the program were confirmed by the significant progress ($p < 0.05$) recorded.

Conclusions. Aerobics can thus be one of the subjects valued by students participating in the course and can bring positive effects on their physical condition.

Keywords: aerobic gymnastic, students, fitness.

Introduction

Aerobics is an extreme agreed discipline among students, especially by the female students. It can be practiced at any age, having positive effects on the development of motor abilities among children [1] and among adults [2].

There are numerous studies that have demonstrated that specific aerobic gymnastics means, properly applied can positively influence your body mass index (BMI) [3,4] thus contributing to maintaining an optimal body mass that ensures good health.

In a research that showed the effects of aerobic dance on body image and physical self-perception, the author [5] cited Chepyator-Thompson and Ennis concluded that aerobic provides a sense of social support, fulfils the participation motives and serves the importance of the attached body image and physical look.

Thus, aerobic exercise can have positive influences on both motor and functional potential. At the bachelor level, the aerobics can be practiced during physical education lessons or in fitness clubs.

Aim of the study

The purpose of the research was to track the effects that aerobic exercise has on some components of physical fitness, especially on strength and body mass.

Method

The experiment was conducted over 12 weeks, during which, aerobics lessons lasting 50 minutes, 2 times per week were performed. The research subjects ($n = 19$, female, aged 19 ± 1 year) were tested before and after implementing the work programs.

To identify the role of specific aerobic gymnastics exercises we evaluated body mass, body mass index and motor tests for evaluating the force abdominal muscles, back and legs.

The tests were held in long jump - strength in the legs, torso bending forward - anterior-posterior mobility; Raising the trunk from lying - abdominal strength, trunk extension forward from lying – back strength lift the legs vertically from lying - abdominal strength.

All the subject agreed to take part at this research. None of them had any healthy problems.

The statistical analysis was performed using SPSS, version 21 and we used mean, average, minimum and maximum values. In order to validate the program, we used Paired T-test for the significant results pre and post intervention. The significance threshold was set at $p<0.05$.

Results

Table 1. Evolution of anthropometrics variables

Variables	Height	Weight T1	Weight T2	BMI T1	BMI T2
MEAN	165	62,92	58,92	22,88	21,43
STDV	0,06	7,11	6,04	1,97	1,62
MINIMUM	1,55	48	48	20	21
MAXIMUM	1,75	74	68	26	24
T value		6,24		6,25	
p		0,001		0,001	

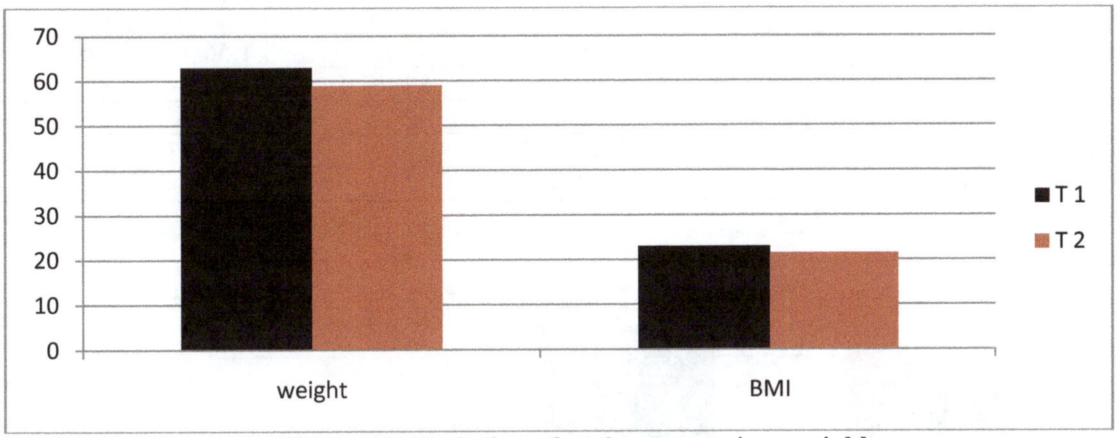

Chart no.1. **Evolution of anthropometrics variables**

On the first testing the body weight (Table 1), subjects experienced a mean of 62.92 (± 7.11) kg, the values were between 48-74 kg. BMI was on the first test of 22.88 (± 1.97). At the end of the experiment, the average body mass decreased to 58.92 (± 60.4kg) values ranging between 48-68 kg. Also, BMI / ul dropped to 21.43 (± 1.62). The efficiency program was confirmed statistically by t-test value of 6.24 / 6.25 at a threshold of $p < 0.001$.

Table 2. Evolution of the lower limbs strength and flexibility

Variables	Long jumpT1	Long jump T2	Flexibility T1	Flexibility T1
MEAN	151,53	158,54	0,8	4,38
STDV	11,05	9,94	2,7	2,5
MINIMUM	130	142	-4	4
MAXIMUM	166	173	1	8
T value	-8,10		-16,39	
p	0,001		0,001	

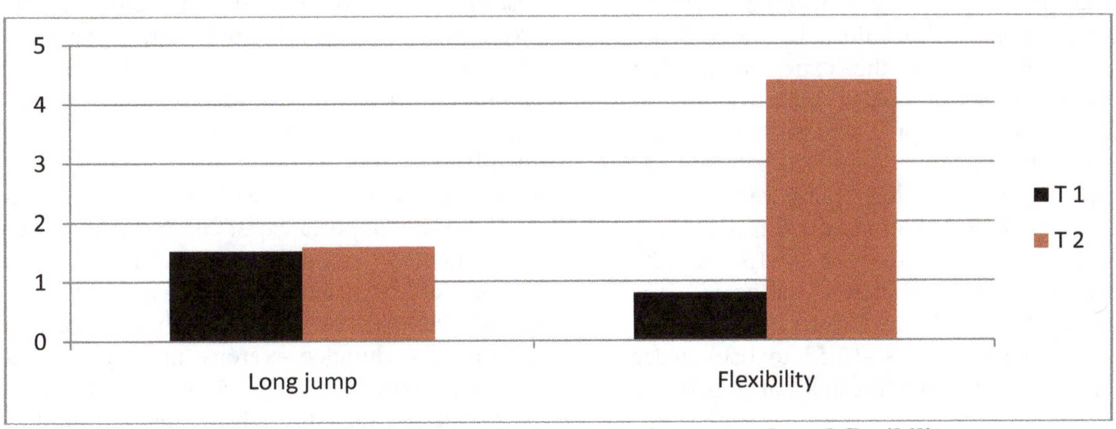

Chart no. Evolution of the lower limbs strength and flexibility

At the first test the lower limbs strength (Table 2), subjects experienced an average of 151.53 (± 11.05cm), the values were between 130-160cm. The antero-posterior Flexibility in the first test was 0.8 (± 2.7cm). At the end of the experiment, the average flexibility increased at 4.38 (± 2.5cm) being comprised between 4-8cm. Also, lower limb strength rose to 158.54 (± 9.94cm). The Efficiency of the program was confirmed statistically by the t-test value of 8.10 for abdominal strength and flexibility t = -16.39 for the anteroposterior values standing at a threshold $p<0.001$.

Table 3. Evolution of the abdominal and back strength

Variables	Abdominal strength T1	Abdominal strength T2	Back strengthT1	Back strengthT2	Leg lift T1	Leg lift T2
MEAN	26,15	30,92	33,15	37,15	7,54	10,69
STDV	2,99	2,95	3,99	3,23	1,56	1,6
MINIMUM	22	28	27	32	6	8
MAXIMUM	32	36	40	42	11	14
T value	-13,922		-12,538		-12,653	
p	0,001		0,001		0,001	

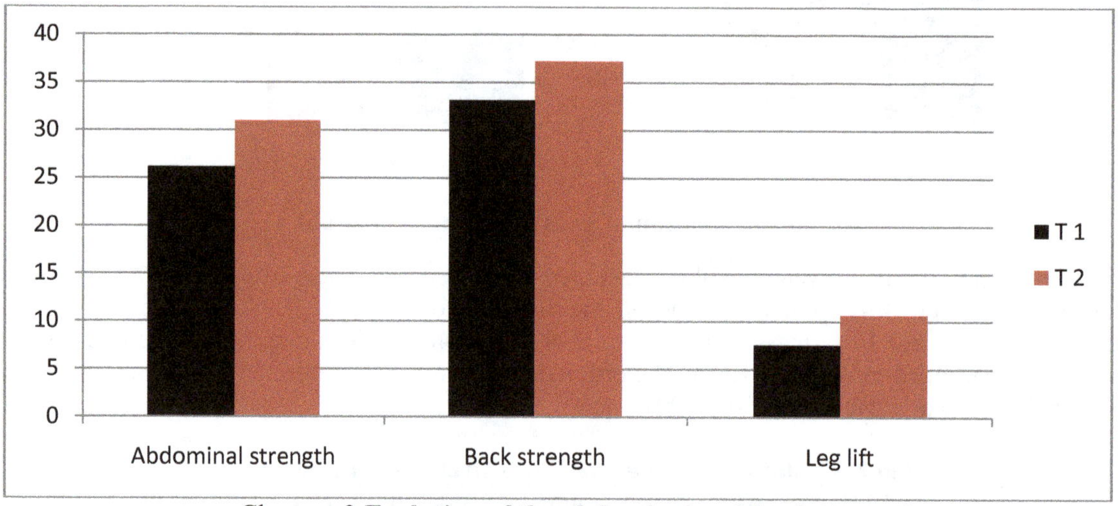

Chart no.3 **Evolution of the abdominal and back strength**

At the first abdominal strength test (Table 3), subjects experienced a mean of 26.15 (± 2.99 repetitions) with values that were between 22-32 reps. Raising legs from sitting at the first test was 7.54 (± 1.56 repetitions). Strength in the back of the first test registered 33.15 (± 3.99 repetitions) with values between 27-42 reps. At the end of the experiment, after applying specific aerobic gymnastics means, media crunch executions increased to 30.92 (± 2.95 repetitions) being comprised between 28-36 reps. And lifting legs lying recorded an average of 10.69 evolution (± 1.6 repetitions). Also, back strength rose to 37.15 (± 3.23 repetitions). The efficiency program was confirmed statistically by t-test 13.92 value for abdominal strength, t = -12.53 to back force the values standing at a threshold of $p<0.001$.

Discussion and conclusions

Regarding the lower limb strength a progress of 4% was registered, most means used targeting this segment. Valuable progress has been registered in anteroposterior flexibility testing, the evolution of the end of the experiment is about 4 cm better. Abdominal strength has also registered an 18 percent improvement in crunch execution and 43% for raising the legs from lying, the latter requiring mainly the lower abdomen.

Our study is consistent with other studies that highlight the importance of aerobic gymnastics in obtaining an optimal physical fitness. Aerobics or aerobic dance rhythmic gymnastics has ways by which the positive effects of endurance exercise and gymnastics can be combined. [6]. Also, it has been demonstrated that through aerobic gymnastics can improve a number of physical parameters that influence mental health later. [7,8].

The research results validated the work program, so after participating in sessions of aerobic exercise there have been significant advances in the parameters targeting muscle strength in the legs, abdomen and back, but positive results have been recorded on the impact of aerobic exercise on BMI.

Acknowledgement
All authors have equal contributions.

References

[1] Mehrtash M., Rohani H., Farzaneh B., Nasiri R., (2015), The effects of 6 months specific aerobic gymnastic training on motor abilities in 10-12 years old boys, *Science Gymnastic Journal*, vol.7, issue 1. pp.51-60

[2]. Hartmann A., Murer K., de Bie Ra, de Bruin ED, (2009), The effect of a foot gymnastic exercise programme on gait performance in older adults: A randomized controlled trial, *Disability and rehabilitation*, vol.31, issue 25, pp.2101-2110

[3]. Cuceu D., Cuceu M., Dumitrescu M., 2014, Study on the influence of exercise on the body mass index in first year students, *Palestrica of the Third Millennium Civilization & Sport*, vol.15, issue 2, pp.127-130.

[4]. Lei Y, Zang D., Zhou Q, (2007), Effects of aerobic exercise on obese female students in college, *Journal of Nanjing Institute of Physical Education* (Natural Science), 2007-04.

[5]. Burgess G., Grogan S, Burwitz L., (2006), Effects of a 6-week aerobic dance intervention on body image and physical self-perceptions in adolescent girls, Body Image, vol.3, issue 1, pp.57-66

[6]. Viru A., Smirnova T., (1995), Health promotion and exercise training, *Sports Medicine*, vol.19, issue 2, pp.123-136

[7]. Yan C., (2004), Effects of aerobic exercise on BMI, WHR, and psychological health of the college girls-students, *Journal of Neijiang Teachers College*, 2004-06

[8]. Ilieva I., (2015), Guidelines for forming healthy habits in female students in aerobic classes, *Activities in Physical Education & Sport*, vol.5, Issue 2, p.211-213.

12

ISSUES ON LAPEL LEARNING METHODOLOGY WITH TWO HANDS IN TENNIS TO CHILDREN

Claudiu Cristian TEUŞDEA

Faculty of Physical Education and Sport, Spiru Haret Spiru Haret

Abstract: In the early executed tennis backhand with one hand.
With the increasing speed of the game, was looking for a solution to meet the blows coming fast on the backhand; thus the two-handed backhand.
This process evolves constantly perfected techniques, tactics, methods and materials for the game.
Keywords: tennis, methodical, backhand with two hands, kids, technique.

Introduction

The current tennis backhand with two hands is used by players and especially the players, because it has greater certainty and precision kicking the ball away.

At the children this technique complements the lack of force in the arm, wrist and difficulties encountered in changing socket rocket.

Material and method

Tennis

Game that takes place between 2-4 players or players who send the ball over the net with rockets, namely arranged on land, split into two by a net .

Technical

Engineering a branch of sport: includes all actions executed driving ideal in terms of their effectiveness. [1]

Technique sport is a process or set of processes, learned through the exercise, in order to solve more economic, more rational and with maximum effectiveness a task-based movement (in other words a problem motive). [2]

Technique playing tennis is a set of motor skills specific form and content, characterizing how the handling of the racket hitting the ball and movements specific field, all being carried by the laws of higher nervous activity and the biomechanics in order to realize maximum efficiency in game. [2]

The tennis technique means all specific procedures used in order to practice the game with maximum efficiency.

Backhand

Two-handed backhand technique that consists in sending the ball over the net after contact with the ground on the opposite side of the hand that holds the racket.

The right-handed backhand with two hands running down the left side of the body and the left-handed running on the left side of the body.

Two-handed backhand is the second blow to learn in the game of tennis, right after the coup.[3]

Technical backhand include:

-fundamental position;

-outlet;

-preparation, impact and end the coup.

The techniques are composed of four basic points, ensuring their development:

- preparation mechanism;

-training mechanism for kicking the ball away;

-the mechanism of hitting the ball;

-completion mechanism of actions of hitting the ball. [4]

Grip the backhand racket with two hands can hold as follows:

- grip backhand (semi-open) with basic arm placed first hand on the handle of the racquet and a second grip right (semi-closed) the opposite arm with his hand resting on the handle of the second rocket;

- grip backhand (continental hand-arm basic hand resting on the handle rocket first and a second grip right (semi-closed) the opposite arm with his hand resting on the handle of the second rocket.

Hands are placed side by side on the handle of the racket without overlapping .

Holding hands at different players handed to left-handed players (figure 1, figure 2).

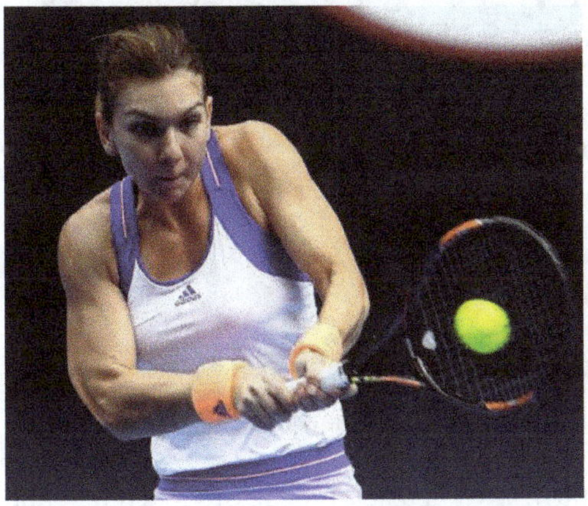

Figure 1. Grip for the right-handed [5]

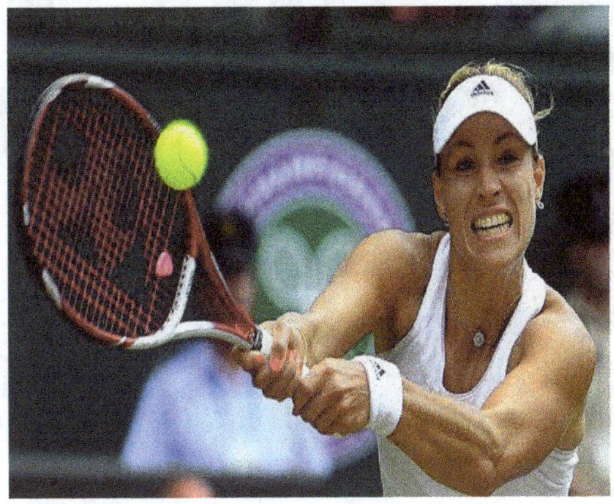

Figure 2. Grip for the left -handed [6]

Two-handed backhand can run through the following techniques:
- stepping off place (figure 3);
- shift to ball (figure 4);
- spin (figure 5);
- flat (figure 6).

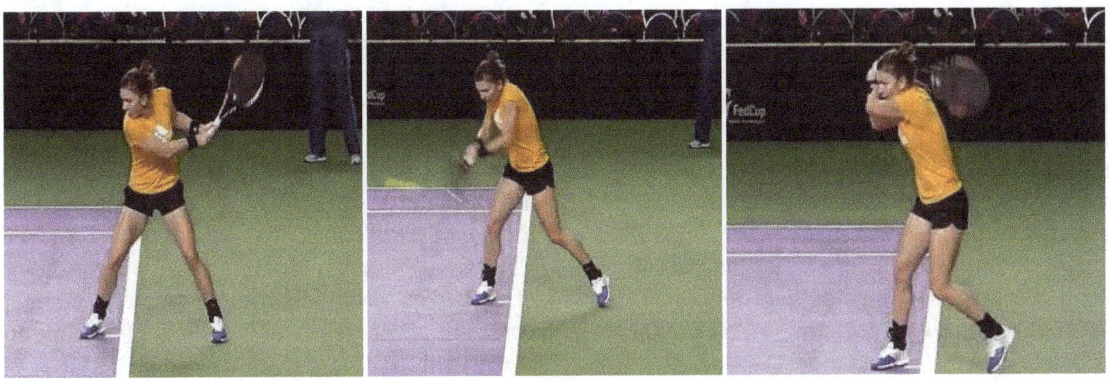

Figure 3. Two-handed backhand in place [7]

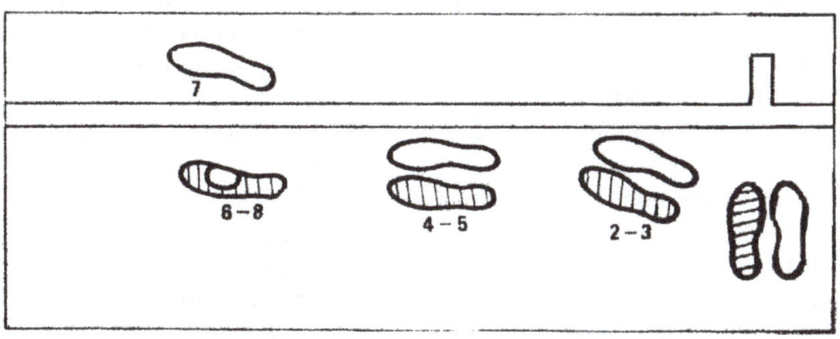

Figure 4. Moving to backhand with two hands

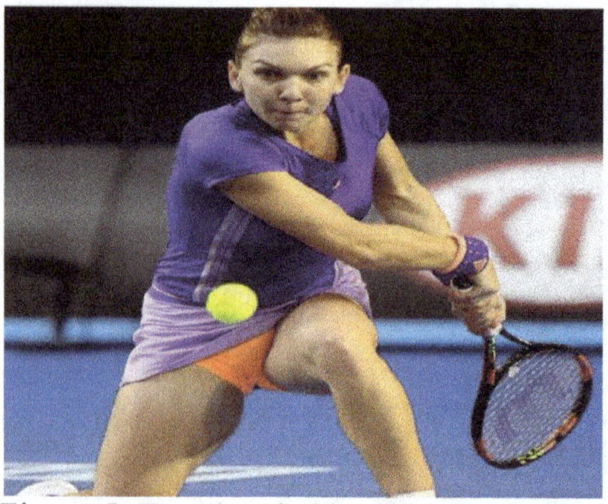
Figure 5. Two-handed backhand spin [8]

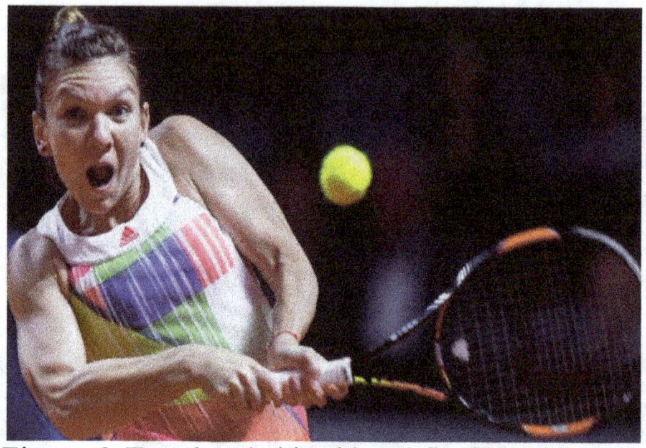
Figure 6. Two-handed backhand flat [9]

Children

Tennis is sport accessible for children, regularly practiced it provides many health benefits associated with physical and mental development.

Children up to 10 years, as required practiced tennis Play and Stay T10 concept developed and applied by the International Tennis Federation (ITF) from 2012.

Method

With the work we used the method of ascertaining study, bibliographic study method and the method of video movie about the coup learning techniques and methods right, taken from the "You Tube" processed by Freemake Video Downloader Defragmenter.

Learning Methodology

The methodology is the science method, which enables the teacher to better meet the educational objectives set for a particular lesson.

The method involves presenting things in an orderly manner, it is a set of rules that should be followed to achieve specified learning objectives. [10]

The main objectives of teaching are:
- accelerating the learning process;
- learning a greater number of students;
- teaching in order of progressive difficulty;
- teaching use of all the possibilities, facilities and systems.

Teaching is what makes coach, is what makes student learning.

If the coach wants to facilitate the teaching of pupil learning it is important to concentrate on the following issues:
- teaching objectives and content ;
- the teaching methods and teaching styles used;
- teaching tools available.

I know two basic types of teaching and learning:

Own teaching (learning by substitution):
- scholar and teacher are the same person;
- can be productive if the curriculum is organized a good observer;
- if not, it may cause errors in production and kick following a delay in the learning. [10]

Formal teaching :
- two sides: the teacher and scholar;
- it is most useful when schoolboy wants to learn a sound technique in a short period of time, under appropriate progression. [10]

Tennis players learn skills through a process of first learning the technique, and its development situations in conditions of increasing difficulty. [10]

The final stage involves using technology effectively in situations match game, combining reception and technical execution decision. [10]

Learning stages of a technical process are:
- step training plan or step verbal / cognitive.
- step practice / repetition or associative:
- step autonomous / differentiated. [10]

In Tennis applied the following learning styles:

STYLES OF CONTROL used in the pre-impact:
- command;
- exercise / assignment;
- reciprocity / learning friendly;
- own verification;
- involvement. [10]

STYLES OF EXPLORATION used in stage impacts:
- guided discovery;
- problem solving (divergent);
- individual program;
- student initiatives;

- own training. [10]

In tennis there are three main methods of teaching:

Global Approach: When the coach demonstrates and teaches a free kick to break up into its constituent parts.

Analytical Method: When coach shot separates into its component parts to facilitate learning.

Mixed method uses both methods above.

When choosing a method of teaching, the coach should take consider the following:

- the level of the players;
- complexity ability;
- the manner of manifestation of ability;
- combinations.[10]

Learning backhand

Learning methodology backhand two hands in children pursues the following tasks:

- knowledge of rocket grips;
- analytical and global learning coup;
- learning processes;
- directing the blows;
- exchanging blows.

Learning backhand depends on the following factors:

Order learning: second blow.

Place execution: by age on the field red, orange and green.

Structure movement: analytical; overall.

Teacher actions: given the ball thrown and released.

Condition of practice: relieved, with coach; with a partner.

Structure motor : the place; walking, running.

Number of subjects: in groups, with partner, individually.

Effect ball: spin, flat, cut.

Direction coup: median; long line; long diagonal and short diagonal.

Learning the backhand with two hands is done in stages with specific means:

1. Step preparatory exercises with the ball and racket:

- preparatory exercises with the ball and racket.

The objective of the exercise:

- learning backhand grip ;
- accommodating backhand grip (figure 6, 7,8).

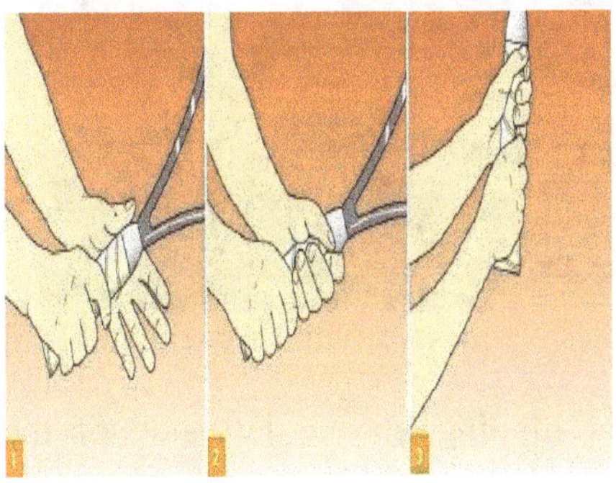

Figure 6. Backhand grip [11] on racket

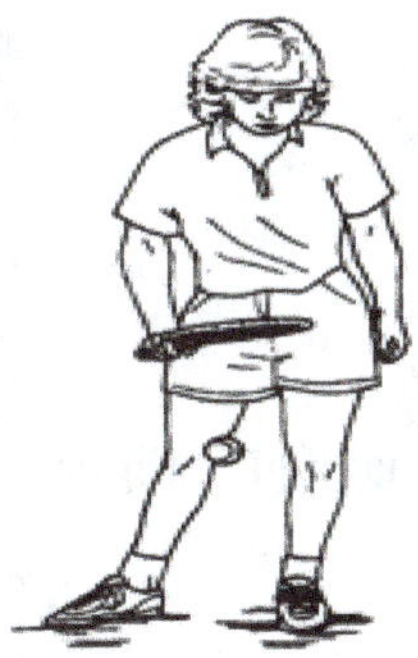

Figure 7. Striking the ball

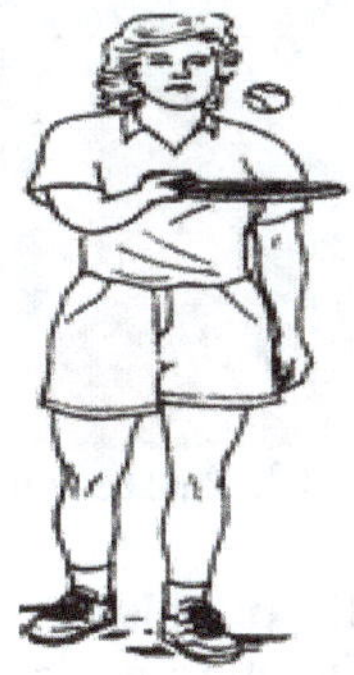

Figure 8. Keeping the ball

2 .Step imitation exercises:

- exercises imitation of the coup.

The objective of the exercise:

- learning to grip backhand;
- learning the backhand technique coup ((figure 9).

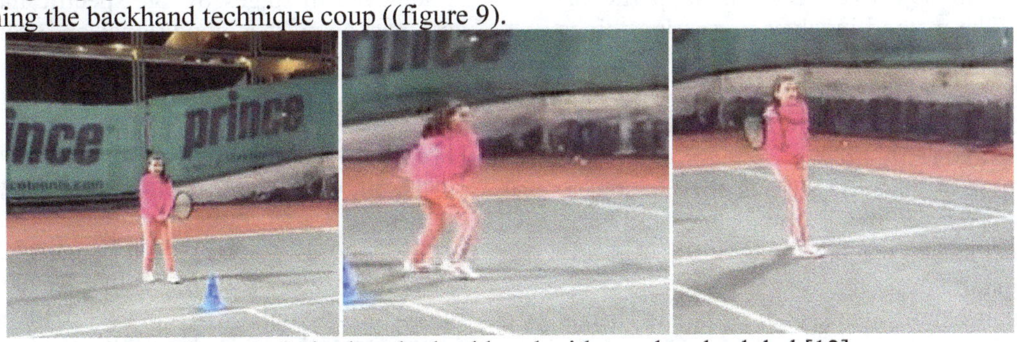

Figure 9. Imitating the backhand with two hands global [12]

3. Step exercises of hitting the ball:
- the ball provided (figure 10);
- the ball thrown (figure 11) ;
-launched the ball (figure 12);
- passes with two-handed backhand (figure 13).
- contest with two-handed backhand (figure 14).

The objective of the exercise:
- learning to grip backhand;
- learning the backhand technique coup.

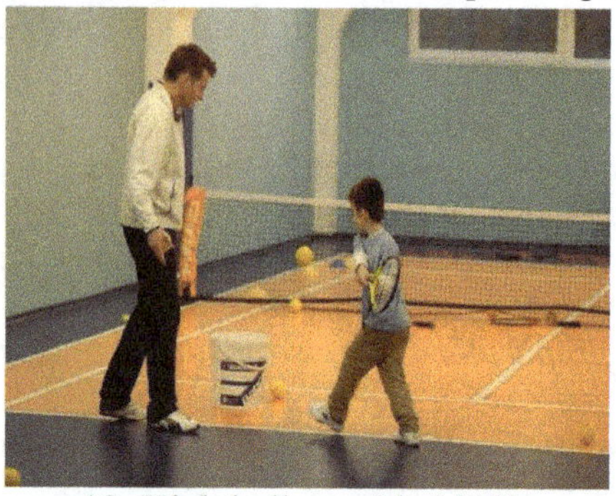

Figure 10. Kick ball provided [13]

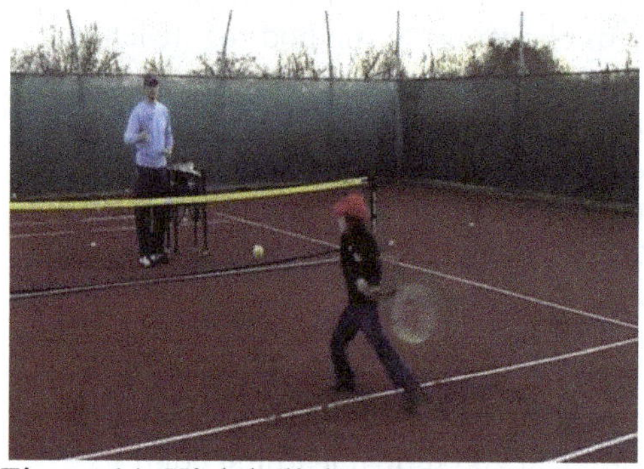

Figure 11. Kick ball thrown[14]

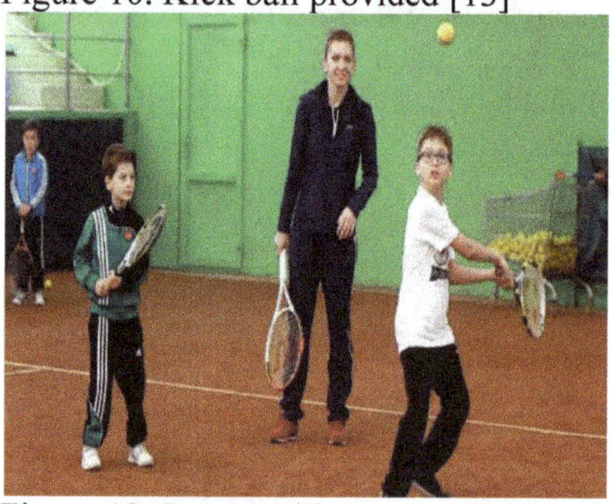

Figure 13. Passes with two-handed backhand [15]

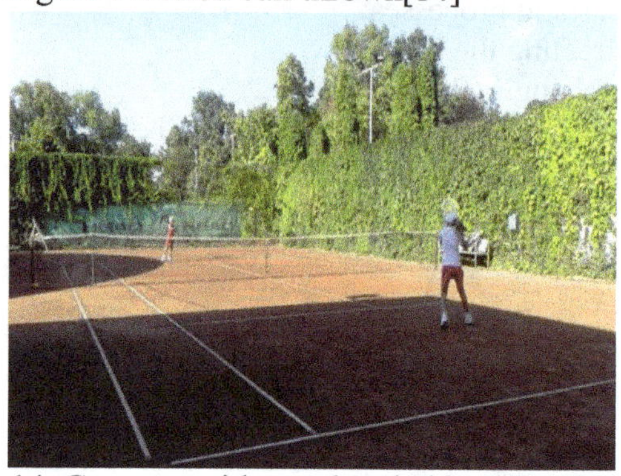

Figure 14. Contests with two-handed backhand [16]

Results and discussions

The literature on learning backhand with two hands in tennis to children is extensive.

Technical backhand include:-fundamental position, outlet, preparation, impact and end the coup.

The methodology is the science method, which enables the teacher to better meet the educational objectives set for a particular lesson. The method involves presenting things in an orderly manner, it is a set of rules that should be followed to achieve specified learning objectives. I know two basic types of teaching and learning.

Learning a technical process is done in stages. In Tennis applied two learning styles and three main methods of teaching.

Conclusion

The right-handed backhand with two hands running down the left side of the body and the left-handed running on the left side of the body.

Backhand is done in three sequences linked unit whit various actions of body segments.

Learning backhand two-handed strokes is preceded by learning the right, thus driving skills will be transferred from blow right at the two-handed backhand.

Is achieved in stages by age-specific methods and means and it is conditional on a series of factors.

References

[1]. Dragnea A. (1996) *Antrenament sportiv* Bucureşti, Editura Didactică şi Pedagogică, pag 14.

[2]. Manno R. (1992) *Bazele teoretice ale antrenamentului sportiv,* Edit. Revue EPS Roma,1992. Traducere rom.CCPS în Sportul de performanţă nr.371-374,1996, pag 28.

[3]. Gh. Moise, D. Moise, Ş. Doboşi (1995). *Tenis pentru începători* Cluj Napoca:Editura Garamond, pag.29.
[4]. Dan George Moise, Gheorghe Moise (1999) . *Tenis Modele de lecţii de antrenament pentru pregătirea tehnico-tactică de performanţă* Constanţa:Editura Leda Muntenia, pag.25, 26.
[5].http://observator.ro/cdn/wp-content/uploads/2015/02/halep-muschi.jpg
[6].https://constative.com/wp-content/uploads/2016/01/Angelique-Kerber.jpg
[7]. https://youtu.be/nIKKiq14XKU
[8]. http://www.telegrafonline.ro
[9].http://deschide.md/images/cms-image-000039778.jpg
[10].http://www.frt.ro/_public/resources/files/ManualulAntrenorilorAvansati.pdf. pag 24, pag 25, 26, 28,33.
[11].http://www.edituracasa.ro/img/cms/casa/regi_hirek_kepek/3tenis.jpg
[12]. https://youtu.be/GWDOFddtVWg
[13].http://www.miciiasi.ro/userfiles/image/galerii/sala/cursuri-tenis-copii-009.jpg
[14]. http://youtu.be/dTRAqFuJz9Y
[15].http://www.cugetliber.ro/imagini/mari/simonahalep-1417626345.jpg
[16].http://sportfit.ro/static/images/clase-copii-tenis.jpg

13

DETERMINATION OF THE HANDBALL PLAYERS' PROBLEM SOLVING SKILLS IN TERMS OF SOME VARIABLES

Ali GOK, Sefa Sahan BIROL, Elif USTUN, Mehmet Ali HOROZOGLU

Karamanoglu Mehmetbey University, Physical Education and Sports High School, Karaman, TURKEY

ABSTRACT: Purpose: This research was done with the aim of revealing whether problem solving skills differ in terms of different variables or not. Descriptive method, one of the quantitative research methods, was adopted as the search model.

Materials and Methods: Research group consisted of 64 male athletes who participated at the third sports UNIKOP handball competition. In this study, "Problem Solving Skills Inventory" developed by Heppner and Petersen (1982) and the adaptation work of this scale to Turkish was conducted by Şahin, Şahin and Heppner (1993) and "Personal Information Form" which was developed by researcher in order to determine personal characteristic of athletes, were used as data collection tool. The unique Kolmogorov Smirnov Test was used in order to determine whether measures were suitable for normal dispersion or not. Kruskal Wallis-H test and Mann Whitney-U test were used on analyzing and evaluating the data and meaningfulness was obtained as P<0,05. SPSS (Statistical package for social sciences) package programme was used on evaluating data and finding calculated values.

Findings: It could be said that problem solving total point average of the athletes, participated in the research, with (Mean=110,1719), considering approach point average with (Mean=14,7656), Evuluator Approach point average with (Mean=9,5469), Self-confidence approach point average with (Mean=22,9219) and planned approach point average with (Mean=12,63) were low, but impetuous approach point average with (Mean=33,9219) and avoidant approach point average with (Mean=16,3594) were high.

Results: Meaningful difference was found in terms of personal characteristic on problem solving total and sub dimensions of the problem solving skills of participants' "class which they study at", "school which they study at", "department which they study at", "father occupation" and "mother education" variables whereas meaningful difference was not found on "age", "place in which they spend most of their life", "mother occupation", "father education" and "position which they play" variables.

Key Words: Problem Solving, Athletes, Handball, University

INTRODUCTION

Problem solving is a skill that is necessary for human life and even beyond that it is the most frequently used skill to overcome the problems encountered. [14]. Heppner ve Petersan have used the terms "to cope with problems" and "problem solving" in the same meaning.[8].

D'Zurilla ve Nezu have defined the problem solving as cognitive, affective and behavioral processes formed and developed to overcome the difficulties faced by individuals effectively.[5] [9] have also explained the problem-solving phenomenon as an important feature which is closely related to success in the social and professional life.[9],[15].

Problem solving ability is an important factor to create a favorable environment for the life of the individual [20]. Being a social existence, human life must continue by performing different status and taking on different roles in the community. Individuals determine their status and the roles they have acquired during their life with the help of problem-solving skills. It is contemplated that the individuals with better problem solving skills will reach a higher level status and will assume important roles in social life[3]. It is determined by Şahin and his colleagues that the individuals who cannot effectively solve the problems are more anxious and insecure when compared with those who have effective problem-solving skills [13].

Problem solving method requires creative and scientific thinking skills. This method also requires a six-stage process which can be summarized as follows: to feel the difficulty, to recognize and classify the difficulty, to express the difficulty as a problem, to determine observable truths and to develop a hypothesis, to put into this hypothesis into practice and to evaluate the whole process [21].

Sports develops creative thinking, supports problem solving skills and conceptual change, and activates cognitive skills. It also develops social competency skills and sense of emphaty, supports positive self-development. Thus, an individual gets much more stronger in dealing with the problems. Sports also improves people's social life skills such as collaboration and teamwork. [15].

In this day and age, there are many factors that affect the level of sportive performance. The psychological state and performance of the athletes are closely related to the level of their problem-solving skills. For example; to train a lot or to have very high condition alone is not enough for an athlete to be successful. It can be said that the ability to make the right decisions as soon as possible provides an advantage in reaching success more quickly for an athlete. Consequently, problem solving skills of an athlete can be considered as an important factor in achieving success [10].

According to Koray and Azar problem solving is a social activity [12],[7]. Taken in this context, it is possible to say that those who engaged in sports trust themselves more and they are less impressed by stress. When the individuals engaged in sports faced with a problem, they are trying to solve their problems through problem-solving thinking on the basis of thinking schemes arises depending upon experience. With the idea of problem solving athletes can use their existing talents and skills to reach their goals. Although the problems faced in real life are valid for all individuals, it can be said that individuals engaged in sports are more flexible and comfortable when they encountered the problems compared those who do not [1].

METHODS

In this chapter there is information about the model of research, the research group, the collection of data, the data collection tools and the transactions in the process of analysis of data.

The Model of Research

This research is a descriptive study. Descriptive statistics is a statistical process that allows the collection, depiction and presentation of the numerical values related to a variable [2].

The Research Group

The research group is consisted of 64 male handball players who participated in the handball competitions in the 3rd UNIKOP Games.

The Collection of Data

Firstly, the current information about the purpose of the study is given in a systematic manner by scanning the literature. Thus, a theoretical framework has been created about the topic. Secondly, "Problem Solving Inventory (PS-A)" developed by [8] has been applied over the participants through random sampling.

The Data Collection Tools

The data collection tools needed to achieve the desired goals related to research are given below in order:

The Personal Information Form

An information form consisting of 10 questions has been prepared by researcher in order to create arguments of the research topic and to gather information about the personal characteristics of the players who participated in the handball competitions in the 3rd UNIKOP Games.

The Problem Solving Inventory (PSI)

The Problem Solving Inventory has been developed by [8] to determine the dimensions of the problem-solving methods and to determine how the person perceive himself about the competence to solve problems. On this inventory such problem-solving stages as "general tendency", "the definition of the problem", "develop alternatives", “decision making” and "evaluation" have been taken into account [16]. Within the framework of the Turkish version works, translation studies have been done by [6,18,19],and validity and reliability studies have been done [18,19,3]. As a result of the factor analysis conducted by [18], it is stated that the scale consists of six factors. These factors are as follows:

1. Impetuous Approach: Articles 13, 14, 15, 17, 21, 25, 26, 30 and 32, α = 0.78,
2. Considering Approach: Articles 18, 20, 31, 33 and 35, α = 0.76,
3. Avoidant Approach: Articles 1, 2, 3 and 4, α = 0.74,
4. Evuluator Approach: Articles 6, 7 and 8, α = 0.69,
5. Self-Assured Approach: Articles 5, 11, 23, 24, 27, 28 and 34, α = 0.64,
6. Planned Approach: Articles 10, 12, 16 and 19, α = 0.59

The answers are scored from 1 to 6. The 9th, the 22nd and the 29th articles have been kept off the scoring. Scoring has been carried over 32 articles. The Article 1, 2, 3, 4, 11, 13, 14, 15, 17, 21, 25, 26, 30 and 34 have been scored as reverse. The score range which can be taken from inventory is between 32 and 192. If the total points received from the scale is high, it means that the individual is feeling himself inadequate in the matter of problem-solving skills. If the total points received from the scale is low, perception of problem-solving skills are considered to be positive. In the scoring of the sub-dimensions, as the scores of the sub-dimensions that measure problem-solving approaches decreases (Considering Approach, Assuredapproach, evaluatives approach, planned approach) it has been seen that more use of the relevant approaches. And as the scores of the sub-dimensions that measure problem-solving approaches (Impetuous Approach and avoidant approach) it has been seen that less use of the relevant approaches [6]. This scale is aiming to measure problem-solving skills of physical education and sports teachers. Internal consistency reliability coefficient was found as 0.72 (Cronbach Alpha).

The Analysis of Data

Kruskal Wallis-H ve Mann Whitney-U tests have been used in the interpretation of the datas, and meaningfulness has been taken as P<0,05. SPSS 21 (Statistical package for social sciences) and a package software has been used to evaluate the data and to find the calculated value.

FINDINGS

Table 1. Kruskal-Wallis Test Results Regarding to the total score and Problem Solving Skills Sub-Dimensions According to the Father's Occupation of the participants

		n	Mean rank	Sd	X^2	p	Meaningful Differences
TOTAL POINT	Officer	23	112,13	60	1,089	,361	-----
	Artisan	18	110,44				
	Farmer	10	105,60				
	Self employment	13	109,84				
IMPETUOUS APPROACH	Officer	23	35,17	60	1,363	,263	-----
	Artisan	18	31,77				
	Farmer	10	34,90				
	Self employment	13	33,92				
CONSIDERING APPROACH	Officer	23	15,00	60	,120	,948	-----
	Artisan	18	14,38				
	Farmer	10	14,70				

	Self employment	13	14,92				
AVOIDANT APPROACH	Officer	23	17,56	60	1,103	,355	-----
	Artisan	18	15,05				
	Farmer	10	16,50				
	Self employment	13	15,92				
EVALUATOR APPROACH	Officer	23	9,60	60	2,048	,117	-----
	Artisan	18	10,50				
	Farmer	10	8,20				
	Self employment	13	9,15				
SELF ASSUREI APPROACH	Officer	23	22,13	60	3,218	,029*	2-3
	Artisan	18	25,22				
	Farmer	10	21,00				
	Self employment	13	22,61				
PLANNED APPROACH	Officer	23	12,65	60	2,299	,087	-----
	Artisan	18	13,50				
	Farmer	10	10,30				
	Self employment	13	13,30				

*p<0,05

In Table 1, it was analyzed by Kruskal-Wallis test if the problem solving sub-dimensions and the total scores of the average of players are changed or not according to the occupation of the fathers of the participants. In the study results; no significant differences in any other sub-dimensions, there were statistically significant differences in the self-assured sub-dimensions scores according to the father's occupation (X^2 =3,21 P<0.05).

Table 2. Kruskal-Wallis Test Results Regarding to the total score and Problem Solving Skills Sub-Dimensions of participants According the school which they study at

		n	Mean rank	Sd	X^2	p	Meaningful Differences
TOTAL POINT	Karamanoğlu Mehmetbey University	18	112,44	60	,833	,481	-----
	Niğde University	17	107,35				
	Selçuk University	14	110,71				
	Aksaray University	15	110,13				
IMPETUOUS APPROACH	Karamanoğlu Mehmetbey University	18	34,38	60	,587	,626	-----
	Niğde University	17	34,76				
	Selçuk University	14	34,07				
	Aksaray University	15	32,26				
CONSIDERING APPROACH	Karamanoğlu Mehmetbey University	18	14,44	60	,113	,952	-----
	Niğde University	17	14,82				
	Selçuk University	14	15,14				
	Aksaray University	15	14,73				
AVOIDANT APPROACH	Karamanoğlu Mehmetbey University	18	18,88	60	3,617	,018*	1-3
	Niğde University	17	15,17				
	Selçuk University	14	14,35				
	Aksaray University	15	16,53				
EVALUATOR APPROACH	Karamanoğlu Mehmetbey University	18	9,33	60	1,832	,151	-----
	Niğde University	17	8,88				
	Selçuk University	14	10,85				
	Aksaray University	15	9,33				
SELF ASSUREI APPROACH	Karamanoğlu Mehmetbey University	18	22,88	60	,714	,548	-----
	Niğde University	17	22,00				
	Selçuk University	14	22,78				
	Aksaray University	15	24,13				
PLANNED APPROACH	Karamanoğlu Mehmetbey University	18	12,50	60	,849	,473	-----
	Niğde University	17	11,70				
	Selçuk University	14	13,50				

Aksaray University	15	13,13	

*p<0,05

In Table 2, it was analyzed by Kruskal-Wallis test if the problem solving sub-dimensions and the total average scores of the players are changed or not according to the school which they study at. In the study results; there were no significant differences in any other sub-dimensions, there were statistically significant differences in the avoidant approach sub-dimensions scores according to the school which they study at (X^2 =3,61 P<0.05).

Table 3. Kruskal-Wallis Test Results Regarding to the total score and Problem Solving Skills Sub-Dimensions of participants According to the class which they study at

		n	Mean rank	Sd	X^2	p	Meaningful Differences
TOTAL POINT	1.class	15	109,53	60	,435	,728	-----
	2.class	14	108,28				
	3.class	12	112,50				
	4.class	23	110,52				
IMPETUOUS APPROACH	1.class	15	33,13	60	2,962	,039*	2-3
	2.class	14	30,85				
	3.class	12	36,83				
	4.class	23	34,78				
CONSIDERING APPROACH	1.class	15	16,00	60	1,050	,377	-----
	2.class	14	14,85				
	3.class	12	14,00				
	4.class	23	14,30				
AVOIDANT APPROACH	1.class	15	14,33	60	1,421	,246	-----
	2.class	14	17,07				
	3.class	12	17,41				
	4.class	23	16,69				
EVALUATOR APPROACH	1.class	15	10,33	60	1,058	,374	-----
	2.class	14	8,71				
	3.class	12	9,33				
	4.class	23	9,65				
SELF ASSUREI APPROACH	1.class	15	22,40	60	,614	,609	-----
	2.class	14	23,21				
	3.class	12	21,83				
	4.class	23	23,65				
PLANNED APPROACH	1.class	15	13,33	60	1,667	,184	-----
	2.class	14	13,57				
	3.class	12	13,08				
	4.class	23	11,43				

*p<0,05

In Table 3, it was analyzed by Kruskal-Wallis test if the problem solving sub-dimensions and the total average scores of the players are changed or not according to the class which they study at. In the study results; there were no significant differences in any other sub-dimensions, there were statistically significant differences in the impetuous approach sub-dimensions scores according to the class which they study at (X^2 =2,96 P<0.05).

Table 4. Kruskal-Wallis Test Results Regarding to the total score and Problem Solving Skills Sub-Dimensions of participants According to the department which they study at

		n	Mean rank	Sd	X^2	p	Meaningful Differences

TOTAL POINT	P.E.Teaching	21	110,04	60	,383	,684	-----
	Coaching	20	108,85				
	Sports Management	23	111,43				
IMPETUOUS APPROACH	P.E.Teaching	21	34,71	60	2,330	,106	-----
	Coaching	20	35,35				
	Sports Management	23	31,95				
CONSIDERING APPROACH	P.E.Teaching	21	14,66	60	1,609	,208	-----
	Coaching	20	13,85				
	Sports Management	23	15,65				
AVOIDANT APPROACH	P.E.Teaching	21	17,00	60	2,364	,103	-----
	Coaching	20	17,50				
	Sports Management	23	14,78				
EVALUATOR APPROACH	P.E.Teaching	21	8,85	60	3,843	,027	1-3
	Coaching	20	9,00				
	Sports Management	23	10,65				
SELF ASSUREI APPROACH	P.E.Teaching	21	21,95	60	3,418	,039	3-1 3-2
	Coaching	20	21,95				
	Sports Management	23	24,65				
PLANNED APPROACH	P.E.Teaching	21	12,85	60	3,315	,043	3-2
	Coaching	20	11,20				
	Sports Management	23	13,73				

*p<0,05

In Table 4, it was analyzed by Kruskal-Wallis test if the problem solving sub-dimensions and the total average scores of the players are changed or not according to the department which they study at. In the study results; there were statistically significant differences in the sub-dimensions scores of evuluator approach (X2=3,84 P<0.05), self-assured approach (X2=3,41 P<0.05) and planned approach (X2=3,31 P<0.05) according to the class which they study at. But there were no significant differences in any other sub-dimensions.

Table 5. Kruskal-Wallis Test Results Regarding the total score and Problem Solving Skills Sub-Dimensions According to the educational level of the mothers of the participants

		n	Mean rank	Sd	X^2	p	Meaningful Differences
TOTAL POINT	Non-literate	10	108,00	60	2,039	,139	-----
	Primary school	32	108,59				
	High school	22	113,45				
IMPETUOUS APPROACH	Non-literate	10	37,50	60	2,548	,087	-----
	Primary school	32	33,46				
	High school	22	32,95				
CONSIDERING APPROACH	Non-literate	10	14,30	60	2,627	,080	-----
	Primary school	32	14,03				
	High school	22	16,04				
AVOIDANT APPROACH	Non-literate	10	16,90	60	,124	,884	-----
	Primary school	32	16,40				
	High school	22	16,04				
EVALUATOR APPROACH	Non-literate	10	7,50	60	4,828	,011*	2-1
	Primary school	32	10,15				
	High school	22	9,59				
SELF ASSUREI APPROACH	Non-literate	10	19,80	60	7,221	,002*	3-1
	Primary school	32	22,43				
	High school	22	25,04				
PLANNED APPROACH	Non-literate	10	12,00	60	1,892	,159	-----
	Primary school	32	12,09				
	High school	22	13,77				

*p<0,05

In Table 5, it was analyzed by Kruskal-Wallis test if the problem solving sub-dimensions and the total average scores of the players are changed or not according to the educational level of the mothers of the participants. In the study results; there were statistically significant differences in the sub-dimensions scores of evuluator approach (X2=4,82 P<0.05), and self-assured approach (X2=7,22 P<0.05) according to the class which they study at. But there were no significant differences in any other sub-dimensions.

DISCUSSION and RESULTS

It can be said that the total scores of problem solving skills of the participating athletes and the sub-dimensions such as Evuluator Approach, self Assuredapproach and planned approach are also low. But it can be clearly understood from the study that the average scores of Impetuous Approach and avoidant approach are high. The reason there are higher average scores in the hasty and avoidant approach compared to the other sub-dimensions of the problem-solving skills is that people tend to move in line with the first idea that comes to their mind to solve problems and people think that they cannot succeed if they act in accordance with their planned solution.

According to the variable of the father's occupation of the participants; the scores of those whose fathers are tradesmen in the sub-dimension of self-Assuredapproach are higher than those who are farmers. It can be said that those whose fathers are tradesmen have much more self confidence because they are able to express himself more comfortably and they imitate their fathers to overcome the problems they faced.

According the variable of school which they study at; the avoidant approach scores of the students of Karamanoğlu Mehmetbey University are higher than the students of Selçuk University. It is believed that the province where the university is located and the social structure of the province have significant effects on overcoming the problems encountered and dealing with the problems.

According the variable of the class which they study at; Impetuous Approach scores of the students of the third class are higher than the students of the second class. The reason why people act without taking into account various factors on coping with problems is because they are closer to professional life. By doing so they increase the possibility of sudden and accurate decisions.

According to the variable of department which they study at; it is seen that the Evuluator Approach scores of the students of management department are higher than the students of schoolteaching department, the self-Assuredapproach scores of the students of management department are also higher than the students of schoolteaching and coaching department. Similarly, it is seen that the planned approach scores of the students of management department are higher than the students of coaching department. It is believed that the reason of the findings match the qualifications required to have an administrator is because each and everyone of the participants is an adminastor candidate.

The Evuluator Approach scores of the participants whose mothers are graduated from the primary school compared to the participants whose mothers are illiterate. The self-Assuredapproach scores of the participants whose mothers are graduated from the high school compared to the participants whose mothers are illiterate. The educational level and mother's education level are effective in self-confidence and the ability of making decision of the participants.

References

[1]. Barut Y., Yılmaz M. (2000) "Beden Eğitimi ve Spor Bölümüne ve Eğitim Fakültesine Devam Eden Öğrencilerin Problem Çözme Becerilerinin Çeşitli Değişkenler Açısından İncelenmesi", Uluslararası 1. Spor Bilimleri Kongresi Bildirileri, Gazi University, Ankara, 290-297.

[2]. Büyüköztürk, Ş. (2010) Sosyal bilimler için veri analizi el kitabı. Ankara: Pegem Akademi Yayınları.

[3]. Çam, S., (1995) Öğretmen Adaylarının Ego Durumları ile Problem Çözme Becerisi Algısı İlişkisinin İncelenmesi. Psikolojik Danışma ve Rehberlik Dergisi. 6(2), 37-42.

[4]. Dönmez, KH., Kaçar F., (2015) "Giresun University Beden Eğitimi ve Spor Bölümü Öğ-rencilerinin Sosyal Öz-Yeterlik ve Problem Çözme Becerilerinin İncelenmesi",İnternational Journal of Social Sciences and Education Research, 1(2), 655.

[5]. D'Zurilla TJ, Nezu M. (1990) "Development and preliminary evaluation of the social problem solving", Psychological Assessment: A Journal of Consulting and Clinical Psychology, 2(2), 156-163.

[6]. Ferah, D., (2000) Kara Harp Okulu Öğrencilerinin Problem Çözme Becerilerini Algılamalarının ve Problem Çözme Yaklaşım Biçimlerinin Cinsiyet, Class, Akademik Basarı ve Liderlik Yapma Açısından İncelenmesi. Yayınlanmamış Yüksek Lisans Tezi. Hacettepe University, Sosyal Bilimler Enstitüsü, Eğitim Bilimleri Anabilim Dalı, Ankara.

[7]. Gökkurt B., Örnek T., Hayat F., Soylu Y. (2015) "Öğrencilerin Problem Çözme ve Problem Kurma Becerilerinin Değerlendirilmesi", Bartın University Eğitim Fakültesi Dergisi, 4(2), 752.

[8]. Heppner PP., Petersen CH. (1982) "The development and a implications of a personal problem solving inventory", Journal of Counseling Psychology, 29(1), 66–75.

[9]. Heppner PP., Anderson WP. (1985)"The Relationship Between Problem Solving Self –Appraisaland Psychological Adjustment", Cognitive Therapy and Research, 4, 415-427.

[10]. Karabulut O., Kuru E. (2009) "Ahi Evran University P.H.Teaching Bölümü Öğrencilerinin Problem Çözme Becerileri İle Kişilik Özelliklerinin Çeşitli Değişkenler Bakımından İncelenmesi", Ahi Evran University Eğitim Fakültesi Dergisi, 10(3), 120.

[11]. Kiremitci O., Canpolat M (2014) "Beden Eğitimi ve Spor Yüksekokulu Öğrencilerinin Çoklu Zekâ Alanlarının Üst bilişsel Farkındalık ve Problem Çözme Becerilerini Belirlemedeki Rolü", Spor Bilimleri Dergisi, 25 (3), 119.

[12]. Koray,Ö., Azar, A. (2008) Ortaöğretim öğrencilerinin problem çözme ve mantıksal düşünme becerilerinin cinsiyet ve seçilen alan açısından incelenmesi. Kastamonu Eğitim Dergisi, 16 (1), 125-136.

[13]. Oğuztürk Ö., Akça F., Şahin G. (2011) "Üniversite Öğrencilerinde Umutsuzluk Düzeyi İle Problem Çözme Becerileri Arasındaki İlişkinin Bazı Değişkenler Üzerinden İncelenmesi", Klinik Psikiyatri, (14)-174.

[14]. Özer B., Gelen İ., Öcal S. (2009) "İlköğretim İkinci Kademe Öğrencilerinin Boş Zaman Değerlendirme Alışkanlıklarının Günlük Problem Çözme Becerilerine Etkisinin İncelenmesi", Mustafa Kemal University Sosyal Bilimler Enstitüsü Dergisi, 6(12), 236.

[15]. Özyürek A., Özkan İ., Begde Z., Yavuz NF. (2015) " Okul Öncesi Dönemde Beden Eğitimi ve Spor", International Journal of Science Culture and Sport, 7(3), 482.

[16]. Savaşır, İ., ve Şahin, N. H. (1997) Bilişsel-Davranışçı Terapilerde Değerlendirme: Sık Kullanılan Ölçekler,

Ankara: Türk Psikologlar Derneği Yayınları, No: 9.

[17]. Schreglmann S:, Doğruluk S. (2012) Bilişim Teknolojileri Öğretmen Adaylarının Problem Çözme Becerilerinin Çeşitli Değişkenler Açısından İncelenmesi, Amasya University Eğitim Fakültesi Dergisi 1(2), 147.

[18]. Şahin N., Şahin NH., Heppner PP. (1993) "Psychometric propoties of the Problem Solving Inventory in a group of Turkish university students", Cogn Ther Res, 17: 379-396.

[19]. Taylan, S. (1990) Heppner'in Problem Çözme Envanteri'nin Uyarlama, Güvenirlik ve Geçerlik Çalışmaları, Yayınlanmamış Yüksek Lisans Tezi, Ankara University, Sosyal Bilimler Enstitüsü, Ankara.

[20]. Türkçapar Ü. (2015) " Üniversite Öğretmen Adayı Öğrencilerin Problem Çözme Becerilerinin Farklı Değişkenlere Göre İncelenmesi" , Niğde University Beden Eğitimi ve Spor Bilimleri Dergisi, 9(2), 236.

[21]. Üstün A., Bozkurt E. (2003) "İlköğretim Okulu Müdürlerinin Kendilerini Algılayışlarına Göre Problem Çözme Becerilerini Etkileyen Bazı Mesleki Faktörler", Kastamonu Eğitim Dergisi, 11(1), 14

14

COMPARATIVE STUDY OF WUSHU HITTING AND KICKING TECHNIQUE FOR JUNIORS 14-18 YEARS

Mihai Cristian NEGOESCU, Sanda Toma URICHIANU

candidate PhD. USEFS, of Moldova, Prof. PhD. Ecologic University of Bucharest

Abstract. In this paper was aimed at improving technique blows arms and legs wushu martial arts specific to the semi contact at juniors 14 - 18 years. For it was considered that the comparative analysis techniques blows arms and legs specific wushu -his juniors of 14-18 years, we will highlight if there are significant differences between them and influence means training on improving the technique of execution.

This scientific approach has led to organizing a study Sports Club "Jad" in Bucharest on a group of junior athletes aged 14-18 years, from wushu station.

In the study we used the following research methods: bibliographical study method, pedagogical observation method, the method of testing, pedagogical experiment method, method of mathematical statistics and graphical representation.

Technique for highlighting specific strokes arms and legs wushu - samples were used to control the penetrating hits and snap hits. Also during the course of the study was implemented a program of exercises for improving technique blows both arms and legs.

The results of the study highlight the significant differences between arms and legs kicks wushu specific - his juniors 14 - 18 years of training means and influence on improving the technique of execution.

Key words: wushu, qinda, technical training, stripes, competition, performance.

Introduction.

Chinese martial arts have great diversity and variety of fighting styles. All these styles have the same aim, namely victory in battle, making it resulted centralize their four internal martial arts and several hundred external martial arts. The link between these two classes is represented variants competition for sports competitions to test the technical and tactical training of fighters. Thus appeared the wrestling sport as arbitrated by Sanda Sanshou (full contact fighting), Qinda (semi contact fighting), Shuai Jiao (free fighting melee), and Chi Sao (box in enclosed spaces). Of these Qinda believe that competition is best adapted to beginners who have no experience and no driving skills developed [1, 2, 3, 4].

After Dragnea A. and S. Mate - Teodorescu (2002) sport training is a "complex process systematically and continuously developed gradually adapting athlete body to intense physical and mental effort involved in participating in competitions" . Qinda Wu Shu competition is specifically designed for groups of beginners, they did not have sports experience nor developed body to withstand and absorb the blows they receive. An important feature is that all the fighting techniques with speed and then apply the force reduced to only 10% of the maximum potential athletes for the body to adapt accordingly requests the real battle. In addition linear blows to the head are prohibited because Beginners properly appreciate the distance of struggle and do not have time to beware of direct hits[5]. Performance in sport aims to destroy each other but do not assume the existence of communication relations between opponents in the spirit of fair play - acquis [6]. Technical any sport branches include driving the set of all actions carried out with maximum accuracy and efficiency envisages principle with minimal effort. Wu Shu sport technical branch Qinda include [7]:

- Strokes and blockages in the arms;
- Strokes and blockages in the legs;
- Trips, falls and tumbles, slits, dodge and sockets on the opponent;
- Throws, projects and slamming the opponent.

Techniques for influencing psychological battle cries represented by discharge energy; we remark that all these classes of important techniques must be present to be effective. The importance of technical and tactical training is vital for harmonious and sustainable development, but in the area of sports wushu has a major characteristic Qinda general physical preparation and physical preparation specific technical working simultaneously with tactical training [8, 9].

According to A. Dragnea (adapted) have a basic rule in working with novice athletes namely to ensure constant availability under the required physical properties of the new elements and it is through a large number of repetitions in front of the mirror for self-correction. This type of training we call "shadow boxing". Briefly illustrate the art of Wu Shu Qinda components:

Technical element is a fundamental structure underlying motive of practicing sports industry is represented by various kicks and blocking with his arms and legs. Technical processing is a specific and complex motor structure is a particular way of making technical element, here we illustrate the action of specific technical counter attack. Attack with direct kick back with your right hand to the body (you chong quan) and against the attack lateral right foot shot from behind the body (you ce chuai tui).

The basic mechanism of any techniques is the natural and logical sequence of motor acts needed to ensure objective.

Here we give an example: any kicks will be start first on ball of the foot pivot to avoid stress and tear over the ligaments foot support.

Personal style comes as a culmination of three technical components above, and is in fact what defines a particular sport namely by way of personal footprint by conducting a technical process.

This subtly visible only for specialists in the field. Morphological, functional (blocking execution recent injury) and mental form personal style that gradually grow stronger with the passage of time in sports practice.

From the historical perspective Qinda Wu Shu competition is the newest and adopted with the spread of global sports industry wushu, but athletes who began attending the Wu Shu sports competitions have greater longevity Qinda performance in sporting competitions. This is due to the fact that they learned to avoid injuries through technical and tactical execution speed and low power. Qinda Wu Shu competitions are local, national, European and international.

The main features of the rules of competition are:

- Strength and speed are reduced to 10% of capacity;
- Two rounds of 2 minutes with a minute break between them;
- Fighting area rug is an elastic 8x8 m without being high on a platform;
- Athletes before competition should come with a health certificate and annex electro-cardiogram and electroencephalogram (not to exceed 20 days from the date of issue);
- Competitive system allows direct elimination, double elimination tournament and system.

Tournament consider most useful system because it offers more opportunities for promotion and affirmation of future champions. The tournament is the type used in meetings friendlies verification. Athletes are necessarily equipped with braces, helmet, jacket, gloves, shin guards and protectors testes in boys and girls breasts protection;

- Valid striking areas are the sides of the head, torso, legs and back sides.

The techniques are prohibited:

- Hitting or even reaching the opponent's face;
- Direct attack on the joints and limbs;
- Header, elbow, knee;
- Throws, projections, sweeping dangerous;
- Buying time;
- Using fingers as gun attack;
- Bottlenecks and choke;
- Wresling specific ground fighting;
- Young passive (clinch) more than 3 seconds;
- Joint actions;
- Hitting opponent from the socket;
- Scratching, hair pulling, spitting
- Hitting series continue or what part of the body;
- Pushing - pulling opponent more than 1 meter;
- Prohibited attack areas are the face, neck, eyes and throat, testicles, spine, knees, elbows and other joints.

Criteria scoring enumerate them as follows:

- 2 points are awarded when (an athlete out of the fighting area, design safe and clean, and the performer remains standing right foot shot on a valid area (head or body, the opponent is penalized).
- 1 point is awarded when (kick right arm over a zone valid; kick right leg on the thigh side, the opponent is warned; if the athlete that is above simultaneous fall, when the opponent is counted.

The main purpose of the work is to improve the technique blows arms and legs wu shu martial arts specific to the sample level juniors 14 - 18 years.

Hypothesis work.

We believe that by conducting comparative analysis techniques specific strokes arms and legs-his junior wushu of 14-18 years, we will highlight if there are significant differences between them and influence means training on improving the technique of execution.

Research methodology and organization. This scientific approach has led to organizing a study Sports Club "Jad" in Bucharest on a group of junior athletes aged 14-18 years, from wushu department. The research was conducted over a 6 month period (January 2015 - June 2015).

In the study we used the following research methods [10]: bibliographic study method, pedagogical observation method, the method of testing, pedagogical experiment method, mathematical statistical method and graphical representation.. Technique for highlighting specific strokes arms and legs Wushu were used as control samples, the penetrating hits and reportisante.

Control samples applied:

1- sample directly hit the front left hand to the body (zuo chong quan);

2- proof direct hit from behind with his right hand to the body (you chong quan);

3 - circular kick with his left hand in front of the body (zuo guan quan);

4 - kick back with your right hand circular to the body (you guan quan);

5 - direct kick with the left foot in front of the body (zuo deng tui);

6 - direct kick with the right foot back to the body (you deng tui);

7 - side kick with the left foot in front of the body (zuo ce chuai tui);

8 - side kick with the right foot back to the body (you ce chuai tui);

9 - circular kick with the left foot in front of the body (zuo ce tan tui);

10 - circular kick with the right foot back to the body (you ce tan tui).

Content means used in training:

Exercises for arms

1. Exercise "with direct bunnies".
2. Exercise "bunnies with clubs".
3. "Zhanxiong Kunda" - swinging / swaying horizontal arms.
4. "Swimming virtual".

Leg exercises (dynamic stretching):

5. Zhen ti tui - kick straight forwards balance - leg stretched forward.
6. Xie ti tui - kick forward obliques - swaying leg stretched diagonally.
7. Ce ti tui - straight kick to the side - balance right foot to the side.
8. Lihe tui - inward crescent kick straight: balance with outstretched leg inward.
9. Wai bai tui - straight outward crescent kick - balance with leg stretched out.
10. "Shadow Boxing with the mirror".

The results and their interpretation. Comparative analysis techniques specific strokes arms and legs Wushu's juniors 14-18 years was conducted upon registration at the match fighting Semi blows penetrating initial testing and final testing. Table 1 presents the results of specific techniques kicks Wushu's arms juniors 14-18 years, the average error of the arithmetic mean and the Half penetrating strokes 1, 2 and their total.

Table 1. Results arms kicks techniques juniors 14 - 18 years

Statist. Indic. samples		Initial testing (x±m)			Initial testing (x±m)		
		1 st half	Round 2	Total	1st half	Round 2	Total
1 (No. Repet.)	T	5,70; 1,32	5,40; 1,18	11,10; 2,49	9,10; 0,53	8,90; 0,66	18,00; 1,17
	S	4,70; 1,17	4,50; 1,18	9,10; 2,35	8,50; 0,72	8,40; 0,76	16,90; 1,46
2 (No. Repet.)	T	5,60; 1,06	5,10, 0,79	10,70; 1,81	7,10; 0,43	6,60; 0,6	13,70; 1,02
	S	3,20; 1,38	3,30; 1,20	6,50; 2,56	6,50; 0,62	6,30; 0,76	12,80; 1,36
3 (No. Repet.)	T	4,40; 1,27	4,80; 1,2	8,20; 1,61	8,40; 0,70	8,10; 0,66	16,50; 1,34
	S	2,40; 0,72	2,20; 0,65	4,60; 1,33	7,60; 0,81	7,10; 0,86	14,70; 1,65
4 (No. Repet.)	T	6,10; 1,53	6,50; 1,51	12,60; 3,03	7,50; 0,52	7,20; 0,44	14,70; 0,94
	S	2,50; 0,87	2,60; 0,83	5,10; 1,68	6,70; 0,47	6,40; 0,4	13,10; 0,86

Note: T - shot thrust penetrating arms; S - shot snap arms; x - arithmetic average; m - the average error; No. I repeat. - Number of repetitions effective

Table 2 presents the results averages differences arms kicks specific techniques wushu's juniors 14 - 18 years between tests, the penetrating hits and reportisating between collisions, initial testing and final testing.

Table 2. Results of differences means, techniques specific strikes wushu's arms, juniors 14 - 18 years

Statist. Indic. samples		(t; p)		
		1st half	Round 2	Total
1 (No. Repet.)	T	2,684; <0,05	3,158; <0,05	2,925; <0,05
	S	2,752; <0,05	2,467; <0,05	2,678; <0,05
	T-S initial	0,565; >0,05	0,537; >0,05	0,583; >0,05
	T-S final	0,674; >0,05	0,496; >0,05	0,588; >0,05
2 (No. Repet.)	T	1,964; >0,05	2,875; <0,05	2,497; <0,05
	S	2,073; >0,05	2,033; >0,05	2,084; >0,05
	T-S initial	1,381; >0,05	1,249; >0,05	1,338; >0,05
	T-S final	0,794; >0,05	0,309; >0,05	0,529; >0,05
3 (No. Repet.)	T	3,207; <0,05	2,664; <0,05	4,655; <0,01
	S	6,867; <0,001	5,444; <0,001	6,252; <0,001
	T-S initial	1,366; >0,05	1,907; >0,05	1,721; >0,05
	T-S final	0,784; >0,05	0,922; >0,05	0,846; >0,05
4 (No. Repet.)	T	0,875; >0,05	0,482; >0,05	0,694; >0,05
	S	3,372; <0,05	3,217; <0,05	3,315; <0,01
	T-S initial	2,043; >0,05	2,256; <0,05	2,162; <0,05
	T-S final	1,136; >0,05	1,341; >0,05	1,252; >0,05

Note: No. I repeat. - Number of repetitions effective; T-S - the difference between strokes

Table 3 presents the results of specific techniques kicks wushu's, juniors 14-18 years on average and arithmetic average error of blunt and penetrating in Half reportisating 1, 2 and their total.

Table 3. Results techniques kicks juniors 14 - 18 years

samples Indic. statist		Initial testing (x±m)			Initial testing (x±m)		
		1st half	Round 2	Total	1 st half	Round 2	Total
5 (No. Repet.)	T	4,30; 1,14	5,50; 1,33	9,80; 2,41	7,50; 0,48	6,70; 0,42	14,20; 0,89
	S	1,40; 0,34	1,80; 0,29	3,20; 0,55	6,50; 0,62	6,10; 0,60	12,60; 1,19
6 (No. Repet.)	T	4,70; 0,65	4,40; 0,56	9,10; 1,18	7,40; 0,52	7,20; 0,44	14,60; 0,93
	S	1,80; 0,25	1,70; 0,3	3,50; 0,45	7,00; 0,45	6,60; 0,37	13,60; 0,79
7 (No. Repet.)	T	2,40; 0,81	2,30; 0,77	4,70; 1,57	4,90; 0,53	4,30; 0,45	9,20; 0,96
	S	1,10; 0,69	1,10; 0,69	2,20; 1,38	3,40; 0,45	2,70; 0,42	6,10; 0,85
8 (No. Repet.)	T	2,50; 0,98	2,70; 1,13	5,20; 2,08	4,40; 0,58	3,50; 0,5	7,90; 1,07
	S	0,90; 0,50	0,70; 0,47	1,60; 0,96	3,20; 0,59	3,00; 0,63	6,20; 1,19
9 (No.Repet.)	T	6,70; 1,34	6,50; 1,16	13,20; 2,48	8,00; 0,67	7,50; 0,48	15,40; 1,12
	S	2,10; 0,71	2,50; 0,89	4,60; 1,57	7,00; 0,47	6,70; 0,37	13,70; 0,79
10 (No. Repet.)	T	7,10; 0,84	6,50; 0,78	13,60; 1,58	6,70; 0,33	6,70; 0,42	13,40; 0,70
	S	2,30; 0,78	2,00; 0,83	4,30; 1,58	6,30; 0,54	6,00; 0,49	12,40; 0,97

Note: T – thrust kicks; S – snap kicks; x - arithmetic average; m - the average error; No. I repeat. - Number of repetitions effective

Table 4 presents the results of differences of averages kicks specific techniques Wushu's juniors 14 - 18 years between tests of thrust penetrating kicks and snap flicks between initial testing and final testing.

Table 4. Results of differences of averages kicks techniques to juniors 14 - 18 years

Statist Indic. Samples		(t; p)		
		1st half	Round2	Total
5 (No. Repet.)	T	3,012; <0,05	0,847; >0,05	1,848; >0,05
	S	9,328; <0,001	6,286; <0,001	7,938; <0,001

	T-S$_{initial}$	2,427; <0,05	2,724; <0,05	2,667; <0,05
	T-S$_{final}$	1,279; >0,05	0,814; >0,05	1,073; >0,05
6 (No. Repet.)	T	2,793; <0,05	3,441; <0,01	3,127; <0,05
	S	9,097; <0,001	12,043; <0,001	10,787; <0,001
	T-S$_{initial}$	4,162; <0,001	4,239; <0,001	4,436; <0,001
	T-S$_{final}$	0,583; >0,05	1,039; >0,05	0,817; >0,05
7 (No. Repet.)	T	2,142; >0,05	1,917; >0,05	2,043; >0,05
	S	2,501; <0,05	1,986; >0,05	2,273; <0,05
	T-S$_{initial}$	1,225; >0,05	1,156; >0,05	1,195; >0,05
	T-S$_{final}$	2,162; <0,05	2,596; >0,05	2,413; <0,05
8 (No. Repet.)	T	1,696; >0,05	0,706; >0,05	1,207; >0,05
	R	3,632; <0,01	2,725; <0,05	3,146; <0,05
	T-S$_{initial}$	1,451; >0,05	1,637; >0,05	1,568; >0,05
	T-S$_{final}$	1,446; >0,05	0,629; >0,05	1,062; >0,05
9 (No. Repet.)	T	0,908; >0,05	0,819; >0,05	0,837; >0,05
	S	5,301; <0,001	3,953; <0,01	4,648; <0,01
	T-S$_{initial}$	3,303; <0,01	2,746; <0,05	2,928; <0,05
	T-S$_{final}$	1,225; >0,05	1,329; >0,05	1,242; >0,05
10 (No. Repet.)	T	0,446; >0,05	0,215; >0,05	0,115; >0,05
	S	4,000; <0,01	3,561; <0,01	4,067; <0,01
	T-S$_{initial}$	4,209; <0,001	3,955; <0,001	4,157; <0,001
	T-S$_{final}$	0,631; >0,05	1,076; >0,05	0,829; >0,05

Note: No. I repeat. - Number of repetitions effective

The results of the comparative analysis on the gender specific media coups Wushu's arms juniors 14-18 years highlight significant differences (Table 2): the direct kick with his left hand to the body from the 1st, 2nd and total between tests blows thrust and snap ($p < 0.05$); Direct kick back with your right hand to the body in round 2 and the total penetrating shot ($p < 0.05$); circular kick with his left hand to the body of the half 1, 2 and totally blows penetrating between tests ($p < 0.05$, $p < 0.01$) and snap ($p < 0.001$); circular kick back with your right hand to the body in half 1, 2 and totally snap blows between tests ($p < 0.05$; $p < 0.01$) and between 2 and Half blow to the total ($p < 0.05$). The results of comparative analysis differences of averages kicks specific Wushu's juniors 14-18 years highlight significant differences (Table 4): the direct kick with the left foot in front of the body between tests with blows penetrating the 1st ($p < 0.05$) and hits the Half snap 1, 2 and total ($p < 0.001$); the direct hit to right hind leg in between tests both body blow to 1st, 2nd and total ($p < 0.05$; $p < 0.01$; $p < 0.001$) and between blow to initial testing in Half 1, 2 and total ($p < 0.001$); Side kick with his left foot from the front kick to the body between tests with the Half snap 1 and total ($p < 0.05$); the side kick with the right foot back to kick snap body between tests with the 1st, 2nd and total ($p < 0.05$; $p < 0.01$); the circular kick with the left foot front kick to the body between tests with Half snap at 1, 2 and total ($p < 0.05$; $p < 0.01$) and between blow to initial testing in Half 1, 2 and total ($p < 0.05$, $p < 0.01$); the circular kick with the right foot back to kick snap body between tests with the 1st, 2nd and total ($p < 0.01$) and between blow to initial testing in Half 1, 2 and total ($p < 0.001$).

Conclusion.

The comparative analysis of results of specific arms kicks wushu's highlights increasing the number of effective shots in final testing, 1 Half higher values in both testing and greater number of shots penetrating on both tests. Comparative analysis techniques specific arms and legs kicks his junior wushu-14 - 18 years highlights the significant differences between them and influence means training on improving the technique of execution.

References

[1]. Deliu, D., [2014], Combat courses for students, Discobol Publishing, Bucharest, pp.68;

[2]. Deliu, D., [2008], Methodology combat disciplines, Bren Publishing, Bucharest, pp.132;.

[3]. Gălan, D., [2014], Martial arts instructor training course, Riso print Publishing, Cluj Napoca, pp.42; .

[4]. Triboi, V., Păcuraru, A., [2013].,Theory and Methodology of Sport Training, PIM Publishing, Iaşi, pp.162; .

[5]. Todiriţă, A. B., [2008], Chinese shaolin kung fu, Domino Publishing, Bucharest, pp.14; .

[6]. Dragnea, A. Mate-Teodorescu, S., [2002], Theory of sports, FEST Publishing, Bucharest, pp.155;.

[7]. Ionescu, M. L., [1998], Chinese Sanda Sanshou full contact, Garell Publishing House, Bucharest, pp.63; .

[8]. Bompa, T. O., [2001], Theory and methodology of sports training, Ex Ponto Publishing, Constanţa, pp.168;

[9]. Bompa, T. O., [2003], Skills development biomotric, Ex Ponto Publishing, Constanţa, pp.74;.

[10]. Epuran, M., [2005], Research methodology bodily activities, FEST Publishing Bucharest, pp.49.

15

DYNAMIC BALANCE DEVELOPEMENT TO FOOTBALL PLAYERS

Florin ŢURCANU

Universitatea de Medicină şi Farmacie Tîrgu Mureş

Abstract: The role of unstable surfaces is to intensify muscular activity, particularly the neuromuscular component associated with static balance at the expense of the mechanical load. By the introduction of unstable surfaces in the training process the proprioceptive feedback is weak on account of the permanent stimulation on the balance controlling mechanism, maintaining balance becoming difficult. The correct and timely use of unstable surface procedures during training sessions, when compared to classical football training methods, clearly lead to a better development of static and dynamic balance. The use of static and dynamic unstable surface procedures influences the appropriate space and time orientation indicators as well as balance. The research was carried out during one sport season on two groups: experimental and control, each comprising ten players. The training of both groups was executed based on the same anual training plan, the difference being that on the experimental group unstable surface procedures were used, while on the control group procedures specific to football training. The following tests were applied: stability test with multiple single leg jumps (right and left), two-leg balance with legs close together, eyes open and closed. After applying the tests there was visible improvement in results for the experimental group, while there was no obvious change in the results of the control group. The procedures used on the experimental group proved to be more effective than the procedures specific to football training. The results of the experimental group in both tests, following the use of unstable surface procedures, shows an improvement in balance compared to control group subjects.

Key words: balance, unstable surface, optimization, football, training.

Introduction

On a high level, football players have a vast technical repertoire backed by their skills, like coordination, balance, or reaction and execution speed [1].

One of the current trends is to introduce specific elements of proprioceptive development into frame of training programmes, meant to improve the specific indicators of static and dynamic balance, as well as neuromuscular coordination, starting from an early age [2].

The programmes meant to develop neuromuscular control often include balance exercises whose purpose is optimizing training, prevention of and recovery from injuries [3].

Posture control or balance can be defined as the ability to maintain a foothold with minimal movement, as well as the ability of executing a task while preserving a stable position. This is maintained by way of a dynamic integration of forces and both internal and external factors involving the environment [4, 5]. Adjusting balance dependson visual, vestibular and proprioceptive stimuli [6, 7].

Maintaining posture control includes integrating information from neurosensors of three types, vestibular, visual and somesthetic, into the vestibular nuclei, to generate a motoric response in a certain context which leads to control of the anti-gravitational activity [8].

The authors Freiwald, J. and Gstöttner, M., underline the importance of training balance based on scientific programmes on coordination to prevent lesions and improve performance [9, 10].

Various studies show that developing balance may lead to improving posture and neuromuscular control. The same studies show that, from a clinical point of view, developing balance leads to improving static and dynamic postural balance.

Periodical evaluation and monitoring of static and dynamic balance in young athletes may be an important instrument the correct layout and alternation of training programmes, depending on the sport in question, the improvement rate of balance scores in time and athlete's age. This would allow, in each period of the athlete's development, the creation and optimization of a large, well rounded set of fundamental motoric skills [11].

Hypothesis

This research was started from the idea that the optimization of the training of men football players, can be achieved with greater efficiency when developing balance by way of utilising unstable surfaces.

Materials, methods, procedures

Period and location of research

This research was carried out during 2014-2015 sport season, on two groups: a experimental group and a control group. The athletes from the experimental group were players of Stadium GAZ Tirgu Mures. The members of the control group were players of the Stadium ASA Tirgu Mures.

Research subjects

The subjects of this research had the age of 18 to 22 and were a total of twenty (15 for the experimental group and 15 for the control group).

Both groups had ten training sessions per week, each of a duration of an hour and half, based on the training plan devised by the two coaches. Traditional training methods were used, specific to the game of football and adapted to the level of training of the two groups. In addition to these specific procedures of football training, the experimental group, during individualised training, was subjected to specific balance developing procedures on unstable surfaces, with elastic bands, on gym balls and with TRXs, three times a week, for thirty minutes each.

Procedures

The procedures proposed by us were adapted to the game of football, having the purpose of static and dynamic balance development.

The proposed programme aimed at the development of the following skills: force, speed, balance and leg control. The procedures used were aimed at improving posture and neuromuscular control.

Ex.1. Forward movement on 10 lined-up balance fits.

Ex.2. Backward movement on 10 lined-up balance fits.

Ex.3. Standing on two balance fits in basic position specify football players (facing the ball), with defender's opposition.

Ex.4. Elastic band around hip, drawn, lateral movement to intermediary defenders' area.

Tests applied

The efficiency of the procedures used during this research was verified by applying the following tests:

Two-leg balance with legs close together, eyes open (15 seconds recording time)

Two-leg balance with legs close together, eyes closed (15 seconds recording time)

Aim: evaluating static balance through marking the average displacement.

Before the start of the training programme and at its end measuring sessions (Table 1) were held by means of AMTI BP400600 force plate (www.AMTI.biz).

Table 1 **Two-leg balance with legs close together, eyes open**

Group	Avg.	Avg. diff.	Median	Minimum	Max.	Variation coeff.	Mann-Whitney		Effect size
							Z	P	
Experimental	0.254	-0.065	0.227	0.172	0.419	35.0%	-2.268	0.023	0.51
Control	0.319	-20.5%	0.321	0.274	0.379	10.8%			

Upon testing two-leg balance with legs close together and eyes open, a 0.065 (20.5%) cm lower average value of displacement was found for the experimental group. This difference shows an increase of static balance for the experimental group. The average values are 0.254 for the experimental group and 0.319 cm for the control group.

The data dispersion is inhomogenous with the experimental group and homogenous with the control group. The difference is statistically significant according to the Mann-Whitney significance test, for $z = -2.268$ and $p = 0.023 < 0.05$. The effect size index (0.51) shows a high to very high difference between the two groups (see Table 1).

Table 2 **Two-leg balance with legs close together, eyes closed**

Group	Avg.	Avg. diff.	Median	Minimum	Max.	Variation coeff.	Mann-Whitney		Effect size
							Z	P	
Experimental	0.299	-0.144	0.279	0.253	0.485	22.9%	-3.214	0.001	0.72
Control	0.443	-32.6%	0.455	0.356	0.532	12.6%			

The test for two-leg balance with legs close together and eyes closed showed a 0.144 (32.6%) cm lower average value of displacement for the experimental group. This signifies a better static balance of the experimental group.The average values are 0.299 for the experimental group and 0.443 cm for the control group. The data dispersion about the average is relatively homogenous with the experimental group and homogenous with the control group. The difference between the two average values is statistically significant according to the Mann-Whitney significance test, for z = -3.214 and p = 0.001 < 0.05. The effect size index (0.72) shows a high to very high difference between the two final testings (see Table 2).

Stability test with multiple single leg jumps

Aim: evaluating control over body position and balance during functional performance with repeated jumps.

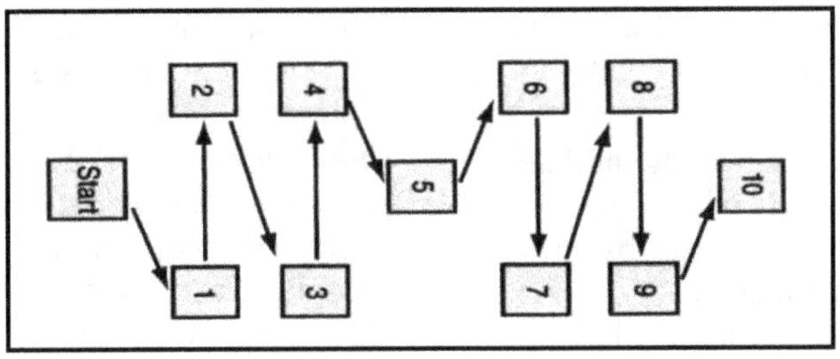

Figure 1.

Table 3 **Stability test with multiple single right leg jumps**

Group	Avg.	Avg. diff.	Median	Minimum	Max.	Variation coeff.	Mann-Whitney		Effect size
							Z	P	
Experimental	21.20	-29.90	20.50	6	36	53.1%	-3.100	0.002	0.69
Control	51.10	-58.5%	52.00	21	73	38.6%			

The multiple single right leg jumps stability test showed a 29.90 (58.5%) point lower average value of execution errors for the experimental group. The average values are 21.20 for the experimental group and 51.10 points for the control group. The data dispersion with both groups is inhomogenous. The difference is statistically significant according to the Mann-Whitney significance test, for z = -3.100 and p = 0.002 < 0.05. The effect size (0.69) shows a high to very high difference between the two final testings (see Table 3).

Table 4 **Stability test with multiple single left leg jumps**

Group	Avg.	Avg. diff.	Median	Minimum	Max.	Variation coeff.	Mann-Whitney		Effect size
							Z	P	
Experimental	23.60	-26.40	22.0	6	43	55.8%	-2.879	0.004	0.64
Control	50.00	-52.8%	42.0	28	79	35.9%			

The multiple single left leg jumps stability test showed a 26.40 (52.8%) point lower average value of errors made by subjects from the experimental group. The average values are 23.60 for the experimental group and 50.00 points for the control group. The data dispersion with both groups is inhomogenous. The difference is statistically significant according to the Mann-Whitney significance test, for z = -2.879 and p = 0.004 < 0.05. The effect size (0.64) shows a high to very high difference between the two groups (see Table 4).

Discussion

The results recorded in this research indicate the emergence of significant differences between the two groups from the initial to the final testings, on account of, as we believe, the procedures carried out on unstable surfaces, proposed by us. After applying the Two-leg balance tests with legs close together, eyes open and closed (15 seconds recording time) and the Stability test with multiple single (right and left) leg jumps, a significant progress can be observed with the experimental group as compared with the control group.

It is recommended that with young athletes training balance be started with exercises aiming static balance, followed later by more complex ones for dynamic balance.

It is also recommended that training balance should start on a stable surface with a wide base for foothold and visual feedback. For increased efficiency the difficulty level of execution can be raised: narrow base for foothold with eyes open; wide base fro foothold with eyes closed; narrow base for foothold with eyes closed.

The complexity of movements involved as well as the execution of exercises on different types of surfaces (sand, lawn, grass, various devices etc.) lead to the facilitation of the balance training process.

The role of unstable surfaces is to intensify muscular activity at the expense of mechanical load. By introducing unstable surfaces the proprioceptive feedback is unreliable due to the fact that the control mechanism responsible for maintaining balance is being permanently stimulated, its task thus becoming more difficult.

Conclusion

In view of the results of this study we can conclude that implementing programmes that include procedures on unstable surfaces can have a considerable impact on performance by creating and optimizing a wide array of fundamental motor skills.

The role of unstable surfaces is to intensify muscular activity at the expense of mechanical load. By introducing unstable surfaces the proprioceptive feedback is unreliable due to the fact that the control mechanism responsible for maintaining balance is being permanently stimulated, its task thus becoming more difficult.

These exercises, carried out in special conditions (on balance fits, using TRXs, gym balls), stimulate proprioception and may lead to an increase in athletic performance both in case of a high stress game and of technical performance demands in particular situations: imbalance, shooting, passing etc.

References

[1]. Starosta,W., (2006) *The concept of modern training in sport*, Physical Culture And Tourism, 13(2), pp. 9-23;

[2]. Acsinte, A., Alexandru, E., Guiterrez a Quilar, O., (2012);*Neuro-muscular coordination and balance skills development in young female handball players,* 2nd EHF Scientific conference women and handball scientific and practical Approaches, pp. 28-32

[3]. Zech, A., Markus Hubscher, M., Vogt, L., Winfried Banzer, W., Hansel, F., Pfeifer, K., (2010) *Balance training for neuromuscular control and performance enhancement: a systematic review,*Journal of athletic training, 45(4), pp. 392–403;

[4]. Lee, A., Lin, W., Huang, C., (2006) *Impaired proprioception and poor static postural control in subjects with functional instability of the ankle*. J Exerc Sci Fit 4, pp. 117–125;

[5]. Bressel, E., Yonker, J.C., Kras, J., Heath, E.M., (2007) *Comparison of static and dynamic balance in female collegiate soccer, basketball, and gymnastics athletes,* Journal of Athletic Training, 42, pp. 42-46, [Abstract];

[6]. Subasi, S.S., Gelecek, N., Aksakoglu, G., (2008) *Effects of different warm-up periods on knee proprioception and balance in healthy young individuals*. J Sport Rehab 17, pp. 186–205,;

[7]. Gribble, P.A., Tucke,r W.S., Whit, P.A., (2007) *Time-of-day influences on static and dynamic postural control*. J Athl Train 42, pp. 35–41,;

[8]. Gauchard, G.C., Gangloff, P., Jeandel, C., Perrin, P.P., (2003) *Physical activity improves gaze and posture control in the elderly,* Neurosci Res 45, pp. 409-41;

[9]. Freiwald, J., Papadopoulus, C., Slomka, M., Bizzini, M., Baumgart, C., (2006) ;*Prävention im fußballsport.* Sportorthopädie Sporttraumatologie, 22, pp. 140–150,

[10]. Gstöttner, M., Neher, A., Scholtz, A., Millonig, M., Lembert, S., Raschner,C., (2009)

Balance ability and muscle response of the preferred and nonpreferred leg in soccer players,motor control, Human Kinetics,13, pp. 218-231,;

[11]. Ilić, D., Drašković, V., Marković, S. (2009) *.Selection of students for handball gifted teaching physical education* . In Book of Abstracts 5-th FIEP Euoropean congress, 2- nd Serbian congress of P.E. Teachers (52). Niš: Ministry of youth and sport, Minisrty of science and technological development ministry of education, pp 152

16

CONSIDERATIONS ABOUT THE PLANNING AND THE DYNAMICS OF THE TRAINING PROCESS

Glicheria DĂIAN
University of Craiova

Abstract
The sport training must be well planned in order to achieve high performances. The programs are according to the physical and functional possibilities of the athletes.
The training it self represents the fundamental method of practice of the athlete, based on the use of the exercises in a specific sequence, repeated a specific number of times, with specific intensities, at specific time intervals. The paper aim was to determine the importance of planning the training in order to obtain the performance in sport.
Keywords: *training, adaptation, planning, results.*

Introduction
The realization of a sports activity implies making efforts of different complexities. The practical results, the effects of these activities depend primarily on the exigencies of the respective activity and on the individual's possibilities.

Planning dynamics, records and analysis of the training represent the means to ensure a scientific management of the training process.
Aim and premise of the research

The high exigencies of performance sports lead to a high degree of improvement of the motor skills. Achieving performance is the result of a training process spread out over several years, during which the athlete, through an integrative system, perfects his/her motor skills, techniques, physical and volitional abilities, and consolidates his/her knowledge and health condition.

The training it self represents the fundamental method of practice of the athlete, based on the use of the exercises in a specific sequence, repeated a specific number of times, with specific intensities, at specific time intervals.
Their fusion in various proportions leads to the global or differentiated development of the motor skills which directly condition the athlete's possibilities. [1]

From intention to achievement there is the action, the daily sport training. Within it, the coach-athlete relationship is in a tight interdependency (Figure 1a, 1b).

The intensity of the effort represents the fundamental element which permanently strains and leads to the improvement of sports efficiency. [2]
This progression refers to two parameters:
- the athlete's momentary possibilities
- the demands of the proposed performance objectives.

The parameters draw between them the general curve of effort and training.
In terms of the first parameter (the momentary potential), performing another training involves taking into account several aspects:
1. The effort does not reach the momentary-limit possibilities of the athlete, thus resulting in decreasing the degree of training.
2. The effort reaches the threshold of momentary-limit possibilities of the athlete, resulting in maintaining the degree of training.
3. The effort exceeds the limit threshold of possibilities, resulting in the increase of the degree of training.
4. The effort greatly exceeds the athlete's threshold of possibilities, resulting in overtraining.
Materials and methods

The balance between the intensity and the volume of the stress during the training, on the one hand, and the possibilities of adaptation of the organism, on the other hand, can be expressed by the correlation between the results obtained in the Ruffier effort functional test and by the control test of 600m run, with two middle-distance runners as subjects.

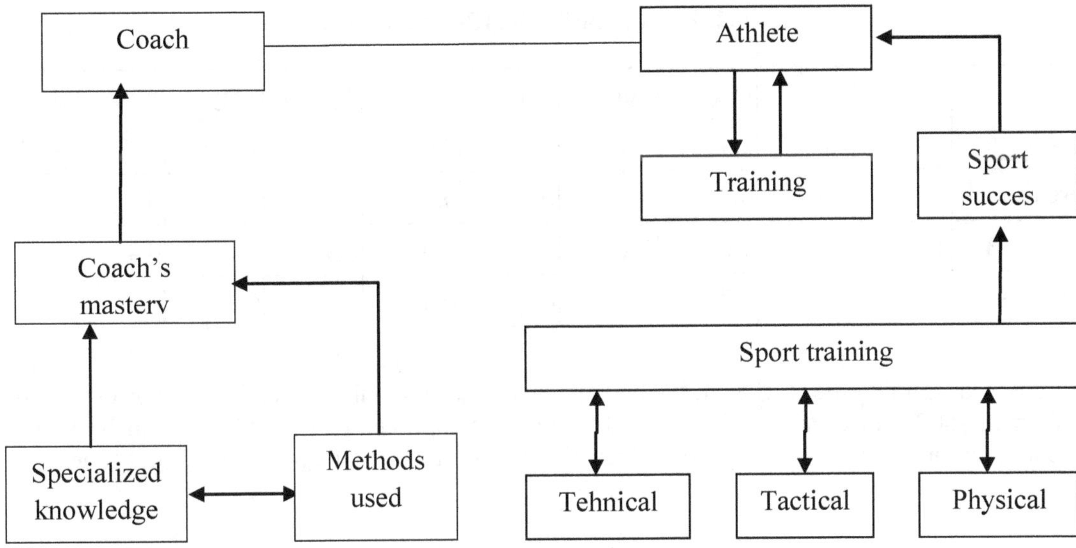

Figure 1a. Coach-training-athlete interrelationship [3]

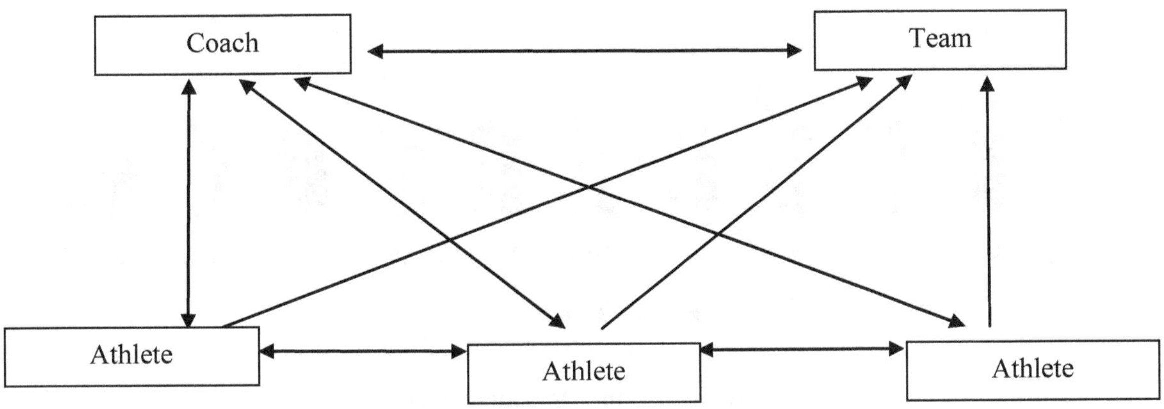

Figure 1b. Coach-training-athlete interrelationship [3]

Results and interpretation of data

The result of functional test is expressed by an index in the form of a figure, and the result of the 600m race in minutes, seconds and tenths allowing an immediate easy appreciation of the effort.

Tabel no.1. Results in the 600m race

	Oct.	Nov.	Dec.	Jan.	Feb.	Mar.	Apr.	May	Jun.	Jul.
Values for A	1:28.5	1:26.4	1:26.2	1:26.0	1:25.8	1:25.1	1:24.7	1:24.5	1:24.3	1:23.8
Differences		2.1	0.2	0.2	0.2	0.7	0.4	0.2	0.2	0.5
Values for B	1:30.5	1:28.1	1:27.2	1:27.0	1:26.6	1:26.5	1:26.0	1:26.1	1:26.6	1:25.3
Differences		2.4	0.9	0.2	0.4	0.1	0.5	0.1	0.5	0.3

Tabel no.2. Results in the Ruffier functional test

	Oct.	Nov.	Dec.	Jan.	Feb.	Mar.	Apr.	May	Jun.	Jul.
Values for A	3	1.6	1.4	1.4	1.2	0.6	0	-1	-1.2	-1.4
Differences		1.4	0.2	0	0.2	0.6	0.6	1	0.2	0.2
Values for B	4.2	2.4	1.6	1.4	1.4	0.6	0	0	0.4	0.4
Differences		1.8	0.8	0.2	0	0.8	0.6	0	0.4	0

Over a one-year training the Ruffier index had an increase of 4.4 units for subject A, corresponding to 4.70.00 in the 600m race, and subject B – 3.8 units corresponding to 5.20.00. It can be noticed a significant relationship between the two indices, the lowest values correspond to the best times.

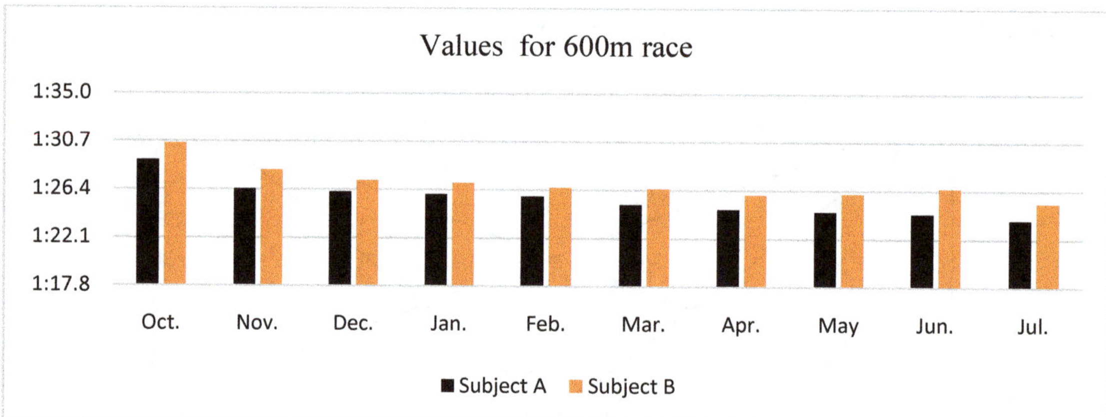

Figure 2. Values for 600m race

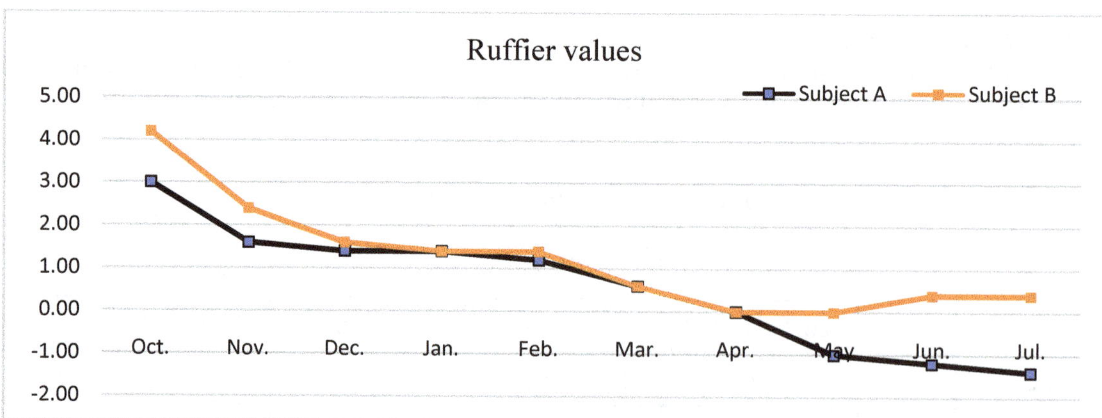

Figure 3. Ruffier values

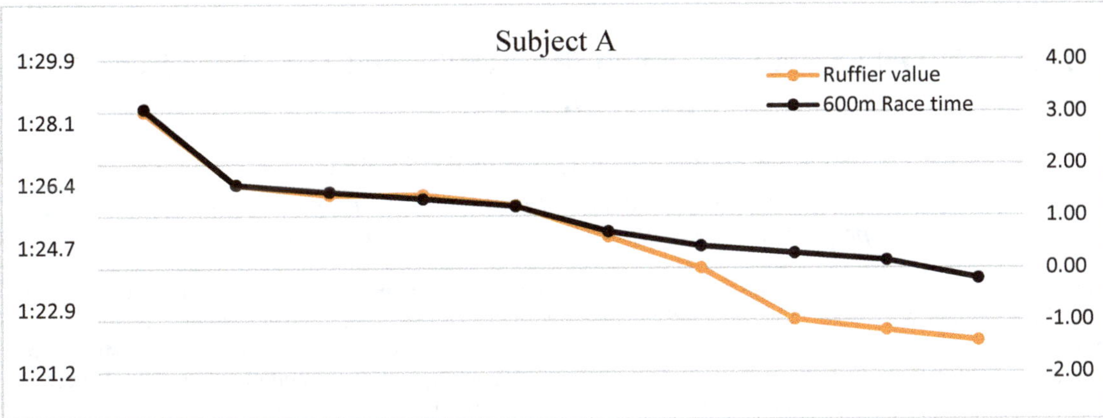

Figure 4. Subject A

We may notice in subject A a big difference between the progress realized in April (2" in the control test) and the qualitative leap of the values of the Ruffier index in the same period. The same finding is valid also for subject B in February, a 1" progress in the control test compared to 0.8 in the functional index.

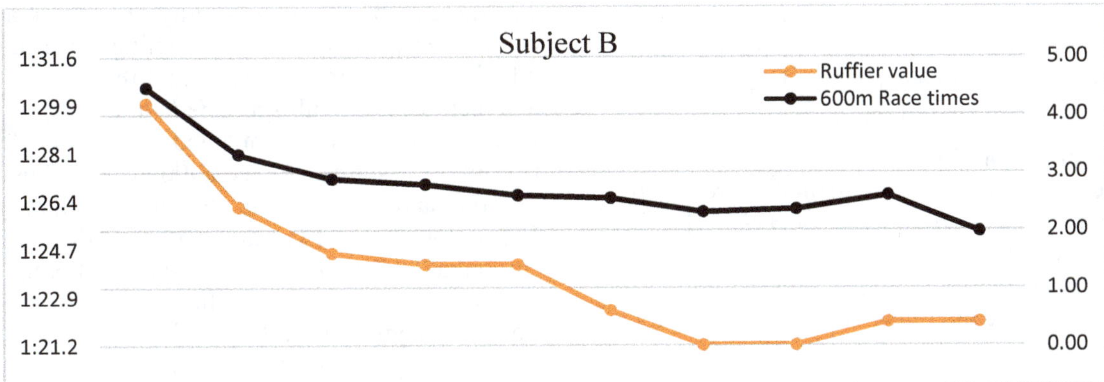

Figure 5. Subject B

The momentary possibilities of the athletes in those periods were higher than the stress during the training.

Conclusions

The comparative estimation of the data resulted in new guidelines for the planification of the training for the next work stage in terms of the workload, the intensity of the effort and the means to be used. We wanted to reassessment of the data and to bring new rescheduling of the parameters so that to eliminate the discrepancies between the values obtained during certain periods of the training year.

References

[1]. Dragnea A., Mate-Teodorescu S. (2002). *Teoria sportului*, Editura FEST, Bucureşti, p.75

[2]. Nicu A. (1993). *Antrenamentul sportiv modern*, Editura EDITIS, Bucureşti, p.38

[3]. Sotiriu R., Marolicaru M. (1977). *Valenţe instructiv-formative ale structurii si dinamicii antrenamentului*, Revista EFS nr. 10/1977.

17

OPTIMIZATION STRATEGIES FOR SPORTS MEDICINE SERVICES IN ROMANIA

Razvan BUSNEAG, Carmen BUSNEAG

"Spiru Haret" University – Faculty of Physical Education and Sport
Specialisation: Kinethotherapy and special motricity

Abstract: The paper aims to provide solutions for optimizing the management of the national system of sports medicine in Romania.We used as a qualitative research method the structured interview, being set-up evaluation questionnaires for medical staff but also for the sport personnel . By processing the questionnaires, we were able to draw a number of conclusions concerning the specialty of sports medicine but also its network and its financing and issues of national and international research programs in sports medicine.

Key words: sports medicine, management, Romania, Europe

Introduction

The purpose of the research was driven by the need of stremline the objective causes and methods of optimization strategies of the national sports medicine.

This paper seeks to optimize business performance management strategy in the Romanian system of sports medicine and, especially, to implement strategic policies in the specific structure of this system

Research Methodology

In the study was used a qualitative research method, namely *structured interview* [1,2]. The choice of this method and the quantitative waiver was dictated by the impossibility of creating a comprehensive database for sampling [3].

Material and method

Were developed two evaluation questionnaires with 10 questions first for the medical staff and the second with 11 questions for people in sport [3,4,8,9].

There were four questions that were common to the two questionnaires.

Questionnaires were sent to 400 (150 in medical and paramedical staff working in sports and 250 people working in sport). They received responses from 326 people, including 96 medical and 230 of the sports field. These responses were statistically processed and will be subject to critical discussion and conclusions.

The first batch who answered the survey consisted of 96 people working in sports medicine clinics in 37 counties in Romania, less the 6 counties where there are no sports medicine cabinets. Thus answered 50 doctors, 27 nurses, 13 physiotherapists and 6 masseurs .

The second lot that answered the survey consisted of 230 people working in the national sports federations such [4]; 170 athletes, 41 coaches, 19 members of federations.

In this case, the choice of this type of research was dictated by the impossibility of creating a comprehensive database for sampling covering all athletes (junior and senior), all the coaches and members from all sports federations [8].

Questionnaires were sent rated 30 of the 60 national sports federations. Thus, questionnaires were sent to the Romanian Federation of Martial Arts, Athletics, Basketball, Biathlon, Bob-Sleigh, Boxing, Canoeing, Rowing, Cycling, Equestrian, Football, Gymnastics, Rhythmic Gymnastics, Weightlifting, Handball, Ice Hockey , Judo, Wrestling, Swimming, Skating, Water Polo, Bowling, Rugby, Skiing, Fencing, Chess, Tennis, Table tennis, Shooting and Volleyball.

The processing of the questionnaires was done in MICROSOFT EXCELL [9.10].

Results and discussions

A. The results of the questionnaire administered to doctors and other personnel from the medical system

Of the 150 questionnaires sent, 96 questionnaires were obtained which are analyzed below.

1. When asked about the institution that should belong to sports medicine ("You want to keep sports medicine: a. Ministry of Health b. Ministry of Youth and Sport c. Romanian Olympic and Sports Committee") most of those questioned (79 %) replied that the Ministry of Health.

2. When asked about sports medicine financing ("Financing of sports medicine services to be: a. Budget, b. Mixed - Subsidies

from the state budget and its own revenues, c. Own resources") the views of respondents were divided: over half of them (51%) were of the opinion that funding must be budget, a quarter of them (25%) think it should be mixed, while about a quarter of respondents (24%) stated that funding must be made from own funds.

3. When asked about equipping sports medicine cabinets ("Are you satisfied of endowment of your cabinet of sports medicine a.Yes b. Partially c. No"), most (79%) of those surveyed decleared they are not satisfied with current equipment that exist within sports medicine.

4. Looking for athletes locally circuit ("circuit for local athletes will be made to: a. 3 months, b. 6 months. C. 12 months") about three-quarters (72%) believes that local circuit for athletes should be 6 months.

5. When asked about the specialty of sports medicine ("Sports medicine is: a. Speciality independent b. Embedded in recovery. C.Embedded in other medical specialities , if so specified that") almost two thirds (64%) of respondents said they want sports medicine be an independent specialiry, over one third (34%) will be embedded in medical rehabilitation and only 2% (only 2 people) think that should be embedded in a orthopedics.

6. Analysis of responses to the question of payment for Sports Medicine ("Who must pay the sports medicine services : a. All athletes b. Professionals athletes and private sports clubs" c None) more than half of those surveyed (59%) say that the payment should be done by professionals and private clubs, 21% say that no athlete should not pay 20% say the contrary, that all athletes should pay.

7. When asked about medical visa ("Medical visa – able for training and competition - a. Mandatory b. Depending on the case c. Optional") most of those questioned (88%) responded that the current system of mandatory medical visa it is the most indicated .

8. Analysis of responses to the question on the staff ("In the clubs / sporting lots need: a.Personal continuum - full time b. Partially - Part time. c.Occasionally - matches and competitions") showed that the majority of respondents (86%) believe that the clubs / lots sports requires medical staff working part time meaning that is working in a medical office or other structures, and to prepare the team / batch involving a few hours a day or a few hours a week.

9. On the question of training medical staff ("The medical staff are made up of people with: a. Universitary degree – medical doctor, physical therapist, etc. b. Secondary Education - nurse, massage therapist, dietician etc c. Complex teams – universitary degree and secondary education and others - psychologist, methodologist etc. ") most of those questioned (90%) stated that the medical team must be a complex, multidisciplinary, ensuring the health and / or obtain great performance.

10.The question on getting a medical visa ("Getting a sports medical visa to make in : a. Medical Individual Sports Medicine Cabinet b. Ambulatory Specialized County c. Regional Centers") about half of those interviewed (40%) want to done in regional centers, probably better equipped with interdisciplinary checkups with specialists better prepared.

B. The results of the questionnaire applied to athletes, coaches and members of the associations

Of the 250 questionnaires sent 230 questionnaires were obtained which are analyzed below.

1. Responses to the question about how satisfied are of the quality of care in professional sports ("Are you satisfied of the quality of care in professional sports: a. Yes b. Partially c. Not") showed that most many (72%) of those surveyed are satisfied. This proves that the activity of sports medicine is considered to be of good quality, the beneficiaries are satisfied with the performance of medical staff.

2. The views of respondents to the question of gaps sports medicine ("What do you think is missing in sports medicine: a. The number of human resources b. Specialized knowledge c. Endowment ") showed that the majority (82%) admit an insufficient technical equipment and performance parameters required by the third millennium.

3. Analysis of responses to the question of payment of Sports Medicine Services ("Who must pay the sports medicine services : a. All athletes b. Professionals and private clubs c. No athletes ") : majority of respondents (82%) believe that no athletes should pay any sports medicine services

4. When asked about medical visa ("Medical visa – able for workouts and competitions – must be: a. Mandatory b. Depending on the case c. Optional") most of those questioned (84%) responded that they should be mandatory

5. Analysis of responses to the question on the staffing ("In the clubs / sporting lots need: a.Medical personnel continuously - full time b. Partially -Part time. c. Occasionally - matches and competitions") three-quarters (75%) of respondents believe that the number in the clubs / sports need lots of medical staff working part

6. When asked about training of the medical staff ("The medical staff are made up of people with: a. University degree – medical doctor, physical therapist, etc. b. Secondary Education - nurse, massage therapist, dietician etc, c. Complex teams -stud higher education , secondary education and others - psychologist, methodologist etc. ") showed that the vast majority of respondents (87%) think it takes a complex team composed of staff with higher education, secondary education and others.

7. On the question of selection ("Where is your sports medicine more useful: a. In the primary selection b in the secondary selection. c.in the tertiary selection ") more than three quarters (78%) of those questioned replied that sports medicine is to use them in the primary selection.

8. On the question of medical examination ("What medical examination satisfied you most: a. Locally b. To the clubs performance c. To the national and olympic teamns level ") the vast majority of respondents (87%) were of the opinion that most take satisfaction from the medical control on Olympic and National teams.

9. Analysis of responses to address medical-sporting act according to age ("Did you feel any qualitative difference in addressing medical and sporting act according to age: a. Yes b. Partially c. Not") revealed that around three quarters (71%) of those surveyed believe that there are some qualitative differences in approach to sports medical act based on age.

10.There have been selected only people who said they had noticed qualitative differences in approach to sports medical act based on age and analyzed their answers to the question of people who were involved ("If YES who was involved: a. Persons 25-40 years, b. Individuals 40 -60 years c. People over 60 years "). Thus were obtained the following results: 37% of them showed people over 60 years, 36% of people 25-40 years and 27% of people 40-60 years of them.

11.The question reffering to the medical specialty that takes the most satisfied respondents ("What medical specialty satisfied you more: a. Sports medicine b. Orthopaedic Traumatology c. Medical Rehabilitation and Balneology d. Others : appointed") the following results in order of frequency weew obteined: Sports Medicine for 42% (96 persons), Orthopaedics-Traumatology for 25% (57 people), Family Medicine for 20% (45 persons), Rehabilitation for 9% (20 persons), Emergency Medicine 3% (7 persons), cardiology for 1.3% (3 people) and Internal Medicine 1% (2 people).

C. results emerged from the responses of medical and sports personnel at 4 common questions and a different question with the common conclusion

The first common question. Who must pay sports medicine services

Responses to this question are the most divergent of all study can be considered emblematic for the slightly confused situation of sport in the year 2016. Like all areas of economic and social life and sports medicine existence depends on funding sources. After Romania joined the European Union is putting extremely acute the problem of areas where they will collect funds to improve the quality of medical and sports and smooth and efficient functioning of the network of sports medicine.

The second common question . Medical visa – able for training and competition

Answers to this question are about the same. This shows that healthcare professionals and sports professionals are aware of the crucial importance of the existence of sports medical opinion. This is a fundamental part of sports medicine wich is often a preventive medicine par excellence.

The third common question. Needs offs in clubs / sporting lots

Answers to this question are similar, but not identical. The vast majority of both the physicians (85.4%) and the athletes and technicians deemed partially sufficient medical presence. Although somewhere similar. answers are somewhat surprising.

The fourth common question .Medical staff qualification

The answer to this question emerges on the team complex; doctors, nurses , psychologists, methodologists, physiotherapists, dieticians. This time the answers are almost identical, is very clear for all participants in sports phenomenon that only a super team determines the success of a competition and a good physical and mental state of the individuals

Different question with the common conclusion

For physicians and other health personnel question was: Are you satisfied with the current equipment?

For athletes and other staff in their entourage question was: What do you think is missing sports medicine?

Unfortunately, one of the great problems of sports medicine in Romania, at present, is purchasing the equipment and specialized equipment. Often equipment is insufficient (quantitative), obsolete (qualitative) and inconsistency with the latest news worldwide.

Conclusions

Following the responses to questionnaires sent were the following conclusions:

1. Sports medicine is a specialty in itself, with its own content;
2. Network of sports medicine (National Institute of Sports Medicine, Ambulatory specialized offices of Sports Medicine) must belong to the Ministry of Health;
3. National Institute of Sports Medicine activity should be supported financially in parameters of excellence;
4. The territorial network of sports medicine must be properly framed and fitted with proper equipment and know how to improve the medical act;
5. It is needed Emergence Regional Centres of Sports Medicine and the growing number of Specialty Ambulatory County of Sports Medicine ;
6. Funding to the State Budget;
7. Professional athletes and private clubs must pay the sports medicine services ;
8. Increased quality sports medicine is a goal that required the involvement in the medical act with the same determination of all age groups;
9. Network of sports medicine facilities is totally insufficient and needs to increase the quantity and quality of medical devices;
10. Increasing the number of specialists in sports medicine network;
11. Medical team from the National and Olympic teams and / or professional clubs must be a complex team (doctors, nurses, masseurs, physiotherapists, psychologists, dieticians, etc.);
12. Medical complex team staff should be involved in sport;
13. Medical visa ("able for training and competition") to be made compulsory in competitive sport;
14. Medical circuit for local athletes to make every 6 months;
15. Sports Medicine to be heavily involved, especially in primary selection;
16. Sports medicine does its duty abundantly present in Romania, both sporting performance assessments and direct beneficiaries are relevant in this respect.

Capitalization

Based on the results arising from the research, the existing data and the current situation in the European Union can devise a Decalogue of the Romanian sports medicine with major problems requiring urgent solution:

1 Upgrading number of human resources in the field (at least 20 residents of sports medicine / year of which 10 per post);

2. Reestablishment of Sports Medicine Committee of the Ministry of Health (for the reason that the Minister of Health need to be properly counseled by specialists with expertise that may explain the realities currently in Romania and the need to fully comply with the European and Romanian field - EU directives, documents UNESCO, the International Olympic Committee, the International Federation of Sports Medicine and Sports Law 69/2000 etc.);

3. Reestablishment of the Specialized Clinics in Romania abolished abusive, possibly with the appearance of 8 Regional Sports Medicine Centre in the 8 areas of economic and social development of the country;

4. Increase the number of specialists - Network staff (doctors, nurses, masseurs etc) is far below the minimum level required to perform any specific activities (medical examination, granting of visas, selection and orientation action sports medical treatments, qualified

medical assistance in training actions, workshops, competitions etc.);
5. Honoring the references issued by sports doctors to other specialists and recognize the right to prescribe free recipes / compensated for members of sports lots in case of emergency (1-3 days);
6. Increased endowment with specific equipment (including ambulances) to increase the quality of sports medicine, ie improving athletic performance and preservation of a health condition satisfactory to both the athletes and the rest of the population;
7. The possibility of having its own funds and use them anf to have an own national health program with sufficient amounts;
8. The ability to access research programs (domestic and international), this can be beneficial for the development of sports medicine to improve the quality of services provided and to introduce into the system the large sums of money that may reduce financial pressure from Ministry of health;
9.. Increasing the scale of the current medication with involvement of the specialized Ministry of Health and the National Agency for Medicines in compliance with very hard effect on the anti-doping policy.
10. Regulation of the conditions under which professionals from the National Institute of Sports Medicine and Sports Medicine network can work on lots of sports (delegation, detachment) and the conditions under which the sports bodies (Ministry of Youth and Sports, Olympic and Sports Committee Romanian, national sports federations, clubs etc.) can finance medical and sports activity;

Do not forget that in Romania there are hundreds of thousands of practitioners of sports performance and more than three million young people who practice physical education!

References

[1]. Comes, C.A., Spineni Popescu, S. (2005) - *Research methodology*, Cermaprint Publishing House, Bucharest

[2]. Greenfield 5, T. (1996) - *Research Methods*. Guidance for Postgraduates. London

[3]. Cochran, W.G. (1966) – *Sampling Techniques*. New York, Second Edition, John Wiley and sons

[4]. Comite International Olympique (2015) – *Manuel de Administration Sportive*, Edition Solidarite Olympique

[5]. Everitt, B.S., (1989) – *Statistical Methods for Medical Investigations*. New York, Oxford University Press

[6]. Moser, C.A. (1967) – *Metode de anchetă în investigaţia fenomenelor sociale.* Bucureşti, Editura Ştiinţifică

[7]. Radu, I. (1993) – *Metodologie psihologică şi analiza datelor*. Cluj, Sincron Publishing House

[8]. Helmer, O. (1997) – *Problems in Future Research*, Delphi and Causal Cross Impact Analysis, Futures, 9, 2, 17-31

[9]. Kirkwood, B.R. (1988) – *Medical Statistics*. Blackwell Scientific Publication

1. Rizzi, A. (1989) – *Analisi dei dati.* Roma, NIS

18

THE EFFECT OF AN INCREASED VOLUME OF TRAINING FOR SKI ORIENTEERING OVER THE SUMMER ORIENTEERING PERFORMANCE

Veronica MINOIU

University of Craiova, Faculty of Physical Education and Sports, Romania

Abstract: Objectiv: Elite orienteers must run or ski in different types of terrain at the highest tempo which will still allow them an error free course without lost time. Orienteering tasks are the same for both types of orienteering and up to a point, training for both can be beneficial for the overall performance. This paper examines the relationship between the performance of the athletes specialized in summer orienteering and the volume of training specific to ski orienteering.

Methodes: The analysis has been done on statistical data collected from 56 athletes members of the Romamian National Team in the 2005-2006 competition seazon (data collected for physical fitness optimization) and the specifics of the competition preparedness in the 2015-2016 season from 8 athletes, members of national teams. In the latter time frame,
I have analyzed the effects of an increased volume of training specific to ski orienteering.

Results: The increased volume of training for ski orienteering and simultaneously decreasing the training volume specific for summer orienteering resulted in a significant decrease in performance during the first part of the 2016 competition season due to a reduction in average speed.

Conclusions: This study proves that using training methods specific for ski orienteering has a positive effect in performance for the summer orienteering competitions IF the percentage of these methods does not surpass a certain threshold. Going over this threshold will significantly decrease the speed during the early summer orienteering seson.

Key words: Performance, ski orienteering, volume methods; regression;

Introduction

Ski orienteering, is an endurance sport with International events that include World Championships, European Championships and World Cup events. Ski Orienteering will be introduced for the first time at 2019 Winter Universiade and it has good chances to be introduced at the Winter Olympics as well. This sport combines cross country skiing abilities with orienteering skills. The key to success is the ability to read the map and chose without hesitation the best routes between controls while skiing at a high rate of speed. The classic ski orienteering formula is:

Intelligence x Physical Strength x Skiing Ability

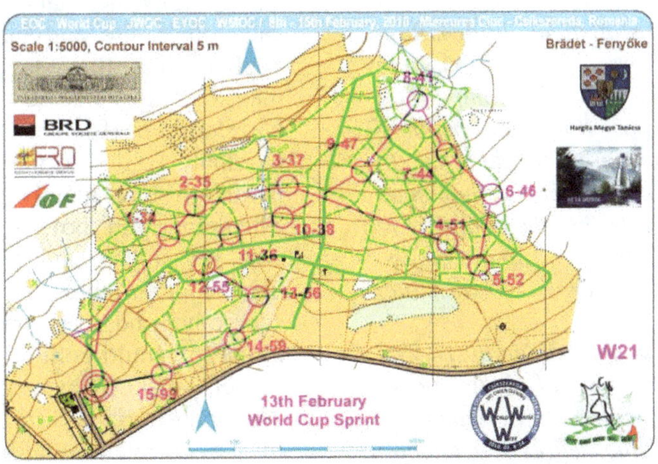

Oja P, Laukkanen RM, Kukkonen-Harjula TK, Vuori IM, Pasanen ME, Niittymäki SP, Solakivi T. [1] in the study „Training effects of cross-country skiing and running on maximal aerobic cycle performance and on blood lipids" suggested that training by cross-country skiing and running of the same duration and intensity at each session for 9-10 weeks improved equally the cardiorespiratory fitness of untrained middle-aged men.

Foster C1, Hector LL, Welsh R, Schrager M, Green MA, Snyder AC [2] in "Effects of specific versus cross-training on running performance" suggest that despite the principle of specificity of training, athletes may improve performance in one mode of exercise by training using another mode. To test this hypothesis they studied 30 well-trained individuals (10 men, 20 women) in a randomized longitudinal trail. Subjects were evaluated before and after 8 weeks of enhanced training (+10%/week), accomplished by adding either running or swimming to baseline running, versus continued baseline running.The authors concluded that "The data suggest that muscularly non-similar XT may contribute to improved running performance but not to the same degree as increased specific training."

In medium and long distance orienteering events, the speed of elite athletes depends on the fitness level of each competitor, but more importantly on the biomechanics of running. By increasing the volume of training methods specific for cross-country skiing and ski orienteering, and dramatically reducing the volume of running in winter, the running biomechanics and the stride frequency are being changed.

The first part of the study will analyze the relevance that the training methods specific to cross-country skiing - parts of the training system - have on the performance level in the running competitions. The analysis was conducted based on statistical information relative to the members of the Romanian national team, in the 2005-2006 competition season. Every sport has its own training workout specifics. Certainly, in addition to training, there are other factors that may impact performance levels (i.e. the competitive experience, the race strategy, innate skills, psychological strength, overall moral state, health, gear, etc.).

For the first part, a graphical analysis was done for the combination of independent variables, coupled with the dependent variables, followed by the regression method which consisted of the construction of linear models for regression for each of the two dependent variables (race speed), in combination with the independent variables and a free term. The analysis will consider the degree of relevance the training methods specific to cross-country skiing - parts of the training system - have on the performance levels in running events.

For the second part, we will analyze athletes' performance after increasing the training methods specific to cross-country skiing above a certain level, volume increased due to athletes' participation at the world ski orienteering championships and cups.

All models have been tested in terms of validity with analysis of variance (ANOVA) method, using the F-test, and it's been confirmed that we are dealing with valid models.

Methods and data source

The analyzed data is based on the author's Minoiu V. [3] and coach's measurements performed on 2005-2006 national teams, athletes of different ages and genders (42 men, 37 women) and eight members of the national teams in 2015-2016 competition season. As a result, the database consists of 40-record data base. The independent variables for which information was collected are as follows: gender, distance (in kilometers), maximum heart rate, average heart rate, and 25 training methods.

From the quantitative methodology point of view, this study will begin with the presentation of the correlation matrix between the analyzed variables. The next section will be dedicated to building regression models to illustrate the relevance (or irrelevance) that different training methods had on the performance levels obtained.

To test how the analyzed variables interact to each other, the correlation method has been applied in a first stage. Thus a correlation matrix was created. The simple linear correlation coefficient of Pearson (r) was used for analysis, due to the fact that the variables involved were mainly quantitative variables. The default threshold of statistical significance was set at 1% and 5%. We find that the dependent variables are highly correlated with each other and, as a consequence, to avoid the effect of multi-colinearity in the regression models that we are going to build, each dependent variable will be analyzed separately. In the correlation table, we will retain the attention in this analysis only through the way the performance variables (speed test 1 and test 2) are correlated (or not) with training methods. At the analysis stage using the regression method, we will include in our models all methods of training.

2.1. Regression Method

This step consists of constructing linear regression methods for each of the two dependent variables (race speed) in combination with groups of independent variables and a free term. The models are expressed by this formula:

$$Y = \beta_0 + \beta_1 X_1 + \beta_2 X_2 + \beta_3 X_3 + \beta_4 X_4 ... + \beta_n X_n + \varepsilon$$

Where

Y denotes the four independent variables

β_0 *is the free term*

X_1 *is the first independent variable*

X_2 *is the second independent variable*

X_3 *is the third independent variable*

X_4 *is the fourth independent variable*

X_n *is the N-th independent variable*

n and ε *are rezidual variables*

Due to the excessive number of independent variables in relation to the number of cases examined (40), the independent variables have been separated in four groups. Each group was placed in the analysis in an area labeled „iteration". Working procedure involved the initial application of the regression method for all the vriables in that group iteration. After analyzing the quality of the resulted regression models, the independent variables that didn't have a significant influence statistically have been removed (basically were removed from the model those variables that showed statistically insignificant regression coefficients). The significance threshold has been set at 5% and in very few cases variables up to 8% significance have been kept.

2.2 Applying the regression method for the „Total Run Time" dependent variable

Models in this iteration that include cross-country skiing as a method of training:

- Orienteering events (training, or sanctioned events) (Km)
- Stretching and aerobic (hours)
- Essential running drills (Km)
- Combined jumps/obstacle jumping (Km)
- Strength exercises (hours)
- Running in snow, sand/rough terrain, swampy/grassy terrain (Km)
- Cross-country skiing (Km)

Table 1. Correlations between the variables of performance and the means of training.

	X1	X2	X3	X4	X5	X6	X7	X8	X9	X10	X11
X1	1	0,86**	0,61**	0,67**	0,67**	0,68**	0,84**	0,56**	0,62**	-0,6**	-0,69**
X2	0,86**	1	0,61**	0,67**	0,67**	0,68**	0,84**	0,56**	0,62**	-0,6**	-0,69**
X3	0,67**	0,82**	1	0,65**	0,7**	0,87**	0,76**	0,48**	0,6**	-0,69**	-0,61**
X4	0,61**	0,71**	0,7**	1	0,71**	0,61**	0,76**	0,44*	0,63**	-0,81**	-0,77**
X5	0,67**	0,83**	0,7**	0,74**	1	0,72**	0,82**	0,47**	0,8**	-0,69**	-0,72**
X6	0,67**	0,87**	0,71**	0,74**	0,7**	1	0,87**	0,37*	0,85**	-0,77**	-0,79**
X7	0,68**	0,86**	0,61**	0,72**	0,7**	0,61**	1	0,6**	0,71**	-0,77**	-0,73**
X8	0,84**	0,97**	0,76**	0,82**	0,87**	0,8**	0,82**	1	0,86**	-0,83**	-0,87**

X9	0,56**	0,54**	0,44*	0,47**	0,37*	0,6**	0,5**	0,45*	1	-0,46*	-0,42
X10	-0,6**	-0,82**	-0,81**	-0,69**	-0,77**	-0,77**	-0,83**	-0,46*	-0,85**	1	0,91**
X11	-0,69**	-0,84**	-0,77**	-0,72**	-0,79**	-0,73**	-0,87**	-0,42	-0,83**	0,95**	1

- ** Correlation is significant at the 0.01 level (2-tailed).
- * Correlation is significant at the 0.05 level (2-tailed).

A. Applying the regression method for the 'total trial speed' dependent variable Regression

Tabel 2. Model Summary

Model	R	R Square	Adjusted R Square	Std. Error of the Estimate
1	,824 [a]	,679	,547	41,7954

a. Predictors: (Constant), Cross-country Skiing (Km), Combined jumps/obstacle jumping (Km), Stretching and aerobic (hours), Essential running drills (Km), Orienteering events (training, or sanctioned events) (Km) Strength exercises (hours), Running in snow, sand/rough terrain, swampy/grassy terrain (Km))

Table 3. Model 1: Speed for Test Run 1 function of Orienteering races, stretching and aerobic, Essential running drills, Multijumps, Strength exercises, Multijumps and cross-country skiing. Regression coefficients: values, standard errors, T test, significance thresholds.

Model		Unstandardized Coefficients B	Unstandardized Coefficients Std. Error	Standardized Coefficients Beta	t	Sig.
1	(Constant)	606,506	53,034		11,437	,000
	Orienteering events, training or Sanctioned events (km)	-6,63E-02	-,116	-,181	-,570	,576
	Stretching and aerobic (km)	-,481	,620	-,184	-,776	-,448
	Essential running drills(km)	-,380	1,185	,083	,321	,752
	Combinet jumps obstacle, jumping(km)	-,791	1,353	-,204	-,584	,567
	Strenght exercices (hours)	1,536E-03	1,607	,000	,001	,999
	Running in snow,sand/rough terrain, swampy/grassy	-,168	,213	-,384	-,790	,441
	Cross –country skiing(km)	1,46E-02	,069	-,036	-,211	,835

a.Dependent Variable:Run 1 speed(sloped terrain)(sec/min)

Table 4. Model 1: Speed for Test Run 2 function of Orienteering races, stretching and aerobic, Essential running drills, Multijumps, Strength exercises, Multijumps and cross-country skiing. Regression coefficients: values, standard errors, T test, significance thresholds.

Model		Unstandardized Coefficients		Standardized Coefficients	t	Sig.
		B	Std. Error	Beta		
1	(Constant)	614,752	38,599		15,919	,000
	Orienteering events, training or Sanctioned events (km)	-5,42E-02	,061	-,156	-,892	,390
	Stretching and aerobic (km)	-,499	,393	-,174	-1,268	,225
	Essential running drills(km)	-,221	,602	,048	-,367	,720
	Combinet jumps obstacle, jumping(km)	-,633	,723	-,167	-,875	,395
	Strenght exercices (hours)	-,196	,973	-,057	,-202	,844
	Running in snow,sand/rough terrain, swampy/grassy	-,252	,130	-,532	-1,936	,077
	Cross –country skiing(km)	3,992E-02	,034	,114	1,171	,264

a.Dependent Variable:Run 2 speed(sloped terrain)(sec/min)

Table 5. Volume of training methods employed in 2005-2006

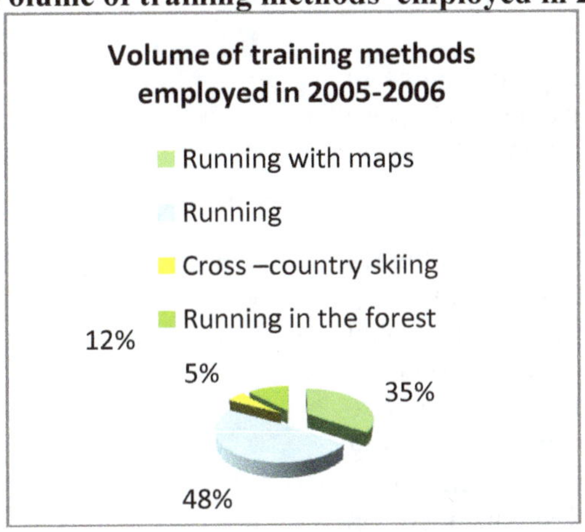

Table 6. Volume of training methods employed in 2015-2016

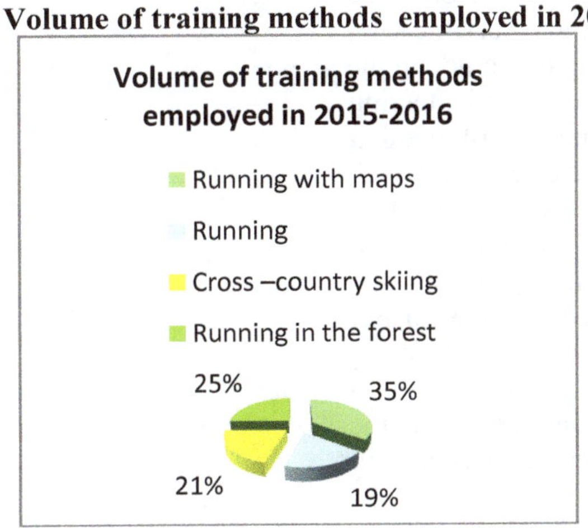

Testing of Statistical Hypothesis

In this section we will analyze how the average performance of the athletes with good results in summer orienteering compares with average performance of the athletes that increased the volume of training by employing methods specific to ski orienteering. The data was collected during the Trial events organized by the Romanian Orienteering Federation. On the next iteration, in case the answer to the first iteration is affirmative, we will be testing if the athletes with better results employed different training methods than others, which may have caused them to have better results.

For this, we have formulated two working assumptions ((Details on how to build, use and interpret tests of hypotheses can be found in Andrei: 2002):

H_0: $\beta = m$

H_1: $\beta \neq m$

Where

β is the average performance of the athletes with the best results

m is the average value of the performance in the comparison group (This is the group of National Team members, which participated in International Ski-Orienteering)

Conclusion. This paper shows that athletes who used in moderation training methods specific to ski orienteering achieved significantly better performance in running events when compared with athletes who have increased drastically the volume of training specific to cross-country skiing. In other words, increasing the training distance on cross-country skis decreases the performance during the nest season's summer orienteering events. It would be interesting to include in the data set the results of the ski orienteering athletes who decrease the amount of running during the summer months and replace it with roller ski training. We consider this analysis very useful for the athletes who are tempted to increase the amount of time spent on skis during the winter with the desire to get better classifications in the National ski-orienteering events, but they have to be aware there is a definite risk that the performance in the upcoming summer orienteering season will decrease.

References

[1] Oja P, Laukkanen RM, Kukkonen-Harjula TK, Vuori IM, Pasanen ME, Niittymäki SP, Solakivi T. *Training effects of cross-country skiing and running on maximal aerobic cycle performance and on blood lipids*, Eur J Appl Physiol Occup Physiol. 1991;62(6):400-4.

[2] Foster C1, Hector LL, Welsh R, Schrager M, Green MA, Snyder AC., Effects of specific versus cross-training on running performance, Eur J Appl Psihol Occup Physiol. 1995; 70(4): 367-72

[3] Minoiu, V., *Optimizarea pregătirii fizice în disciplina orientare sportivă prin raționalizarea și standardizarea mijloacelor*, PhD Thesis, pp 150-183, 2011

19

SELF-ESTEEM IN DECISION MAKING AND DECISION MAKING STYLES OF VOLLEYBALL PLAYERS IN TERMS OF SOME VARIABLES

Elif USTUN, Veysel TEMEL, Sefa Sahan BIROL

Karamanoglu Mehmetbey University, Physical Education and Sports High School, Karaman.

ABSTRACT

Purpose: This research was done with the aim of revealing whether decision making styles differ in terms of different variables or not. Descriptive method, one of the quantitative research methods, was adopted as the search model.

Materials and Methods: Research group consisted of 50 male and 59 female players who play at youth volleyball league in Konya city center. In this study, "Melbourne Decision Making Questionnaire" developed by Mann, Burnett, Radford and Ford (1997) and the adaptation work of this scale to Turkish was conducted by Deniz (2004) and "Personal Information Form" which was developed by researcher in order to determine personal characteristic of athletes, were used as data collection tool. The unique Kolmogorov Smirnov Test was used in order to determine whether measures are suitable for normal dispersion or not. Kruskal Wallis-H test and Mann Whitney-U test were used on analyzing and evaluating the data, and meaningfulness was obtained as $P<0,05$. SPSS (Statistical package for social sciences) package programme was used on evaluating data and finding calculated values.

Findings: It can be said that the self-esteem in decision making making point average of the athletes participated in the research with (Mean=9,0000) and careful decision-making style point average with (Mean=8,4587), sub dimension of decision making styles, were high, but avoidant decision-making style point average with (Mean=4,8716), suspensive decision-making style point average with (Mean.=4,5505) and panic decision-making style point average with (Mean.=4,3670) were low.

Results: Meaningful difference was found in terms of personal characteristic on self-esteem in decision making, careful decision-making style, suspensive decision-making style, panic decision-making style and avoidant decision-making style of participants' team which they play at, gender, education and sport beginning age variables whereas meaningful difference was not found on their parents education, parents occupation, family income and place in which they spend most of their life variables.

Key Words: Decision Making, Self-Esteem, Decision Making Styles, Athletes, Volleyball

INTRODUCTION

Decision-making could be explained as variability of information/interest or both [18]. Decision-making is not only a period to choose and aim the best alternatives for personal value and life style, but also to specify alternatives having regard to various incidents and activities [11].

Individuals should make decisions in every stage of their lifes, both in their professional and their private life. Problems could be very simple and also very complex which are triggered by many factors. Decision-making and problem-solving terms are usually confused with each other. In narrow sense, decision making is a process in which individual choose one thing from many options. On the other hand, problem could be defined as deviation from a standart or aimed performance. Problem-solving; is a detection process in which individual choose essential action, proper reaction for smoothing the problem. Problem-solving includes decision-making; however all decisions does not include problems. On the other hand; almost every decision; is tend to solve a problem or to avoid from problem [16].

Researchers have been studying on relation between sportive success and athlete's decision-making ability and have tried to determine decision-making's effectiveness on sportive performance. It is known that mental factors whose absolute phsyiologic, psychologic and technic-tactic studies are not sufficient, also are effective on the occurence of sportive success. While determining sportive success, the most important ability is the decision-making ability. Decision of the athlete will affect his team's success positively or negatively. Hence, sport researchers and sport trainers makes researchs on development of athletes' decision-making ability. These studies, sportive success is considerably important and necessarily. As a result of application of these studies on workouts, it turns out that athletes' creativities and decision-making abilities improve and become more successful [5].

Decision-making is essential for whole lifespan and it takes place in all incidents from simple to complex. Individual's decisions could lead to his life better or worse way. All these incidents are also valid for athletes. On field, in box-ring or in gym, athlete should adjust his position and move regarding to his team-mates' and opponents' positions and moves. Nowadays, there are so many influencing factors for sportive efficiency level. These are environmental and internal factors [8]. These large number of factors' importance could diversify with respect to conditions and could not form success or failure by itself. For instance, being high-condition is not enough for being successful. It is though that an athlete making sensible and fast decision is an advantage on a sport branch in which people have complex attitudes [6]. Sanchez and ark.. state that plays in almost any sport branch has become faster and is based on more technic and tactic [17]. During competition, athletes should make new decision due to changing dynamics and unexpectable changing on game system, especially on matchs with ball [12].

Decision-making process depends on individual. One's attitude for his reaction in uncertain situation is his strategy for decision-making [10]. Decision-making is composed of different periods. Before decision-making process, individual evaluates the result which could arise from making decision. In decision-making process, individual evaluates his options and eliminates the options but the ideal one. After decision-making process, individual assesses revealed result and interprets [20].

Although, there is not a specific decision-making type in sport, it is considered that sport holds some characterist features. Being natural is the key feature of decision-making in sport. With lots of duties in game, player has multiple potential options. For instance, if he wants to use his decision, responsibility and creativity freely, he can not apply them as it is written on paper, on the contrary, he has to decide during the game in the happenstances. Secondly, most decisions made in sport have external dynamics. In other words, sport has external dynamics changing with time. Due to this dynamic structure, sport requires athlete's ability to create knowledge.

Athlete's dynamic situation is complicated during competition. Thirdly, decisions making during sportive events, are made overt behaviours and under highly time pressure. This pressure is especially about dynamic structure of decision-making. Most moves of athletes in the game are taken evidently [13]. Seiller [19] suggests that decision-making varies in time-limitations [19]. While sports such as; golf, sailing do not have time-limitation, ball games, team games have time limitations that make difficult to decide [21]. Aune and ark. (2008) states that volleyball is one of the main factors that has impose on success by means of making decision fast and reacting fast and accurate to stimulant (Günay, Çelik, Aksu and Çoksevim, 2011).[1],[7].

METHOD

This section is about research model, research staff, data acquisition, data acquisition tools and operations during data analysis.

Research Model

Research, is a descriptional study. Descriptive statistic is a statistic operation which enables to collect, describe and present numerical value related to a factor (Büyüköztürk, 2010).

Research Staff

Research staff consists of total 109 athlete of which 50 men and 59 women players who play in youth volleyball league in Konya.

Data Acquisition

First of all, datas about research are given systematicly after scanning literature. Thus, a theoretical frame of the subject is formed.

Data Acquisition Tool

The necessary data acquisition tool for reach the determinated aims could be seen below:

Personal Information Form

In order to create independant variances of examination on research and to acquire data about personal characterists of 109 players who play in youth volleyball league in Konya.

Melbourne Decision-Making Questionary (MDMQ)

Melbourne Decision-Making Questionary is developped by Mann and ark. (1998), Deniz(2004) adapts the questionary in turkish and exercises reliability study [15],[4]. Melbourne Decision-Making Questionary has two sections:

Section I: It aims to determine self-reliance in decision-making. It is composed of 6 articles and three articles of grade straightly and the other three articles of it grade reversely. Grading measures as 2 points for "True" answer to articles, 1 points for "Sometimes True" answers, 0 points for "Not True" answers. Maximum point for questionary is 12 point. Maximum points stand for maximum self-reliance in decision-making.

Section II: It is composed of 22 articles and measures decision-making styles. It has 4 subfactors [4].

1. Carefully Decision-Making Style: Individual searches for essential data prudentially and evaluates alteranatives carefully before decision-making and then he chooses. This factor is explained in 6 articles [2, 4, 6, 8, 12, 16].

2.Avoidant Decision-Making Style: Individual avoids decision-making, has tendency to give decision-making to someone and thus attempts to get rid of responsibility of decision-making. This factor is explained in 6 articles [3, 9, 11, 14, 17,19].

3.Postponer Decision-Making Style: Individual always postpones, procrastinates and suspends without any reason. This factor is explained in 5 articles[5, 7, 10, 18, 21].

4.Panic Decision-Making Style: Individual is willing to reach fast solutions with hasty actions as a consequence of feeling under pressure when he has to decide. This factor is explained in 5 article [1, 13, 15, 20, 22].

Melbourne Decision-Making Questionary's Reliability

I – II MDMQ 's reliability is calculated with repetition of the test and with internal consistency. With this aim, 56 student of computer systems' and automative teaching in 2002-2003 educational year, in Technical Education Faculty, S. University were tested. With the repetition method of test, reliability parameter obtained from subscale is self-reliance in decision-making r=.85, in carefully decision-making method r=.83, in avoidant decision-making style r=.87, postponing decision-making style r=.68, in panic decision-making style r=.84. When calculating, internal consistency, article analysis is made. Analysis result turns out that 26 articles' correlations out of total 28 articles are over .33 ; other 2 articles' correlations are .26 and .27. This demonstrates that result is statistically sufficient level. Conducted on 154 university student, MDMQ III's internal consistencies are for self-reliance in decision-making Cronbach Alpha=.72, for carefully decision-making in subdimension of decision-making style Cronbach Alpha=. 80, for avoidant decision-making style Cronbach Alpha= .78, for postponing decision-making Cronbach Alpha= .65, for panic decision-making Cronbach Alpha=.71 [4].

Melbourne Decision-Making Questionary's Validity Studies

Content validity and similar scales validity is used for Melbourne Decision Making Questionary's Validity Studies. Content validity occurs consulting an expert's opinion. After examining MDMQ I-II, people who works in this field as experts state that contents and quality of scale articles would calculate related subscales. Similar scales' validity is created with Decision Strategies Scale developped by [22]. MDMQ I-II and Decision Strategies Scale are tested at the same time on students. It is fixed that correlation parameters between MDMQ I-II's subscales and Decision Strategies Scale's subscales varies from r=.15 to r=71 and MDMQ I-II and Decision Strategies Scale have significant relations between 0.01 and 0.05 level. It illustrates that MDMQ I-II is highly valid with this result [4].

Evaluation of Melbourne Decision Making Scale

EMDMS I: It is a scale that aims to determine self-esteem (self-confidence) when making a decision. It is formed by six (6) item and it is scored as the opposite of three items (2, 4, 6). The scoring is done in this way; each "correct answer" that is given for items are 2 points, the answer of "sometimes correct" is 1 point, the answer of "not correct" is 0 points. 12 points are the maximum that an be taken from the scale. High scores are an indicative of high self-esteem in making decisions [4].

EMDMS II: It is formed by twenty-two (22) items. The scale measures the decision-making styles.The questions covering subscales are;

1. Attentive: 2, 4, 6, 8, 12, 16 items
2. Avoidant: 3, 9, 11, 14, 17, 19 items
3. Post poner: 5, 7, 10, 18, 21 items
4. Panic: 1, 13, 15, 20, 22 items

In scoring EMDMS I; the items are evaluted with score range like, attentive (0-12), avoidant (0-12), post poner (0 - 10) and panic (0-10). This scale are answered like EMDMS II. The height of the points indicate that the use of the relevant decision-making style [4].

During scale, the coefficient of self-esteem, decision-making, internal consistency reliability of physical education and sports teachers was found 0.74,8 and the coefficient of internal consistency of decision-making style's reliability was found 0.76.

Data Analysis

While the solution and interpretation of data, with the usage of Kruskal-Wallis H and Mann-Whitney U test, significance was estimated as P<0,05. In the evaluation and the calculation of the data, SPSS 21 (Statistical package for social sciences) packaged program was used.

FINDINGS

Table 1. Sub-dimensions of participants in general problem solving and the results of the total score's average and standard deviation values

	n	Mean	Ss	Min	Max	The lowest and the highest score that can be obtained from the scale
Self-Esteem on Decision Making	109	9,0000	3,17105	,00	12,00	0-12
Careful Decision Making	109	8,4587	3,20165	,00	12,00	0-12
Avoidant Decision Making	109	4,8716	3,05232	,00	12,00	0-12
Post-poner Decision Making	109	4,5505	1,96961	1,00	10,00	0-10
Panic Decision Making	109	4,3670	2,25528	,00	10,00	0-10

In Table 1, it is indicated that, the point average of decision making (Mean. = 9,0000), the point average of careful decision making which is the sub-dimension of decision making skills (Mean. = 8,4587) are in high level, however, the point average of avoidant decision making (Mean. = 4,8716), the point average of post-poner decision making (Mean. = 4,5505), the point average of panic decision making (Mean. = 4,3670) are in low level.

Table 2. The total and sub-dimension results of Mann Whitney U test according to the participants genders related to problem-solving

		N	Mean Rank	Rank Sum	U	Z	P
Self-Esteem on Decision Making	Female	50	74,86	3743,00	482,000	-6,206	,000*
	Male	59	38,17	2252,00			
Careful Decision Making	Female	50	72,19	3609,50	615,500	-5,282	,000*
	Male	59	40,43	2385,50			
Avoidant Decision Making	Female	50	49,24	2462,00	1187,000	-1,779	,075
	Male	59	59,88	3533,00			
Post-poner Decision Making	Female	50	46,01	2300,50	1025,500	-2,790	,005*
	Male	59	62,62	3694,50			
Panic Decision Making	Female	50	44,35	2217,50	942,500	-3,317	,001*
	Male	59	64,03	3777,50			

*p<0,05

In Table 2, it was examined the total and sub-dimension results with Mann Whitney U test according to the participants genders related to decision making. In the study results, there wasn't any sub-dimension substantive for avoidant decision making (U: 482,000 P<0,05), however, in the dimensions of Self-Esteem on Decision Making (U: 482,000 P<0,05), Careful decision making (615,500 P<0,05), Post-poner decision making (1025,500 P<0,05), and Panic decision making (U: 942,500 P<0,05), the differences was founded substantive.

Table 3. The result of Kruskal-Wallis test related to the participant's education factor according to problem-solving total and sub-dimensions.

		N	Mean Rank	Sd	X^2	P	Meaningful Differences
Self-Esteem on Decision Making	High school	48	39,04	2	38,719	,000*	1-3
	University	11	34,36				
	Other	50	74,86				
Careful Decision Making	High school	48	39,88	2	27,978	,000*	1-3
	University	11	42,86				
	Other	50	72,19				
Avoidant Decision Making	High school	48	58,20	2	3,919	,141	-------
	University	11	67,23				
	Other	50	49,24				
Post-poner Decision Making	High school	48	61,32	2	8,232	,016*	2-3
	University	11	68,27				
	Other	50	46,01				
Panic Decision Making	High school	48	63,01	2	11,283	,004*	-------
	University	11	68,45				
	0ther	**50**	**44,35**				

*p<0,05

In Table 3, it was examined the total and sub-dimension results with Mann Whitney U test according to the participants education factor related to decision making. In the study results, there wasn't any sub-dimension substantive for avoidant decision making, however, in the dimensions of Self-Esteem on Decision Making (X^2 =38,719 P<0.05), Careful decision making (X^2 =27,978 P<0.05), Post-poner decision making (X^2 =8,232 P<0.05), and Panic decision making (X^2 =11,283 P<0.05), the differences was founded substantive.

Table 4. According to the team variables of participants , Kruskall-Wallis test results for the total and sub-dimensions in problem solving

		N	Mean Rank	Sd	X^2	P	Meaningful Differences
Self-Esteem on Decision Making	Güneşspor (female)	13	71,08	6	40,355	,000*	**1-6**
	Konya fener (female)	14	63,18				
	Selçuklu belediye (female)	14	65,89				
	Gençlik spor (female)	13	38,12				
	Konya spor (male)	12	31,83				
	Konya büyükşehir (male)	14	32,75				
	Gençlik spor (male)	14	28,43				
Careful Decision Making	Güneş spor (female)	13	70,23	6	26,523	,000*	**1-6**
	Konya fener (female)	14	54,11				
	Selçuklu belediye (female)	14	62,54				
	Gençlik spor (female)	13	45,15				
	Konya spor (male)	12	35,71				
	Konya büyükşehir (male)	14	36,57				

	Gençlik spor (male)	14	27,96				
Avoidant Decision Making	Güneş spor (female)	13	37,38	6	8,065	,233	-----
	Konya fener (female)	14	52,54				
	Selçuklu belediye (female)	14	42,43				
	Gençlik spor (female)	13	47,62				
	Konya spor (male)	12	62,04				
	Konya büyükşehir (male)	14	39,68				
	Gençlik spor (male)	14	52,18				
Post-poner Decision Making	Güneş spor (female)	13	43,31	6	8,841	,183	-----
	Konya fener (female)	14	35,18				
	Selçuklu belediye (female)	14	41,75				
	Gençlik spor (female)	13	48,81				
	Konya spor (male)	12	55,88				
	Konya büyükşehir (male)	14	47,50				
	Gençlik spor (male)	14	61,07				
Panic Decision Making	Güneş spor (female)	13	36,88	6	9,178	,164	-----
	Konya fener (female)	14	42,79				
	Selçuklu belediye (female)	14	39,14				
	Gençlik spor (female)	13	50,92				
	Konya spor (male)	12	54,54				
	Konya büyükşehir (male)	14	46,89				
	Gençlik spor (male)	**14**	**61,82**				

*p<0,05

In Table 4, it was examined the total and sub-dimension results with Mann Whitney U test according to the participant's team factor related to decision making. In the study results, there wasn't any sub-dimension substantive for avoidant decision making, post-poner decison making, panic decision making, however, in the dimensions of self-esteem on decision making (X^2 =40,355 P<0.05) and careful decision making (X^2 =26,523 P<0.05), the differences was founded substantive.

Table 5. The result of Kruskal-Wallis test related to the participant's starting sports factor according to problem-solving total and sub-dimensions.

		N	Mean Rank	Sd	X^2	P	Meaningful Differences
Self-Esteem on Decision Making	5-7	11	82,95	2	14,588	,001*	**1-3**
	8-10	31	61,53				**1-2**
	11-13	67	47,39				
Careful Decision Making	5-7	11	76,45	2	7,977	,019*	**1-3**
	8-10	31	59,52				
	11-13	67	49,39				
Avoidant Decision Making	5-7	11	29,68	2	10,071		**3-1**
	8-10	31	51,35			,007*	**3-2**
	11-13	67	60,84				
Post-poner Decision Making	5-7	11	25,86	2	13,609	,001*	**3-1**
	8-10	31	50,60				
	11-13	67	61,82				
Panic Decision Making	5-7	11	28,64	2	14,959	,001*	**3-1**
	8-10	31	46,71				
	11-13	**67**	**63,16**				

*p<0,05

In Table 4, it was examined the total and sub-dimension results with Mann Whitney U test according to the participant's starting sports factor for volleyball playes related to decision making. In the study results, in the dimensions of Self-Esteem Decision (X^2 =14,588 P<0.05), careful decision making (X^2 =7,977 P<0.05), avoidant decision making (X^2 =10,071 P<0.05), post-poner decison making (X^2 =13,609 P<0.05), panic decision making (X^2 =14,959 P<0.05) the differences was founded substantive.

THE DISCUSSION OF RESULTS

It was indicated that mean total score of decision making of volleyball players and the point average of careful decision making from decision making skills is in high level, however, it can be stated that average scores of avoidant decision making, post-poner decision-making and panic decision scores are low.

According to gender factor, self-esteem decision making, careful decision making, post-poner decision making, panic decision making in total score has been identified as significant in all sub-dimensions. These results are in line with the work that has done by [9].

Education variables; self-esteem decision making and careful decision making in the lower size, the proportion of those with another educational option, educational level seems to be higher than that of high school. In the sub-dimension of post-poner decision making and panic decision making, according toeducational level, the proportion of the university, seems to be higher than those with other educational options. We can state that education level may influence the size of decision making. The finding from the study of Çetin (2009) are showing similarities with our study results.[3].

According to the factor of the team they play volleyball; with related to the sub-dimensions of self-esteem on decision making and careful decision making; the ratio of volleyball player in Gençlik Spor Erkek team is higher than the volleyball players who play in Güneş Spor Kız team. When considering other findings on these results, when decision making, acting together with the team for men is considered efective.

According to the starting age of volleyball factors, it is shown that in the dimension of self-esteem decision making, the rate for starting sport between the ages 5-7 is higher that the age group of 11-13 and the rate for starting sport between ages 5-7, is higher than the age group of 8-10. In this case, we can interpret that self-esteem prevents adolescents from using the opportunities that were given to them. In the sub-dimension of careful decision making, the rate for the age group of 5-7 is higher that the group of 11-13; and in the sub-dimension of avoidant decision-making, the rate for starting sport between the ages 11-13 is higher that the age group of 5-7 and the rate for starting sport between ages 11-13, is higher than the age group of 8-10. and in the sub-dimensions of postponed decision making and panic decision making, the age of starting sports for the age group 5-7 is higher. Leaving the decision making to others, delaying and feeling under pressure in the event of deciding leads to be in thoughtless attitudes and behave in a hurry tend to get solutions, and it is believed that the age period of starting sports may have an effect on behavior model.

REFERANCE

[1.] Aune T.K., Ingvaldsen R.P., Ettema G.J. (2008) Effect of Physical Fatigue on Motor Control at Different Skill Levels. Percept Mot Skills;106:371-386.

[2]. Büyüköztürk, Ş. (2010) Sosyal bilimler için veri analizi el kitabı. Ankara: Pegem Akademi Yayınları.

[3]. Çetin, M. Ç. (2009) Beden eğitimi ve spor yüksekokulu öğrencilerinin karar verme stilleri sosyal beceri düzeyleri ve stresle başa çıkma biçimlerinin bazı değişkenler açısından karşılaştırmalı olarak incelenmesi. Yayınlanmamış doktora tezi, Gazi Üniversitesi, Ankara.

[4]. Deniz, M. E. (2004) Üniversite öğrencilerinin karar vermede öz saygı, karar verme stilleri ve problem çözme yöntemleri arasındaki ilişkinin incelenmesi üzerine bir araştırma. *Eğitim Araştırmaları Dergisi, 4*(15), 25- 35.

[5]. Egesoy H., Eniseler N., Çamlıyer H., Çamlıyer H. (1999) Elit Ve Elit Olmayan Futbol Oyuncularının Karar Verme Performanslarının Karar Verme Hızı Ve Verilen Kararın Doğruluğu

Açısından Karşılaştırılması, BESBD, 3(2), 24.

[6]. Gülşen, D. (2008) Farklı Lig Düzeyinde Oynayan Futbolcuların Oynadıkları Mevkilere, Öğrenim Durumu Ve Spor Yaşlarına Göre Problem Çözme Becerilerinin İncelenmesi, Çukurova Üniversitesi Sağlık Bilimleri Enstitüsü, Yayınlanmamış Yüksek Lisans Tezi, Adana

[7]. Günay E., Çelik A., Aksu F., Çoksevim B. (2011) 14 - 16 Yaş Voleybol ve Tenis Oyuncularının Görsel ve İşitsel Reaksiyon Zamanlarının İncelenmesi, DEÜ Tıp Fakültesi Dergisi, 25(2), 64.

[8]. Gürçay S. S. (1998) Aile ve Arkadaşlardan Algılanan Sosyal Destek, Bireyler Arası İlişkilerde Yeterlik ve Karar Verme ilişkileri. Psikolojik Danışma ve Rehberlik Dergisi, 2 (9), 7-16.

[9]. Gürçay S. S. (2001) Ergenlerde Karar Verme Davranışlarının Öz Saygı Ve Problem Çözme Becerileri Algısı İle İlişkisi, Çukurova Üniversitesi Sosyal Bilimler Enstitüsü Dergisi, 8(8), 116.

[10]. Ersever, H.Ö. (1996) Karar Verme Becerileri Kazandırma Programının ve Etkileşim Grubu Deneyiminin Üniversite Öğrencilerinin Karar Verme Stilleri Üzerindeki Etkileri, Yayımlanmamış Doktora Tezi, Ankara Üniversitesi Sosyal Bilimler Enstitüsü, Ankara

[11]. Harris, R. (1998) Introduction to decision making. Vanguard University Of Southern California, California, USA.

[12]. Kelecek S., Altıntaş A., Aşçı F.H. (2013) Sporcuların Karar Verme Stillerinin Belirlenmesi,
CBÜ Beden Eğitimi ve Spor Bilimleri Dergisi, 8(1), 22.

[13]. Johnson, JG. (2006) Cognitive modeling of decision making in sports. Psychology of sport and exercise,; 7: 631–52.

[14]. Mann L, Burnett P, Radford M, Ford S (1997) The Melbourne Decision Making Questionnaire: An instrument for measuring patterns for coping with decisional conflict. J. Behav. Dec. Mak.. 10: 1-19.

[15]. Mann L, Radford M, Burnett P, Ford S, Bond M, Leung K, Nakamura H, Vaughan, G, Yang K (1998) Cross-cultural differences in selfreported decision making style and confidence. Int. J. Psy.. 33(5): 325-335.

[16]. Rue & Byars (2003) Decision Making Skills, Management skills and application mcgraw hill, 68.

[17]. Sanchez, A.C.J., Calvo, A.L., Bunuel, P.S., Godoy, S. J. I. (2009) Decision-making of spanish female basketball team players while they are competing. *Revista de Psicologia del Deporte,* (18), 369.

[18]. Satman, C. (2005) The Analysis Of Audience Voice On The Decisions Of Football Referees, Publicized M.A. Thesis, Published Master Thesis, Ankara University, The Institute of Educational Sciences, Ankara.

[19]. Seiller, R. (1997) Decision making in sport. International Symposium of the Turkish Association of Sport Psychology, Mersin,10-12.

[20]. Tatlıoğlu, K. (2014) Üniversite Öğrencilerinin Karar Vermede Öz-Saygı Düzeyleri İle Karar Verme Stilleri Arasındaki İlişkinin Bazı Değişkenlere Göre İncelenmesi, Akademik Sosyal Araştırmalar Dergisi, 2(1), 150-170.

[21]. Vural, M. (2013) Spor Genel Müdürlüğü Merkez Ve Taşra Teşkilatında Görev Yapan Spor Yöneticilerinin Düşünme Ve Karar Verme Stillerinin İncelenmesi, Selçuk Üniversitesi Sağlık Bilimleri Enstitüsü, Yayınlanmamış Yüksek Lisans Tezi, Konya, 30.

[22]. Kuzgun Y (1992). Decision Strategies Scale: Development and standardization. VII. National Psychology Congress Scientific Studies. Turkish Psychologists Association, pp. 161-170.

20

STUDY ON EFFICIENCY OF ACTIONS A SERVICE AND RECEPTION SERVICE, YOUTH LEVEL IN THE GAME OF VOLLEYBALL

Adin-Marian COJOCARU, Marilena COJOCARU

Spiru Haret University Bucharest, Faculty of Physical Education and Sport

adincojocaru@yahoo.com

Abstract: By means that we belong, volleyball claims to use their own methods. In this regard, the directions of scientific research is moving towards detailed knowledge and the development of models and micro-models drawn from the work itself.

The chosen theme is, we believe, of the utmost importance because of the work of coaches who prepare teams of cadets, performance varies later. Making a technical preparations in order to achieve higher sports results, occur over time and the clubs divisional A1.

It started the development of science-based operational models that contain standardized means of preparation will lead to a more efficient process at each level of education.

Finally this research attempts to evaluate whether those specific drive systems used in the training of volleyball players were youth, had been successful in shaping the pattern of play and training.

In modernizing education and training to improve the capacity at every level, develop operational models.

Key words: efficiency, skills, service, reception from service, volleyball

Introduction

The variety of techniques, whose materialization is manifested in the plethora of tactical execution of actions has great theoretical and practical learning opportunities and broadening the knowledge base and stimulating the creative initiative, both for players and coaches. As such, it becomes necessary theoretical process or training.

The multitude and variety with successive phases of the game, alternating rapidly situations attack the defense, the opportunities they give players to display their imagination and their ability inventive, attacking in strength or stability of passes executed with great finesse pressure emulation, all offering both players, but especially the audience, moments of great spectacle [1].

The game of volleyball plays an important role in the development of combined speed qualities - strength, particularly the large number of jumps, requests the data from the tare weight of each player, in terms of speed gear [2]

The training of cadets has a number of features mainly due to peculiarities they present different periods of their development [3].

The chosen theme is, we think have, of utmost importance because of the work of coaches who prepare teams of cadets, performance varies later. Making a technical preparations in order to achieve higher sports results occur in the divisional clubs A1.

Research hypotheses

The main purpose of this paper is to highlight the main aspects of the training content and resources to serve the newly specialists as documentary material.

In order to solve these problems we proposed, need to verify the training into practice patterns, with the task:

- Selection and systematization means;
- Quantification of scientific knowledge on the collective capacity;
- Systematization of operations;
- Directions optimization training;
- Verification objectives.

We started from the hypothesis that: the development of science-based operational models that contain standardized means of preparation will lead to a more efficient process at each level of education.

Research tasks

We work in developing methodological several stages, as follows:

- setting goals which arose from the concrete problems that they achieve initial work;
- documentation done by attending specialized bibliography, through discussions with various specialists and methodical selection of findings of its own experience;
- shaping the content elements of the work and methodology development;
- material analysis, interpretation and conclusions detachment;
- structuring content and drafting work.

The object of this research it was preformed group (youth) Sports Club Dinamo Bucharest, which is a homogeneous group, selected well.
Working conditions are good, we mean that is a proper gym, and the base material is acceptable.
During my training researched models presented in this paper is dated 08/01/2015 and until 07/01/2016.

Performance objective for the year we carried out the research were as follows:
- for the team - participating in the final of C.N. the Romanian Federation of Volleyball, occupying a podium place;
- proposal of one or two players to the national team of youth.

Result

Sports included in the study sample were as follows:

Table 1 – Components of the studied sample

Nr. crt.	Nume and surname	Age	Waist	Wingspan	Weight	Position
1	*H.E.*	16	174	176	62	*Setter*
2	*T.R.*	15	170	171	55	*Setter*
3	*V.R.*	15	170	172	54	*Setter*
4	*T.E.*	14	165	166	46	*Setter*
5	*P.L.*	16	183	182	65	*Middle Blocker*
6	*T.R.*	16	182	184	60	*Middle Blocker*
7	*L.M.*	16	179	183	56	*Middle Blocker*
8	*C.D.*	15	177	178	60	*Middle Blocker*
9	*M.A.*	16	176	175	57	*Outside spiker*
10	*R.I.*	16	176	175	58	*Outside spiker*
11	*D.O.*	16	175	180	51	*Outside spiker*
12	*B.M.*	15	175	179	63	*Outside spiker*
13	*B.D.*	15	170	171	55	*Outside spiker*
14	*V.F.*	15	170	172	57	*Outside spiker*
15	*S.R.*	16	165	164	50	*Libero*
16	*T.A.*	15	160	160	51	*Libero*

To determine the physical training of the group, they were used samples Romanian Federation of Volleyball evaluating the potential motor and to assess the technical level were used following control samples:

1. executions service - measure service efficiency;
2. executions reception from service area 1 - measuring the effectiveness of the reception from service zone 1;

executions reception from service area 5 - measuring the effectiveness of the reception from service zone 5.

Table 2 – Technical control samples at the beginning of the preparatory period

Nr. Crt.	Name and surname	Control samples		
		1	2	3
1	**H.E.**	4	3	4
2	**T.R.**	4	4	3
3	**V.R.**	3	3	3
4	**T.E.**	4	4	4
5	**P.L.**	3	3	3
6	**T.R.**	4	4	3
7	**L.M.**	5	5	4
8	**C.D.**	5	5	5
9	**M.A.**	3	3	4

10	R.L.	4	3	5
11	D.O.	3	3	3
12	B.M.	4	4	4
13	B.D.	3	3	4
14	V.F.	4	3	5
15	S.R.	4	4	3
16	T.A.	3	2	3

Table 3 – Technical control samples after of the preparatory period

Nr. Crt.	Name and surname	Control samples		
		1	2	3
1	H.E.	5	5	4
2	T.R.	5	4	4
3	V.R.	4	4	4
4	T.E.	5	4	5
5	P.L.	4	4	4
6	T.R.	4	5	5
7	L.M.	5	5	5
8	C.D.	5	5	5
9	M.A.	4	4	4
10	R.L.	4	5	4
11	D.O.	4	4	4
12	B.M.	5	4	5
13	B.D.	4	4	4
14	V.F.	4	5	4
15	S.R.	4	5	5
16	T.A.	4	3	4

In the interpretation of data (graphic 1) shows that, the arithmetic mean is 3.83 initial effective execution and final arithmetic mean is 4.42 efficient executions; progress is visible 0.59 efficient executions. Due to age close sportsmen and quality training level we find a high homogeneity.

Following the evolution of each player can define the extremes:

- the players 7 and 8 had a constant evolution, recording and initial sample and the final sample maximum effective executions;
- the players 1, 2 and 4 initial testing have been four executions efficient, and the final testing showed five effective executions;
- rest of the players were registered for final testing effective April executions, some with progress of execution.

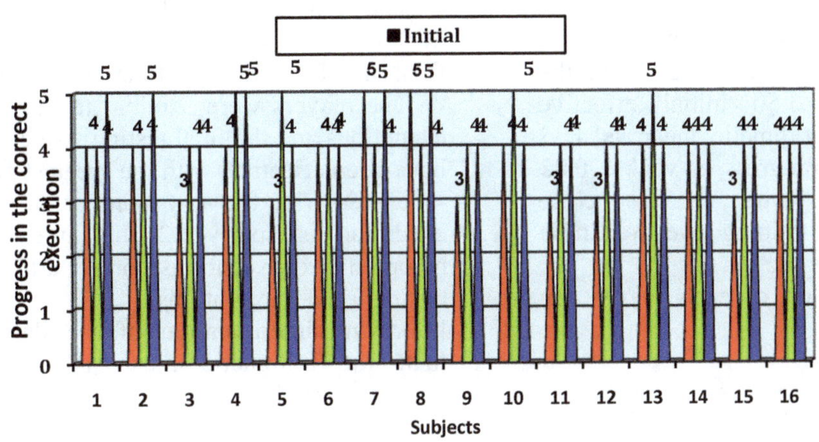

Graphic 1 – Evaluating the efficiency of service

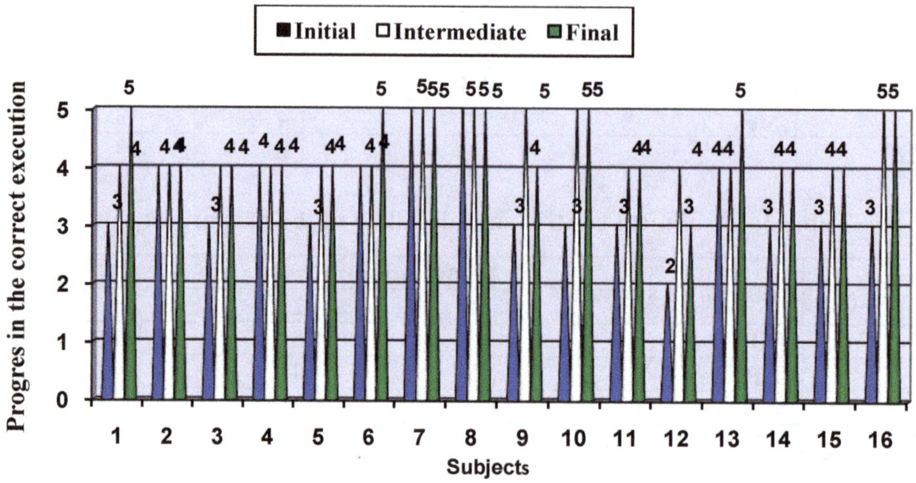

Grafic 2 – Evaluating the efficiency of reception from Z1

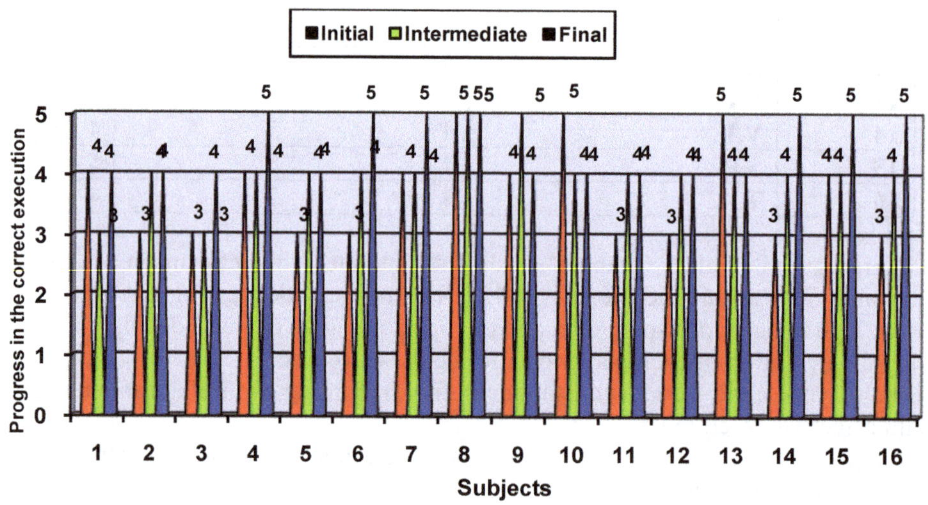

Grafic 3 – Evaluating the efficiency of reception from Z5

Discusions

In the interpretation of data from the reception of services in one area, it appears that the arithmetic mean is 3.50 initial effective execution and final arithmetic mean is 4.33 efficient executions; progress is visible 0,83 efficient executions. Due to age close sportsmen and quality training level we find a high homogeneity (graphic 2).

Following the evolution of each player can define the extremes:

- The players 7 and 8 had a constant evolution, recording and initial sample and the final sample maximum effective executions;
- The players were 3 initial testing efficient executions and the final testing five executions have been effective, with the greatest progress;
- player with the low number of effective execution is sporty 12 that initial testing recorded two executions correct and accurate testing Final 3 executions.

Following interpretation of the data shows that, the arithmetic mean is 3.67 initial effective execution and final arithmetic mean is 4.33 efficient executions; progress is visible 0.66 efficient executions. Due to age close sportsmen and quality training level we find a high homogeneity (grahic 3).

Following the evolution of each player can define the extremes:

- The player 8 had a constant evolution, recording and initial sample and the final sample maximum effective executions;
- he players 4 and 6 initial testing showed executions effective April 3 respectively, and the final testing showed five effective executions;
- player was number 10 had a surprising setback, dropping it from 5 to 4 effective executions.

Service efficiency, action taken as attack is then converted into action by specific tactical attack [4].

It is obvious specialization to take over the service, which is usually performed in the device, with the two players to the service plan and the service of three players jump teams having their structure, 4.3 and even 2 players in reception [5].

Reception gets trajectories medium-high, bouncing ball on lifting, supporting and direct attack, raising the jump, masking intention of lifting and dodge the idea of speeding up construction of attack, the fragment game lifting attack and creating optimal conditions for shooter.

Conclusions

After processing and interpreting data we can conclude the following:

At the beginning of each year the competition, each team will set its own game model in accordance with

individual possibilities and future athletes in that group;

Evidence Control finds that: averages are significant differences due to age and level close to the optimal development of motor skills, group having a high homogeneity;

On preparing specific averages are significant differences due to the evolution of each player. Initial testing only 6 players have achieved scale participation in the championship, and the intermediate testing progress has been very good, the whole team getting points for participation in the competition;

Optimization model of training is achieved by means of selection and systematization of training;

The modernization of education and training to improve the capacity at every level, develop operational models;

To facilitate the improvement of techniques and tactical game play patterns to be used;

After applying the model to fulfill the objective of the team ranking second in National Championship.

Acknowledgement

All authors have equal contribution.

References

[1]. Mârza D.,(2006) - *Volei, bazele teoretice şi metodice*, Editura PIM Iaşi, pg.103.

[2]. Bâc O., (1999) - *Volleyball,* Editura Universităţii din Oradea, Oradea, pg. 67

[3]. Cojocaru, A (2008) – *Voleiul la juniori,* Editura Universitaria Craiova, Craiova, pg. 45

[4.] Niculescu, M. (2002) - *Volei – de la teorie la practică*, Editura Universităţii din Piteşti, Pitesti, pag 79.

[5]. Păcuraru A., Iacob I., Balaiş F., Braharu O., (2000) - *Manualul profesorului de volei,* Editura Helios Iasi, pg.105.

21

STUDY ON DEVELOPMENT SPEED TO EIGHTH-GRADE SCHOOLGIRLS

George Cristian Cătună, Butu Ioana Maria, Simona Teodorescu Anemari

Faculty of Physical Education, Sport and Physical Therapy, Spiru Haret University, Berceni Road, nr. 24, sector 4, Bucharest

Abstract: Introduction The paper entitled "Study on development speed to schoolgirls class VII" wants efficient quality development of basic motor speed, in the use of various means of sports games and athletics as part of secondary education in physical education class and sports.

Material and Methods

The specific methods for the development of the rate applied in this study were:

• maximum application method; Alternative method; exerted on the method handicap pairs of pupils with close; method races or relays; competition distance method gradually increased with intensity.

Obtained results

Develop motor skills are physical education and sports training for one of the major concerns go toward improving the structural and functional parameters of different organ systems of the body.

Following the collection and interpretation of the results of the group subjects improved their general and specific indices of speed, so the means employed and have achieved their goal;

Discussion and conclusions

For physical education, development of motor skills is performed simultaneously with physical development and general consolidation of motion skills and representing an end of the first importance, which is realized in the educational process of physical education and through independent activity of students and does not require special material base.

Keywords: motor quality, speed, gymnasium

Introduction

The paper entitled "Study on development speed to schoolgirls class VII" wants efficient quality development of basic motor speed, in the use of various means of sports games and athletics as part of secondary education in physical education class and sports.

Motor skills development is inextricably linked to physiological changes in the cells, tissues, organs, body organs and systems. Development of motor skills is achieved by gradual improvement of function and anatomy of cells, organs, organs and systems required adequate and targeted to achieve a prolonged adaptation layer enabling driving tasks with maximum efficiency.

"Speed, in the broadest sense refers mainly to the speed of movement or act performing motor unit time. It is determined by the length of the trajectory over time or time to make a movement. It is estimated in m / sec., Or in units of time. "[1]

"With regard to biological factors, some are likely nervous and some are of anatomic, functional:

• the mobility of nervous processes course, the speed of rotation of the excitation of the inhibition and their intensity;

• latency or response time which, in turn, depends on the quality of the nerve, the muscle and the synapse;

• nerve impulse conduction velocity (afferent and efferent) by nervous network;

• speed of muscle contraction following nerve excitation;

• force of muscle entering the contraction;

• length of the segments involved in the activity, joint mobility and muscle elasticity;

• capacity to coordinate muscle groups;

• the type of muscle fibers making up the muscle fibers F. T. White (Fast-Twitchglycolitic fibers - fast fiber) or red S.T. (Slow - Twitch oxidative Fibers - slow fibers);

• macroergic wealth of muscle fiber compounds (CP and ATP). "[1]

In the process of physical education, the factors listed above are subject to the attention of the teacher who put a specific means to improve them. So, following specific programs to increase the speed decreases neuromuscular excitability chronaxi improving, it shortens the latency and increase energy reserves underlying compounds specific efforts to speed.

Speed has various manifestations most important being:

• speed of response;
• speed of execution;

• repetition rate;

In physical activity and sport are distinguished and speed combined forms such as speed acceleration or speed of travel and driving combined with other qualities such as expansion (power-speed) [2]

„In all its forms, speed, as well as resistance in regime of speed, are motric qualities decisive in the game of contemporary handball where to cope with the present level of high performance is required intensive work and sustained" [3]

Speed development is a complex process that depends on other important elements among which highlights the level of technical training in the execution of complex processes or complex motor actions. [4]

Speed is the quality motor whose manifestation is highlighted in particular by the individual genetic treasure, having the spotlight on the quality of the nervous system that facilitates prompt control of movements [5].

To develop all forms of manifestation of speed can act methodically and organized from the age of 10 years. The effect of this operation methodical gradually decreases until final maturity age (approximately 22 years boys and 19 years girls). As comparison of performance between the sexes from the age of about 11-12 years, the boys equals girls that past performance will be superior [6].

Material and methods

Research methods used: literature study, theoretical study and observant, observation, means the application system development, initial and final testing, statistical analysis, and graphic representation.

The specific methods for the development of the rate applied in this study were:

• maximum application method; Alternative method; exerted on the handicap method pairs of pupils with close performance; method races or relays; competition distance method gradually increased with intensity.

For the development and execution speed of reaction and action is taken on other body segments using lightweight materials and exercises sports complex variable, requesting alternative analyzers tactile, visual or hearing.

It was also demonstrated that by acting on the force development by increasing the cross section of muscle and thus force him favoring "sliding" actin and myosin in the muscle fiber, which ultimately results increased speed of contraction and done availability to execute an increased number of repetitions.

Such drives to speed development must fulfill certain conditions:

• exercise are well known and understood, so as to favor execution speed;

• to perform predilection exercises specific for sports events, with technical and tactical actions performed in race conditions, gameplay, stage races, dynamic games;

• dosing should exercise be optimal shape is determined by the speed that is intended to be developed so the speed does not drop to the end.

• to avail the special exercises that lasts from 5-6 seconds until the 50-60 sec., composed mainly by altering the volume and duration of work;

• provide breaks between repetitions must be adequate time for the return of autonomic functions, It has oxygenation muscle, but in order to maintain optimal brain excitation.

Speed development of specific methods applied were:

• maximal request method, which involves performing exercises jersey by completing the rapidly varying distances or running in maximum tempo of the different specific means of sports games;

• alternative method consisting of alternating intensity, for example increasing the speed to maximum, keeping her distance marked beforehand (or time frame), gradually decreasing intensity;

• handicap method exerted on pairs of pupils with close distance between performers may vary

• method races or relays that can successfully address the multiple manifestations of speed;

• method distance contest progressively increased with intensity.

• development and execution speed of reaction and action is taken on other body segments using lightweight materials and exercises sports complex variable, requesting alternative analyzers tactile, visual or hearing.

Results:

Develop motor skills for physical education is one of the major concerns go toward improving the structural and functional parameters of different organ systems of the body pupils.

The experiment was conducted during 2 nd semester education (February-June), with the help of 10 students who were selected on a voluntary basis and the presence of two classes VIII of School 190 in District 4, Bucharest.

I used the following tests of control: speed 30 meters, 30 meters dribbling between landmarks, run in a triangle, Cooper test.

To see the progress of each student testing was conducted on initial and final. Initial testing driving the four samples was performed at the beginning of the experiment in the second week of semester 2 and the final in the last week of it.

Table 1 - The results of the initial and final testing for group of experiment

TEST	GROUP OF EXPERIMENT																			
	T.A.		S.A.		D.M.		S.O.		V.A.		R.C.		T.S.		S.R.		A.A.		B.M.	
	I.T	F.T.	I.T	F.T.	I.T	F.T.	I.T	F.T.	I.T	F.T.	I.T	F.T.	I.T	F.T.	I.T	F.T.	I.T	F.T.	I.T	F.T.
Speed 30 m	5	4,3	5	4,7	4,8	4,4	4,8	4,5	4,8	4,5	4,7	4,5	4,9	4,1	4,6	4,5	4,7	4,6	4,6	4,4
30 metri dribbling	7	6,7	7,1	6,8	6,9	6,3	7,1	6,8	6,8	4,9	7	6,7	6,9	6,7	6,7	5,9	6,7	6,5	6,8	6,3
Move triangle	22,9	21	23,8	23,7	22,5	22,3	22,6	21,2	21,4	20,7	21,3	20,9	24,5	21,5	20,1	20	21,4	21,3	20,4	19,6
Cooper Test	1958	2046	1640	1680	1963	2020	1650	1730	1976	2000	1848	1856	1695	1776	2000	2015	1680	1850	1963	2000

Table 2 - The results of the initial and final testing for control group

TEST	THE CONTROL GROUP																			
	N.E.		H.S.		A.N.		B.R.		D.L.		F.G.		G.E.		R.F.		A.I.		R.S.	
	I.T	F.T.	I.T	F.T.	I.T	F.T.	I.T	F.T.	I.T	F.T.	I.T	F.T.	I.T	F.T.	I.T	F.T.	I.T	F.T.	I.T	F.T.
Speed 30 m	**4,7**	**4,5**	**4,9**	**4,9**	**4,9**	**4,6**	**4,6**	**4,4**	**4,7**	**4,6**	**5**	**4,8**	**4,7**	**4,4**	**4,8**	**4,7**	**4,8**	**4,5**	**4,8**	**4,5**
30 metri dribbling	**7,1**	**7,1**	**6,9**	**6,8**	**7,2**	**7**	**6,7**	**6,4**	**6,7**	**6,5**	**8**	**7,2**	**7**	**6,7**	**6,8**	**6,8**	**6,8**	**6,5**	**7,1**	**6,8**
Move triangle	**23,8**	**23,7**	**22,7**	**22,6**	**21,5**	**21,5**	**20,1**	**20**	**21,4**	**21,2**	**24,9**	**24,5**	**21,3**	**20,9**	**21,3**	**21**	**22,5**	**22,2**	**21,4**	**20,7**
Cooper Test	**1848**	**1856**	**1663**	**1676**	**1886**	**1995**	**2000**	**2033**	**1995**	**2120**	**1628**	**1675**	**1928**	**2000**	**2000**	**1975**	**1685**	**1700**	**1976**	**2000**

In figure 1 and 2 are the results obtained in evaluating the 30m running speed.

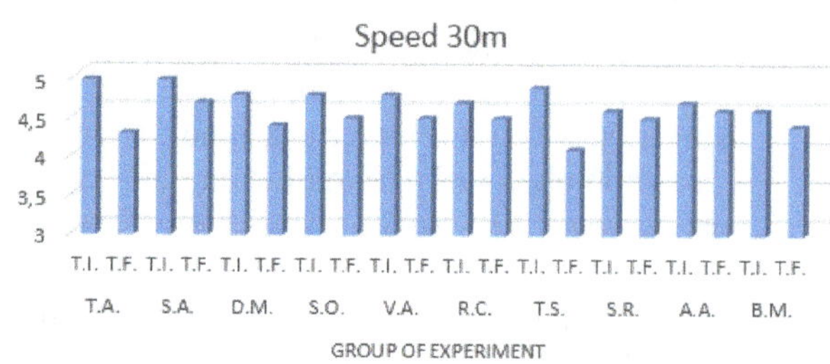

Fig. 1. Group of experiment running speed to 30m

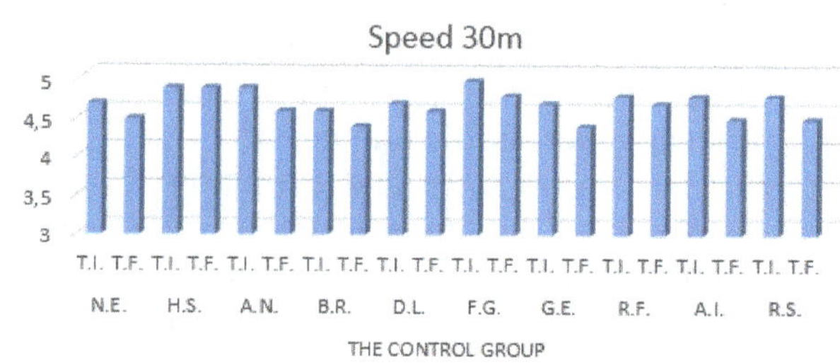

Fig. 2. The control group running speed to 30m

Figure 3 and 4 are the results obtained in the evaluation of speed dribbling between cones on initial and final test.

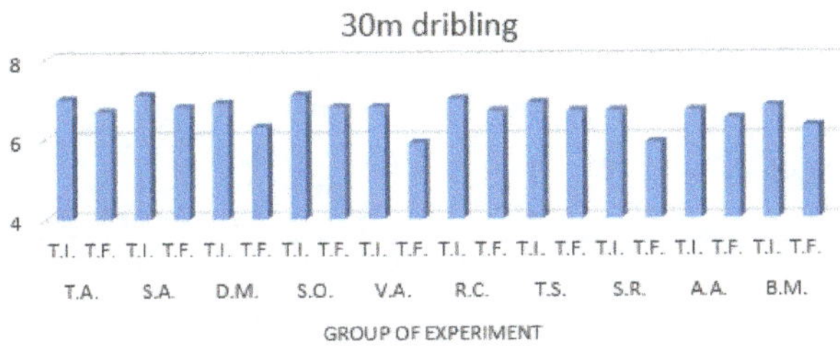

Fig. 3. Speed dribbling between cones on initial and final test for group of experiment

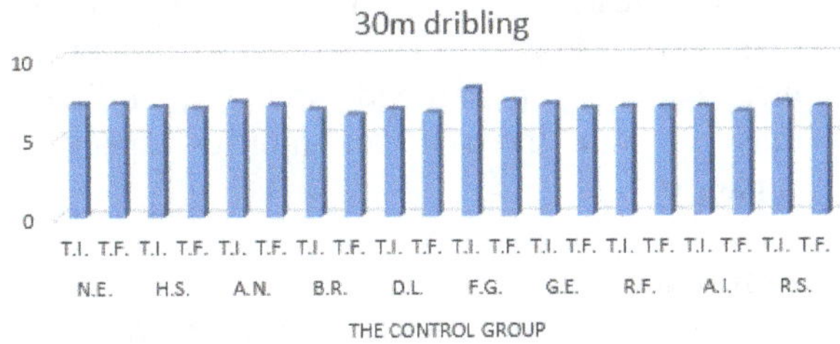

Fig. 4. Speed dribbling between cones on initial and final test for control group

In figure 5 and 6 are the results in the evaluation of displacement delta initial and final testing

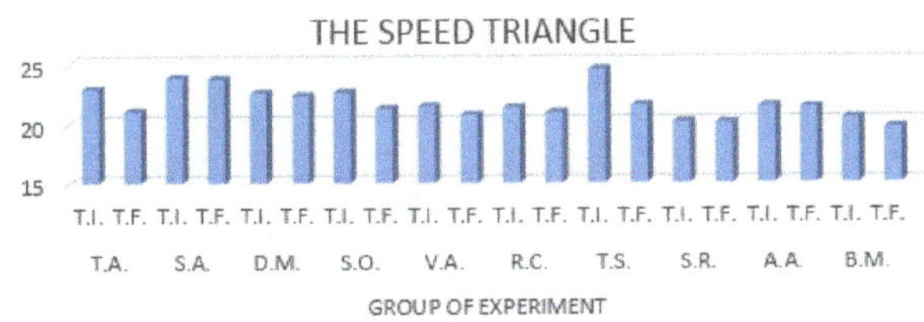

Fig. 5. Moving speed in triangle for group of experiment

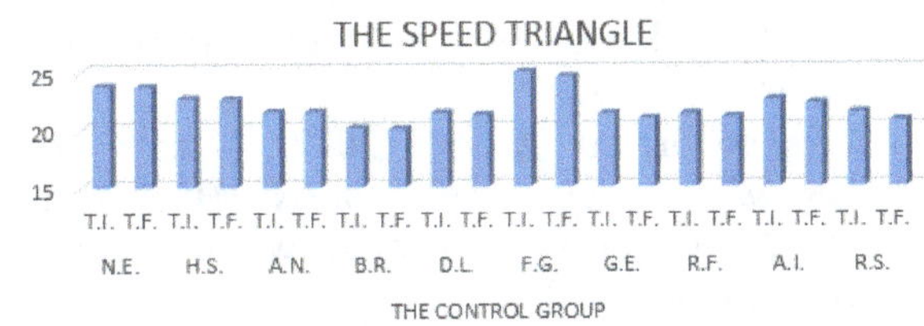

Fig. 6. Moving speed in triangle for the control group

In figure 7 and 8 are the test results obtained in the evaluation of the two tests Cooper

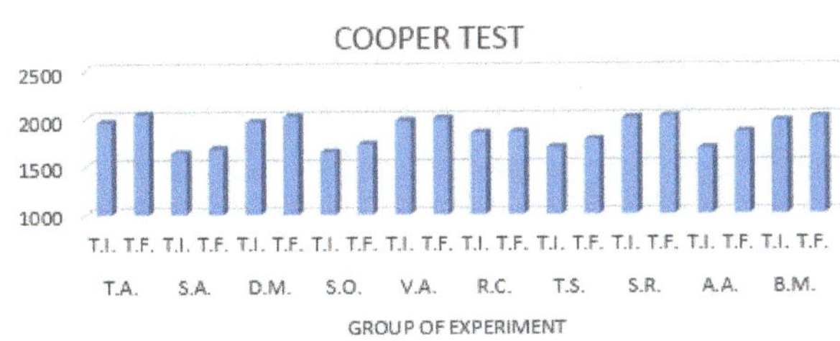

Fig. 7. Cooper test to group experiment

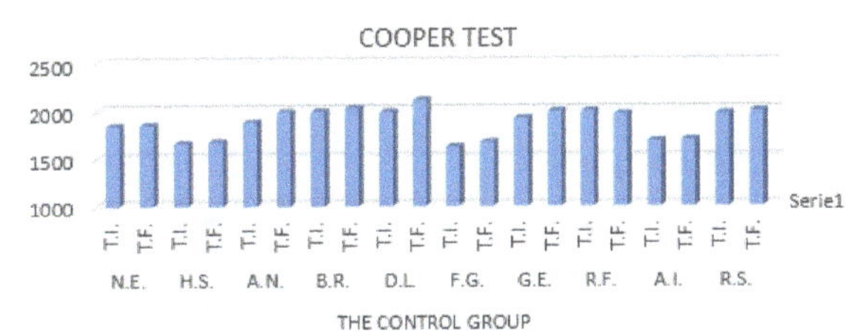

Fig. 8. Cooper test to the control group

Discussion and conclusions

Finally, we conclude the following:

- On initial testing, experimental group and the control group had equal value, but after using after use of the means, values the experiment group increased significantly compared to the control group that grew very little.
- Final testing standard deviation does not increase very much from that initial testing and pursuing the coefficient of variability is observed that homogeneity is greater in the experimental group.

Develop motor skills at primary school is performed simultaneously with strengthening abilities and motric skills, with execute exercises of physical development, as well as through of a particular action system.

Develop motor skills are physical education and sports training for one of the major concerns go toward improving the structural and functional parameters of different organ systems of the body.

After analyzing and interpreting the results of the subjects of the two groups have improved indices of speed, strength, force general and specific with a small surplus for the group of experiment, so the means used and have achieved their goal;

The experiment showed that in terms of somatic, and motrics subjects meet school requirements for this age group.
Specific test results confirm the hypothesis that work using in the workout of training means better streamlined and standardized may get an increase an motrics specific capacity.

References

[1]. Gheorghe I. (2007). *Motric qualities - Theory and Methodology.* Bucharest: Bren, pg. 5-6.

[2]. Acsinte E. (2000). *Handball from initiation to high performance.* Bacau: Media Publishing, pg. 73.

[3]. Catuna C, Alupoaie M. (2014). *Course in IFR Technology - Handball* - Bucharest: Publishing House of Tomorrow Foundation Romania, pg. 53.

[4]. Teodorescu A. S, (2012), *Theory of physical education and sports*, Bucharest: Publishing House of Tomorrow Foundation Romania, pg. 115.

[5]. Ghermanescu K.I. (2000). *Handbal* 2nd edition, Bucharest: Publishing House of Tomorrow Foundation Romania pg. 88.

[6]. Dragnea, A (1996), *Antrenamentul sportiv (teorie si metodica)*, Editura Didactica si Pedagogica, Bucuresti, pg. 105

PHYSICAL TRAINING IN TABLE TENNIS - SOCIOLOGICAL SURVEY

Diaconescu Dragoş, Dragomir Marian
Universitatea din Craiova, România

Abstract: Table tennis is an accessible and performance practicing sport discipline or at the level of sport for all. Table tennis competition has become very fierce, competitors trying to surprise and overcome their opponents, observing changes in the game of table tennis, becoming extremely aggressive. This research aims to identify the views of 43 table tennis coaches in training junior players, the questionnaire referring to the physical training and the weighing of motor skills in training players.
Key Words:table tennis, training, beginners, survey.

Introduction

Getting great performance in sport requires, in addition to a harmonious development of all motor skills, further development of some specific sports skills. Many sports have some technical setbacks when the coaches abandoned totally the use of nonspecific means in performance athletes, attributing exclusive trust to the effectiveness of the specific means.
Literature is relatively "poor" in studies and articles related to the issue of physical training in table tennis, but on the content of sports training, Romanian authors, [1,3,7,8,2] distinguished the following main elements of content, called factors or components of sports training: physical training, technical training, tactical training, psychological training, the theoretical training, which for some sports, add also an aesthetic training.
The dedicated term physical training, sometimes replaced with the physical condition or physical capacity, means the content of the training that ensures the preparedness and physical performance of the athlete consists of a methodical process organized and oriented towards optimal development of human motor skills consistent with the requirements and the specifics of the effort in sports performance of that sport branch.[2,3,4,8]
Thus, our study sought to identify the views of table tennis coaches in Romania, with reference to the physical training of juniors.

Method

The questionnaire based survey method is a method of investigation as written, represented by a succession of questions on the subjects addressed logically sequenced on the studied phenomenon, namely physical training in table tennis sport training. The questionnaire conceived and applied by us, consisted of 18 questions, 7 being closed questions and 11 open questions.
Out of 11 closed questions there was one with two answers, three were with four possible answers and 7 with five possible answers, suitable to statistical approach. There were distributed a total of 50 questionnaires to the same number of specialists. For objective or subjective motives, no more than 43 questionnaires were returned. Out of these, due to answer defects - answers to less than half the questions, three were not taken into account when recording and data processing. We mention that the procedures for transmitting the questionnaire were accompanied by a letter from the doctoral student containing the acceptance request and the purpose, specifying that the information will only be used for processing scientific interest, without disclosing the identity and thanks for the effort to fill in and submit the questionnaires.
When asked about the importance of physical training and the sports training from the data presented in Chart 1, it appears that most experts considered the part of physical training as important (50%) or very important (25%), 25% appreciate the importance of being on average or less, indicating that no specialist considers the importance of this factor as insignificant. It appears that the distribution of the opinions of specialists on the importance of physical training is concentrated in the major proportion - 95% - around great appreciation, with a slight asymmetry to the right and a normal vaulting.

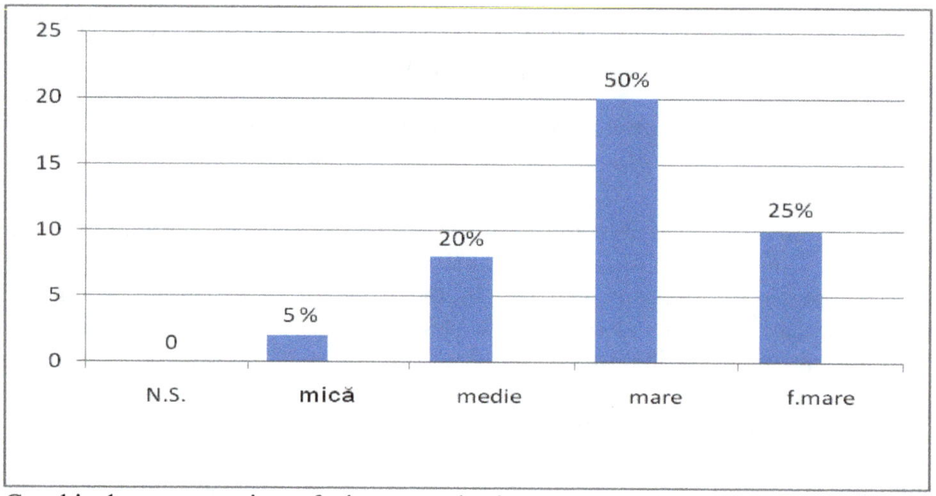

Figure 1. Graphical representation of views on the importance of physical training factor in table tennis

The question which focused on the views on the sports training factor that should be mainly addressed in table tennis. Digital and percentage results are shown in Table 1, revealing that the number of responses - 97 is greater than the persons included in the group investigated, respectively 40.

Table 1. The predominance of emphasis on sports training in actual components and percentages

Training Components	lots	Cumulated lots	Percentage	cumulated Percentage
Physical training	18	18	18,4%	18,4%
Tehnical training	41	59	43,0%	61,4%
tactical training	29	88	29,6%	91,0%
Psychological training	6	94	6,0%	97,0%
Theoretical training	3	97	3,0%	100%

This stems from the fact that they have checked two or three components of sports training, which should focus on specific sports training in table tennis. It appears that most of the specialists' opinions, ie 91% goes to three factors that are addressed mostly through exercise. The order of predominance of emphasis in training within three factors place on the first level, with a significant advance, the technical training - 43.0%, followed by tactical preparation - 29.6% and physical training – 18,4%.

It follows a share of 72.6%, for the technical and tactical component followed by the physical one - 18.4%, the psychological one- and the theoretical one 6% - 3%. We find, however, a non-correlation between opinions on the question of the importance of physical training and regarding the question about the share on the emphasis on training factors, according to the responses, the importance of physical training is at a high and very high rate of 75% while the share resulting from the opinions on the emphasis in preparation, from the next question is only 18.45.

Although we have not requested argumentation views, we believe that these non-correlations expressed in answers to questions are due to a concept that persists in sports games that much of the physical training is done through exercises carried out in technical and tactical preparation. This view was refuted in the practice of activities combated in research papers and topical studies.

A significant aspect in terms of the thesis topic was referred to the proportion of the specific motor skills given by the specific effort in men's table tennis, motor qualities originally listed as top concept and classification. The results of the views expressed by the group researched subjects are presented in Table 2

From the responses of specialists there emerges a model of specific motor skills share in an effort table tennis boys, as well as a model for the formative age-specific second stage.

Table 2. The results the specialists' opinions investigation on the proportion of motor skills in table tennis for boys and training phase two

Motor qualities	The share in boys table tennis	The share in the second training phase
speed	30%	40%
skillfulness	40%	45%
Rezilience/endurance	15%	10%
strength	15%	5%

There is a preponderance of skill and speed characteristics, 40% and 30% in specific boys table tennis effort, plus those of endurance and strength in equal proportions - 15%. In this context we note increasing the share of strength in specific forms of manifestation in table tennis and a broad vision, of the four integrated motor qualities in contrast to views that the table tennis was just a sport skill. As regards the motor skills proportions in the second training phase we believe that they are consistent with the potential development indices of speed, agility, endurance and strength existing in children practicing table tennis in the formative stage in question. Besides a few teachers - coaches have even stated that when talking about development resistance at this age they refer to general endurance as aerobic support and the work for the development of specific indices of work force is made exclusively with the hindering of the body.

Regarding the physical training share in the boys table tennis training effort, as foreseen in the annual training plan

On the share allocated to physical training in the effort of training provided in the annual plan of training of athletes from the phase two training - Chart 2 - the opinion of most coaches is that it should be up to 30% - half of those questioned and up to 40% - 12 subjects. 6 persons stating to allocate physical training up to 50% or even 60% of the work included in the annual plans for physical training, and two subjects ticked other share without specifying what it is.

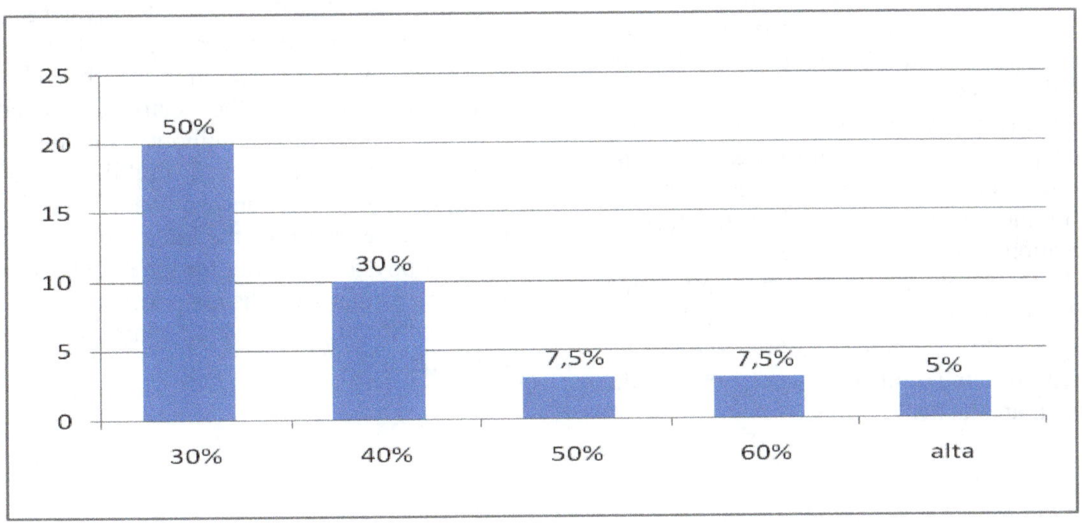

Figure 2. The representation of the share allocated to physical training in the effort of training provided in the annual plan of training - the second training phase

Given the concept of structure of the questionnaire, the opinions expressed on this question should be considered as such. But if we analyze correlative answers to the following questions, you can find some contradictions. For example, most specialists - 30 of 40 consider the importance of physical preparation as large - 20 people or very large - 10 people. Once the answers to another question, it appears that half of experts allocate up to 30% of the annual work training for physical training, although the growth and development of children requires another vision.

The following issues can and should be considered together because they relate to the same set of problems in two temporal phases during the preparatory stages, respectively the first and the second. They covered four problems: the number of lessons- workouts per week, number of lessons workout only physical training topics, the number of topics of physical training and of technical-tactical training and the number of lessons only with technical and tactical topics, all with reference to the children in formative phase two.

We find that the number of training lessons remained constant at 6 per week , aspect that we consider normal, given the program and the children's school obligations. Thus, we see that in the first period part the preparatory workload for the physical component is equal to that assigned to the technical and tactical component. If we take as a benchmark a lesson workout of 120', in the first preparatory phase of the period about 360 minutes is allocated for both physical training component as well as for the technical and tactical training. In the second part of the preparatory period during the time allotted to physical training drops to 240 minutes, while the technical and tactical preparation allocated increase to about 480 min. In the preparatory period from a training workload of about 720' in a week, that averages 300' - about 41.66% allotted to physical training and 420' - 58.33% to the technical and tactical training.

For the preparatory period and the second training cycle, the proportion appears to be functional in what concerns the formative and developmental needs. The condition would be that from which we call technical and tactical most of the time to be allocated to the technical composition, ie at least 80%.

Among coaches, during the competitive period, the average opinion is that only lessons with mixed themes, with physical - technical - tactical nature to be performed, those specialized only in physical training or technical-tactical training disappearing.

Knowing that physical training has two components, namely general physical training and multilateral and specific physical training, we found it necessary to hear the views of experts on their workload in proportions , three times during the annual cycle of training : beginning preparatory period, the end of the preparatory period and during the competition. Specialists shared their opinions via questionnaire outlining the following percentages:

- Beginning of the preparatory period: 80% general and multilateral physical training, 20% specific physical training;
- The end of the preparatory period: 70% general physical training and 30% multilateral specific physical training;
- During the competitive period, the percentage is 60-40%.

We note two significant aspects: greater share of general and multilateral physical training regardless of the preparation phase and the trend of increasing the share of specific physical preparation, without equaling the share of the general and multilateral one. Another matter of concern was that of the experts' assessment of the table tennis players level of physical training for the athletes found in the formative phase two. The views collected through the questionnaire are shown in Graph 3.3.

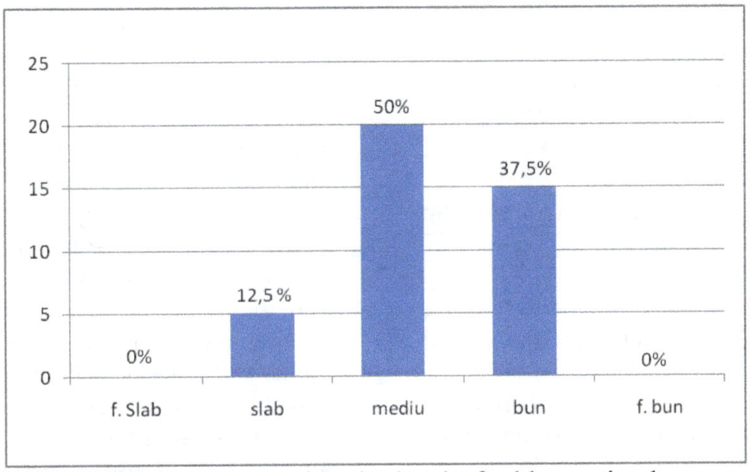

Figure 3. Graphical representation of assessing the level of table tennis players are in the formative phase two physical preparation

Of the five levels of assessment we found that opinions focus on three, excluding the extremes, ie very weak and all too good. If the exclusion of the *very weak* appreciation qualifier is normal, due to the fact that we speak about sports performance, the lack of *very well* qualifier is not a normal one, but they shape both a direction of improvement and a research one. Otherwise half of the interviewed consider physical training on the average level, 37.5% as good and 12.5% as poor. In the context of all questionnaire, recognizing the importance of physical training, mentioning efforts allocations towards the physical training workout, the weak qualifier is less grounded.

The following questions were aimed at motor qualities for which some reservations are expressed, respectively resistance and strength in training and the promotion workout for their development during the formative preparatory phase. In some questionnaires, the answers were double and two of them triple. All were taken so that there were 50 responses. The results are summarized in Table 3.

Table 3. coaches Opinions on physical attributes of strength and resilience in table tennis players in the formative phase two

Degree of recommendation	strength		Resilience	
	number	percentage	number	percentage
Not recommended	-	-	-	-
Slightly recommended	10	20%	6	12%
Necessary	25	50%	25	50%
Highly recommended	8	16%	11	22%
Very highly recommended	7	14%	8	16%

Coaches deem necessary and advisable specific force development to children in the second phase of formative assessment on different levels: in small measure. Seven subjects - 20%, average 25 subjects – 50 highly recommended 8 subjects - 16% and very highly recommended - seven subjects - 14%. We find from the above figures that the majority of coaches - 80% - considers advisable to develop formative force in the second phase from an average recommendation level to a very large one. The same orientation is to be found in the development of resilience when the percentage of recommendation between medium and very large increase to 88%.

The following questions were meant to find views expressed by experts on the possibilities and improvement factors of the two components of interest from the perspective of our work, namely the content of sports training and physical preparation factor therein. Being semi character questions they could mention any fact or possibility up to three options for each person questioned, and only on the content of sports training. Taking into account the 120 theoretical possibilities response and recorded content, the main factors related to the content of sports training whose improvement could lead to increased athletic performance in table tennis were:

- Learning the habit of proper motor technique specific to table tennis - 34.2% / 41 cases;
- Improvement of favored, preferred tactical combinations - 26.6% / 32 cases;
- Development of combined effort in specific forms of table tennis, motor - 22.5% / 27 cases;
- Upgrading methodological tools and training materials promoting modern methods and means - 10% / 12 cases;
- the Rationalization of the means of training, the optimization of their use and promotion of items of advanced knowledge in sports training - 6.6% / 8 cases.

In addition to the items mentioned, related to the content of sports training, about 10% of the responses made reference to issues that do not pertain to the content of sports training, recording the most significant precisely because they can help to improve performance: modernization of sports equipment, better financing, motivating coaches salary and performance, facilities for athletes in social integration.

Discussion and conclusions

The sample of technicians upon who the questionnaire is applied is significant in the light of experience and technique. Subjects are placed in all four time slots considered by some authors as cycles of coach activity.

A quarter of the investigated sample is young and features in development cycle of 10 years of knowledge and practical experiments using the their own and other specialists' experience. We emphasize, however, that the majority of professionals surveyed - 62.5% - 25 cases, fall within the ages of optimal professional performance where advanced knowledge is combined with increased labor power.

The age for initial selection and classification in groups of beginners remains in question as bibliographic sources investigated in our documentation indicate the age of 6-7 years old for initial selection, while 70% of specialists included in research support ages 7-8 years and 8-9 years of age for an optimal selection. Each have their arguments:

- Bibliographic sources authors invoke the 10 years time training to achieve performance levels;
- Practitioners allege losses in the first two formative phase due to the peculiarities of human material development of children 6-7 years old who have not outlined somatic and functional elements to an extent that can be forecast during sports.

It is clear that on this issue, interdisciplinary nature wider debate and research is needed, aspects not covered by our theme.

In the components or factors of sports training, the specialists interviewed appreciate, at a convincing rate - 75%, that physical training is of high and very high importance in table tennis and to be placed among the components that should focus mainly on the sports training. If we correlated the results of questions no. 3 and 4 with those questions no. 7:12 we conclude that the liabilities questions no. 3 and 4 are based to some extent on goals and not on theoretical knowledge derived from learning to take advantage from practice.

Through its design, the questionnaire prepared by us, although not a standardized one, had some control keys able to provide information on the truth claims.

From this point of view we consider as valid the majority of responses and results obtained by processing data, as we consider necessary the research approaches, such as that done by us in a position to argue points of view through specific scientific research instruments.

In what the physical attributes are concerned, they have a meaning insofar only if taken account of the specific effort in table tennis competition, the forms of motor skills and their share in light of the specifics mentioned.

The results of the investigation show that the specialists' opinions on the priority of motor skills in table tennis are skillfulness - a 40% rate - 30% resistance - 15% and power - 15%. If athletes are in the second formative phase, the order is maintained, changing the percentages due to the particularities of age as such: Skillfulness - 45% rate - 40% resistance - 10% and power - 5%. In any vision they recognize the need and importance of physical training and the development of motor skills in specific forms of table tennis and effort adapted to the particularities of age.

The specialists questioned about the weight and share of the general physical training and multilateral physical training, specific to the formative phase two, indicate correct percentage ratios for this age, 80-20%, 70-30%, 60-40% in favor of the first forms of physical training , indicating the orientation towards increasing aerobic capacity. And at the same time, they appreciate the physical training at this age as largely in proportion of 87.5% to the medium and good qualifier, something that argues for improvement, including the experimental research. While some papers mention force as a contributing factor in the performance table tennis, specialists confirmed the views expressing force and strength to be motor qualities with a significant role, being necessary to develop them even at the age specific to the second formative stages.

References

[1]. Angelescu, N., (1977), Tenis de masă, Editura Sport-Turism, Bucureşti

[2]. Bompa, T., (2013), Antrenamentul pentru sporturile de echipă, traducere CNFPA, edit. Ad Point Promo, Bucureşti

[3]. Colibaba – Evuleţ, D., Bota, I., (1998), Jocuri sportive – teorie şi metodică, edit. Aldin, Bucucreşti, pp.

[4]. Dragnea, A.C., Mate-Teodorescu, S., (2002), Teoria sportului, Editura FEST, Bucureşti.

[5]. Nicu, A., (1993), Dezvoltarea calităţilor motrice – element esenţial în programarea antrenamentului sportiv, în Antrenamentul sportiv modern, pp. 310-392, edit. Editis, Bucureşti

[6]. Raţă, G., Raţă, C.B., (2006), Aptitudinile în activitatea motrică, edit. EduSoft, Bacău.

[7]. Simion, Ghe., Mihăilă I, Stănculescu G., (2011), Antrenament sportiv. Concept sistemic, Editura University Press, Constanţa

[8]. Triboi, V., Păcuraru, A., (2013), Teoria şi metodica antrenamentului sportiv, Editura Pim, Iaşi.

23

THE IMPACT OF ARTISTIC TRAINING ON THE EXECUTION OF SOME JUMPS IN AEROBICS

Germina-Alina Cosma, Marian Costin Nanu, Mihaela Păunescu, Forțan Cătălin

Faculty of Physical Education and Sport, Brestei Street, no.156, Craiova, România

Abstract: Aerobic performance requires a combination of technical elements and choreography. For this reason, artistic preparation is extremely important in this branch of sport. The purpose of research is to identify the impact of the means designed for artistic training on the physical and technical preparation of 12 athletes (14-15 years). Thus, for six months they had new operational models with the specific classical dance means, being tested before and after our intervention in training. Following the results achieved, significant changes in the execution of five jumps from group C, the legs force and overall coordination, differences in the initial and final means, falling within an increased significance level $p < 0.05$, were highlighted.

Keywords: group C, *performance, aerobics sport.*

Introduction

The current sport phenomenon, through the level achieved, but also through the social order tends to diversity, to efficiency, shifting the balance pan towards those branches, such as aerobics sport, that may comprise, in their area of maintaining and optimizing the physical condition and state health, broad categories of the population.

The aerobics sport causes the natural temptation of human intelligence of self-knowledge, or the human aspiration to achieve the highest level of self-awareness. The justification is found in man's unceasing desire to overcome and surpass himself in any direction, to fight and win, to find new forms of manifestation of the perfection, of supremacy. This discipline trains the capacity of assessment and self-esteem, particularly important to image the ego.

The means offered by aerobics sport is that it can make them redefine their own body image, social identity, willingness to work towards interpersonal communication. This leads to the complex education of superior moral, physical and psycho-behavioral capacity. [1]

The aerobics sport dynamism creates a special aesthetic dimension and profound and stable emotional satisfactions. Aerobic performance is a competitive sport which captivates the sports enthusiast. It is a unique combination of aerobic choreography and gymnastics elements.

It is a mixed sport, which adjusts at the level of the model, the relationships and communication between boys and girls, because of the particular distinct aspects. sport The aerobics is a useful and pleasant model of collaboration between youth, a universal communication bridge between generations.

The difficulty is one of the essential criteria of assessment and outing exercises in aerobics sports. Exercises must demonstrate a balance between the aerobics specific movements with (combinations of high and low movements) and elements of difficulty. There shall be allowed a maximum of 12 items of difficulty, harmoniously selected from all four groups from the scoring Code: Group A - dynamic force; Group B - static force; Group C - Jumping; Group D - Balance and Mobility. [2]

All the elements in Group C must demonstrate explosive force (expansion) and maximum amplitude. The jumps show the following general characteristics:

- in the air the posture must be well defined;
- while landing, the body segments must present a perfect alignment;
- with landings in push up, the hands and feet must touch the ground simultaneously, in a controlled manner;
- with elements completed in push up, the chest should not touch the ground;
- while landing in string, the hands can touch the ground;
- Landing on one leg or on two legs is considered a variation of the same element; the same is true for the detachment.

Artistic training base is formed in children through exercises borrowed from classical ballet. We opt not to insist on the perfection of technique, because we do not aim to train dancers but gymnasts and the choreographic training will be complemented by specific

physical training components of neuromuscular coordination. [3]
This extremely important aspect involves customizing the artistic preparation of gymnasts with direct influences on postural stability during execution. Stability seen as a tangible force led body control determined by movement, coordination and efficiency involves a complex interaction between sensory, mental and motor elements. [4]
The motor content will be complemented by knowledge of musical training through the basics of theory. These include musical patterns that are organized on an agogic compartment and on a dynamic one.

Materials and methods

To conduct this research, we chose a group of 12 athletes (age 14-15 years) from the National College Sports Cetate Deva, who served in aerobic sport between 3-5 years. The experiment was conducted in the 2013-2014 school year, for 6 months, the subjects were tested before and after the proposed operational models that have the preponderance of specific classical dance means. The tests were: standing long jump (to determine the strength of the lower limbs) and Matorin test (to determine the overall coordination). Also five difficulty jumps from group C (Air turn, turn tuck, pike, street and split to split) were evaluated through scoring, according to FIG scoring code.[2]

Operational Model No.1 at wall bar

1. sitting with the left shoulder to the bar, grabbed by hand on the same side, right hand on the hip: 1-4 - battement tendu forward with the right foot; 5-6 - battement tendu backward with the left foot.
2. sitting to the bar with the left shoulder, grabbed by hand on the same side, right hand on the hip: 1 - right leg bent in passe; 2 - stretching the right leg forward with the tip resting on the ground; 3 is repeated motion 1; 4- comeback.
3. standing position VI, facing the bar, grabbed with both hands: 1-4 - demi-plie; 5-6 - releve; 7 - passe with the right; 8 – return.
4. -standing position VI, facing the bar, grabbed with both hands: 1-4 - demi-plie; 5-6 - releve; 7 - passe the left foot; 8 – return.
5. standing to the bar with the left shoulder, grabbed by hand on the same side, the right arm laterally: 1 - lowering the right arm rounded; 2 - lifting forward the upper right arm, rounded; 3-4 - bending forward trunk; 5-6 - trunk return with rounded forward right arm; 7-8 - carrying forward the right arm laterally.
6. sitting in sixth position, facing the bar, grabbed with both hands: 1 - leap vertically splitting the legs and landing legs split; 2 - jump with legs brought together in the air and landing.

Operational Model no.2at wall bar

1. sitting position I, facing the bar, grabbed with both hands: 1 - bending the knees oriented outward (demi-plie); 2 - return; 3-4 - is repeated; 5-6 - complete bending of the knees (grand-plie); 7-8 - return to start position.
2. standing, position I , left shoulder to the bar, grabbed by hand on the same side, the right arm laterally: 1 - bending the knees; 2 - stretching the right leg forward resting on the tip; 3 - bent return of the right leg; 4 - stretching the knees; 5-8 repeat with the right leg laterally 1-4 - the same with the right leg extention backward; 5-8 - repeat with the right leg laterally stretching.
3. sitting in the second position with the left shoulder to the bar, grabbed by hand on the same side, the right arm laterally: 1 - orienting the right leg resting on tip; 2 - lifting the right leg at 450; 3 - lowering the leg as in time 1; 4 - return; 5-8 - the same laterally 1-4 - same backward; 5-8 - the same laterally.
4. sitting , position I, facing the bar, grabbed with both hands: 1 - bending of the right side of the trunk; 2 - return; 3-4 - the same to the left; 5-6 trunk extension; 7-8 comeback.
5. standing facing the bar, grabbed with both hands: 1 - slight bending of the knees, impulse and vertical jump; 2 - landing with knees slightly bent; 3-4 repeats; 5-6 - movements 1-4 are repeated, making the jump with a slight splitting of the legs brought together in the air and landing still legs split/apart; 7-8 jump _ legs brought together in the air and landing with feet together.

Operational Model No.3at wall bar

1. sitting in the second position facing the bar, grabbed with both hands:1-2 - large bending of the knees (grand-plie); 3-4 - return; 5-8 - 1-4 are repeated;
2. sitting in fourth position with the left shoulder to the bar, grabbed by hand on the same side, the right arm rounded down: 1 - shifting the weight on the left foot, lifting the right heel off the ground, the tip stretched on the ground (temps- lie); 2 - return;

3. sitting in the second position with the left shoulder to the bar, grabbed by hand on the same side, the right arm laterally: 1 - bending the right knee (passe); 2 - stretching it forward (horizontally); 3 - bending the right knee (passe); 4 - return to start position; 5 - bending the right knee (passe); 6 - stretching the right leg backward, horizontally; 7 - bending the right knee (passe); 8 - return to start position;
4. standing position I with the left shoulder to the bar, grabbed by hand on the same side, the right arm laterally: 1 - the right leg forward, resting on tip; 2 - laterally the right leg (tip sliding on the ground) knee taut; 3 - carry it in the same way back to the tip; 4 - return to start position; 5-8 times repeat movements from the 1-4 times; 1-8 - the same movement, starting with the leg backward
5. sitting in the second position with the left shoulder to the bar, grabbed by hand on the same side, the right arm laterally 1-2 - wave with the right arm; 3-4 - lift right arm up; 5-6 - bending the trunk forward, horizontally, 7-8 - return with right arm descent laterally; 1-2 - wave with the arm laterally; 3-4 - lifting the right arm up; 5-6 - trunk extension; 7-8 comeback lowering laterally the arm
6. sitting in the second position with to the bar the left shoulder, grabbed by hand on the same side, the right arm laterally: 1 - small jump on the left leg with the other swinging forward; 2 - small jump on the left leg keeping the right leg forward; 3 - small jump on the left leg with the right foot tapping on the lower back; 4 - small jump on the left leg, keeping the right leg backward; 5 - small jump on the left leg with the right foot tapping away forward; 6 - small jump on the left leg keeping the right leg forward; 7-8 - two small jumps on both feet.

Exercises for artistic jumps

1. Standing: 1 - vertical jump with slightly apart and landing legs slightly apart,with tips outward; 2 - vertical jump and landing, legs close together ;
2. Standing with hands on hips: 1-2 - added step elk, starting with the right foot, impulse on it, vertical jump backward with the left foot balancing, horizontally and landing on the right foot; 3-4 - the same with the left foot; 5-8 - repeat movements from 1-4 times
3. Standing, arms laterally, jump by orienting the arms forward from the baseline, upward, rounded over the head. In landing the arms descend laterally (open jump)
4. Standing with arms laterally 1-2 - changed step with the right foot, impulse on it, vertical shear jump and landing on the left foot; 3-8 - 1-2 idem
5. Standing with hands on hips: 1-4 - Running artistic steps starting with the right foot; 5-6 - impulse on the right foot, vertical shear jump; 7 - small standing vertical jump on both feet; 8 - the same with return in 180 degrees
6. Standing: 1 step on the left foot; 2 - detachment; 3 - bending the free leg, then stretching forward; 4 - return to start position. The same exercise should be performed with the other leg.
7. Fouette jump executed on the ground and jumping.

Results and Discussions

Analyzing the data obtained from Matorin general coordination test, there is a substantial increase in athletes' results from the initial testing to the final one, both in terms of turns to the right (11.9%) and those executed to the left (13%). If with the turns on the right, the string amplitude decreased from 270° (Ti) to 250°(Tf), which means a homogenization of performance around the arithmetic mean, however, the turns to the left, the direction preferred by gymnasts, following the results obtained showed that the amplitude increased slightly, but statistically significant.

Table 1. *Descriptive statistics*

Descriptive Statistics					
	N	Minimum	Maximum	Mean	Std. Deviation
Tiright	12	270.00	540.00	397.50	84.436
Tfright	12	330.00	580.00	445.00	77.518
Tileft	12	330.00	540.00	417.50	74.969

Tfleft	12	360.00	600.00	465.00	73.174
Lung.1	12	171.00	250.00	206.33	21.588
Lung.2	12	178.00	258.00	214.16	22.237
AirTurnT1	12	6.00	10.00	8.16	1.114
AirTurn2	12	7.00	10.00	8.83	.937
TurntuckT1	12	5.00	9.00	7.00	1.128
TurnTuckT2	12	7.00	9.00	7.91	.792
StradleT1	12	5.00	9.00	7.08	1.164
StradleT2	12	7.00	10.00	8.16	.937
PikeT1	12	5.00	8.00	6.16	.937
PikeT2	12	6.00	9.00	7.58	.996
SplittosplitT1	12	6.00	9.00	7.16	.834
SplittosplitT2	12	7.00	10.00	8.41	.900
Valid N	12				

The Matorin Test recorded, with the initial testing, an average of 397.5 (± 84.43 °) with the jump with turn to the right and 417.5 (± 74.96 °) to the left, with the final testing the mean values being 445 (± 77.51 °) with the turn to the right and 465 (± 73.17 °) with the turn to the left (Table 1). Applying the t test for dependent samples, there is a value t (-15.59) for the right and t (-5.39) for the left, both values falling at an increased significance level p <.001. (Table 2).

In the Long standing jump test, there is a 4% increase in performance between the two tests. Analyzing the differences obtained by the 12 athletes from the initial test with the the final one we grasp increases from 2cm to 13cm, the 8cm mean being the final, which seems to be a good value. Applying the t test for dependent samples, there is a value t (-9.61) the average difference falling within a threshold of significance p <.001. (Table 2).

In the test execution of jumps, obvious progress has been made, the differences between the initial and final averages, being statistically significant at a threshold of p <0.05.

Table 2. *Paired Samples Test*

	Paired Differences					t	Sig. (2-tailed)
	Mean	Std. Deviation	Std. Error Mean	95% Confidence Interval of the Difference			
				Lower	Upper		
Tiright - Tf right	-47.50	10.55	3.046	-54.20	-40.795	-15.59	.000
Tieft - Tifleft	-47.50	30.48	8.801	-66.87	-28.128	-5.397	.000
Lung.1 - Lung.2	-7.83	2.82	.814	-9.62	-6.039	-9.612	.000
AirTurnT1 - AirTurn2	-.666	.651	.188	-1.08	-.252	-3.546	.005
TurntuckT1 - TurnTuckT2	-.9166	.668	.193	-1.34	-.491	-4.750	.001
StradleT1 -							

StradleT2	-1.083	.792	.228	-1.58	-.579	-4.733	.001
PikeT1 - PikeT2	-1.416	.996	.287	-2.049	-.783	-4.926	.000
SplittosplitT1 - SplittosplitT2	-1.250	.753	.217	-1.72	-.77	-5.745	.000

The technical jumps (which followed the technique of five major jumps from the scoring code) basically confirmed the results obtained by the athletes in motor tests. More specifically, those who have lower values at lower limb strength testing had difficulties in implementing the proposed jumps. Also the low values obtained by some athletes in The Matorin test were reflected in the wrong execution of turns jumps. However, some athletes managed as with the final testing to correct the executions, which demonstrates that the means we used have been effective in achieving their purpose.

Although artistic training is a difficult aspect of sports training, it should be addressed by appropriate means to improve performance, especially that aerobics is a sub-branch where form is subordinated to the content that generates it. The artistic training results materialize in motor skills practice where performance is achieved with a high degree of expressiveness in order to transmit messages both to the spectators and the referees. [5]

The proposed means proved to be effective, this being readily accepted and practiced by athletes with pleasure, accompanied by a pleasant musical accompaniment. The overall coordination and the force of the lower limbs are capabilities that positively influence the technique of Group C difficulty elements.

Conclusions

The choreographic means training not only contributed to the achievement of a form of motion, which was the basis of expressiveness and correctness, but it also led to improvements in performance indices. The items were made with increased amplitude, which yielded better results in competitions.

Following the results, we believe that these tools need to be addressed with more courage and density in the training, aerobics being a sport of beauty and bodily expression.

References

[1]. HOTTING, K., RODER, B. (2013). *Beneficial effects of physical exercise on neuroplasticity and cognition,* Neuroscience & Biobehavioral Reviews, vol. 37, part.B,pp.2243-2257;

[2]. FIG, Cod de punctaj, 2013-2016, http://www.fig-aerobic.com/accesat la data de 10 octombrie, 2014

[3]. LAFONT, L., MARTIN, L. (2014) *Learning and teaching artistic physical activities: theoretical frameworks empirical researches*, Revue Internationale des Sciences du Sport et de l'Éducation Physique 2014, Vol. 35 No. 103 2014/1 pp. 39-52;

[4]. FORAN B. (2001). *High-performance sports conditioning.* Champaign:Human Kinetic;

[5]. DRAGNEA, A. (1996). *Antrenamentul sportiv*, Bucharest: Publisher Didactică şi Pedagogică, p.234;

STUDY ON TOP 100 ATHLETES IN 800 M DISCIPLINE OUTDOOR ALL TIME

Daniel GHEORGHE, Paula IVAN

Faculty of Physical Education and Sport, Spiru Haret University, Berceni road no 24, Bucharest

Abstract: Introduction. The work is part of the study sports performance, measurement and evaluation. The study is transverse type because the results obtained were collected until 31 December 2015.

Material and methods

This study analyzes the results, age, height and weight of first 100 athletes in the discipline of 800 m outdoor all time. Data were processed on the following statistical indicators: number of cases, the maximum value, minimum value, amplitude, mode, median, average, quartile 1, 3, quartile difference, dispersion, average of absolute deviation, standard deviation, coefficient of variation and correlation. As a research method we had used the case study, observation, statistics and graphics.

Results

After data processing had resulted 2 summary tables and 4 graphs.

Discussions and conclusions

The results were analyzed based on the above parameters. This resulted in the following conclusions:

- The average age is 24.33 years for men and 25.96 years for women.
- The average height is 181.02 cm for men and 168.43 cm for women.
- The average weight is 65.52 kg for men and 57.21 kg for women.

Key words: athletes, performance, statistics

Introduction

The considerable increase athletic performance in this group of disciplines its explanation in training methods, which have continually improved over the years, due to their experience of coaches and athletes and new conquests of science in training [1].

The effort that we provide middle runners fall in mixed type. In this exercise duration is between 1-3/5 minutes, so it than is necessary for anaerobic biochemical processes to provide energy for themselves, but it is shorter than the adaptation requirements of cardiac and respiratory functions, after which it can provide O2 needed just about aerobic energy release [2].

In evaluating athletes we must always take into account two fundamental components of human performance in general: the biological and psychological. In this way the body composition corresponds to the structural components of the human body composed of elements of very different nature and density (bone, fat, water, protein), maintained in constant proportion and functionally integrated [3]. In this way the precise knowledge of the athlete's height and weight and is welcome framing it in a test pattern.

Many times in the sport's practice, while coaches respected the specific training method's guideline, worked with athletes selected by the constitutional model, they did not achieved the expected performance, because they neglected psychological component. The goal of mental preparation for competitions consists in forming for athletes, of a system of attitudes and behavior, with operational and regulative character through which it is flexible and adapts to contest's situations and opponents actions [4].

It is obvious that the main objectives of the training are participating in competitions, challenge other athletes in the competition for a place in the hierarchy of sports and achieve high performance. However, the importance of the competitions passing of these purposes, because they are the most important and specific methods of estimation the progress of athlete [5].

Material and methods

This study analyzes the results [6], age, height and weight of first 100 athletes in the discipline of 800 m outdoor all time [7]. Data were processed on the following statistical indicators: number of cases, the maximum value, minimum value, amplitude, mode, median, average, quartile 1, 3, quartile difference, dispersion, average of absolute deviation, standard deviation, coefficient of variation and correlation. As a research method we had used the case study, observation, statistics and graphics.

Results

In what follows, we present the 2 tables and 4 graphs representative undertaken research.

Table 1. Statistical indicators of women athletes in the discipline 800 m

Indicators	Performance (sec)	Age	Height (cm)	Weight (kg)
N	165	164	101	101
N max	117.52	360.0	182.00	73.00
N min	11328	17.00	159.00	46.00
Amplitude	4,2.4	19.00	23.00	27.00
Mode	116	25	165	63
Median	116.21	26.00	167.00	57,00
Average	116.20	25.96	168.43	57.21
Quartile 1	115.78	23	165	54
Quartile 3	116.7	29	172	60
Quartile difference	0.92	6.00	7.00	6.00
Dispersion	0.617262	17.89452	20.58112	28.34291
Average absolute deviation	0.598841	3.482228	3.719243	4.134889
Standard deviation	0.78566	4.230191	4.536642	5.323806
Coefficient of variation	0.676106	16.29672	2.693556	9.306064
Correlation*	0.04005	-0.31318	-0.03779	-0.1182343

Table 2. Statistical indicators of men athletes in the discipline 800 m

Indicators	Performance (sec)	Age	Height (cm)	Weight (kg)
N	244	244	152	152
N max	103.86	35.00	193.00	84.00
N min	100.91	17.00	163.00	45.00
Amplitude	2.95	18.00	30.00	39,00
Mode	103.38	24	182	63
Median	103.13	24.00	182.00	63.00
Average	103.02	24.33	181.02	65.52
Quartile 1	102.79	22	175	60
Quartile 3	103.34	27	186.25	71
Quartile difference	0.55	5.00	11.25	11.00
Dispersion	0.3082	10.56603	41.26935	46.48645
Average absolute deviation	0.409911	2.605046	5.424775	5.851801
Standard deviation	0.555158	3.250543	6.424122	6.818097
Coefficient of variation	0.538894	13.35914	3.548852	10.40617
Correlation*	0.188175	0.14015	0.029018	0.17355304

* - In order from left to right: correlation between performance and age, the correlation between age and height, the correlation between performance an height, the correlation between performances and weight.

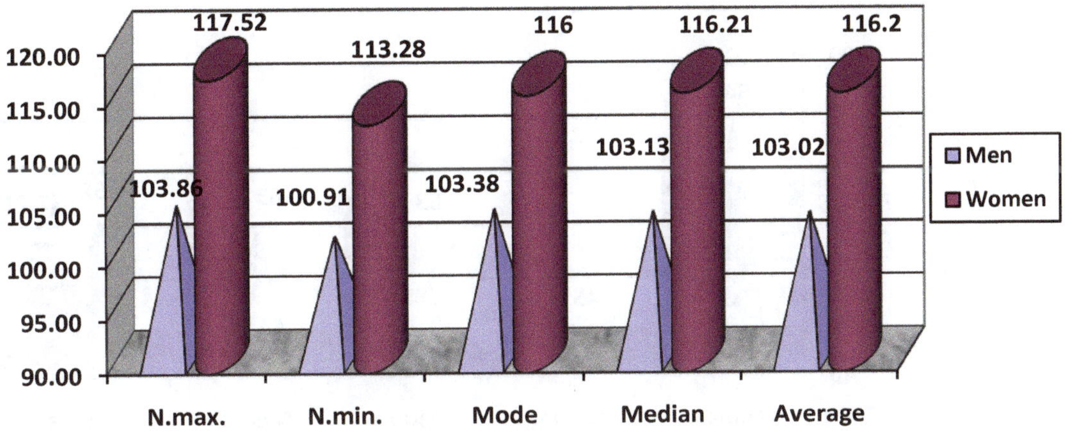

Graph 1 Statistics indicators of performances in the 800 m discipline

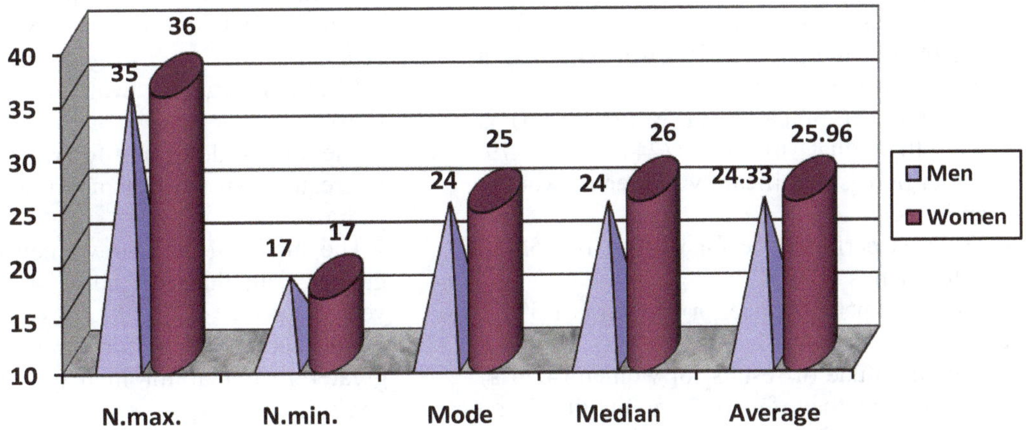

Graph 2: Statistics indicators of age in the 800 m discipline

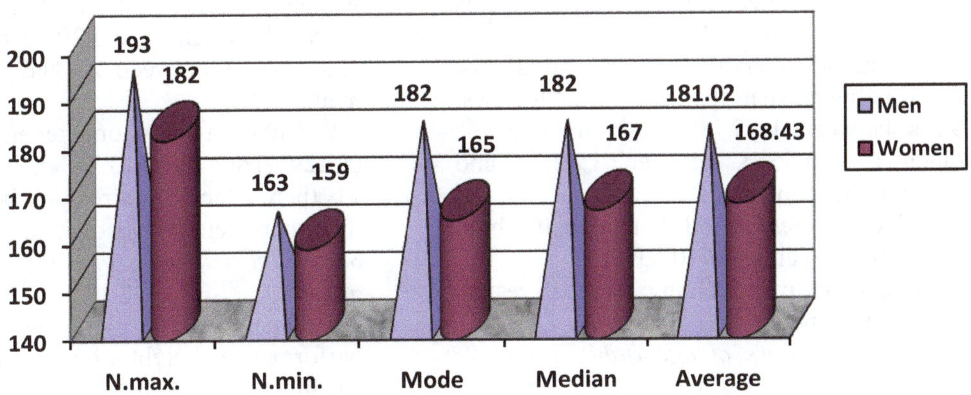

Graph 3: Statistics indicators of height in the 800 m discipline

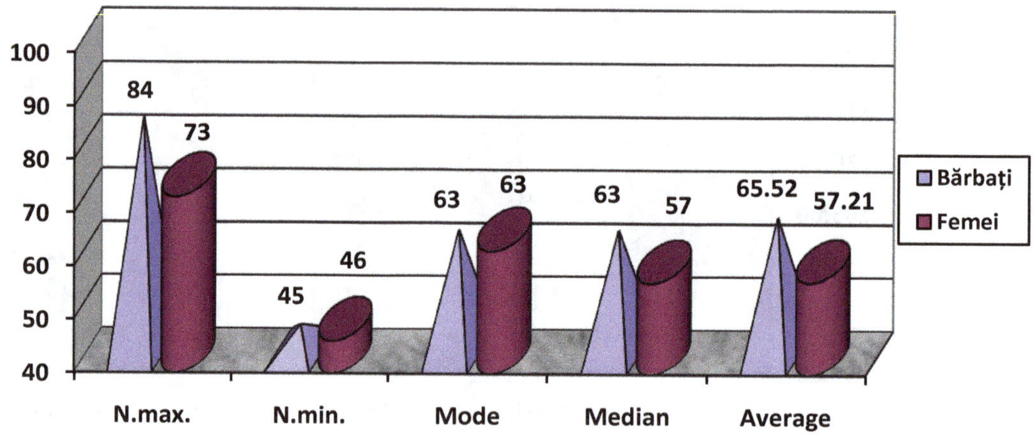

Graph 4: Statistics indicators of weight in the 800 m discipline

Discussions and conclusions

Statistical indicators of results (table 1 and 2; graph 1):

- Compared with older data [8], for best performance, in our study is lower with 0.22 s in women and 2.09 s in men.
- The number of cases for women (165) is lower than that of men (244) with 79. Competition is significantly higher in women than in men.
- The best performance for women is 1:53.28 and for men is 1:40.91.
- The worst performance for women is 1:57.52 and for men is 1:43.86.
- The amplitude of results for women (4.24 s) is greater than that of men (2.95 s) with 1.29 s.
- The mode of performances for women is 1:56.00 and for men 1:43.38.
- The median of performances for women is 1:56.21 and for men 1:43.13.
- The average of performances for women is 1:56.20 and for men 1:43.02.
- The middle interval (half of cases) for women is bigger than that of men, as follows: 0.92 s between 1:55.78 and 1:56.70 at the women and 0.55 s between 1:42.79 and 1:43.34 at the men.
- We have a very good homogeneity both women (0.67%) and men (0.53%).
- Is there a lack of correlation between results and other parameters investigated.

Statistical indicators of age (table 1 and 2; graph 2):

- Compared with older data [8], for best performance, age of women in study is 5.2 years higher (32 years as compared to 26.8 years), and in men is 2.5 years higher (24 years as compared to 21.5 years).
- The number of cases for women (164) is lower than that of men (244) with 80.
- Maximum age for women (36 years) is greater than that for men (35 years) with 1 year.
- Minimum age for women and men is 17 years.
- The amplitude of age for women (19 years) is greater than that for men (18 years) with 1 year.
- The mode of age for women (25 years) is greater than that for men (24 years) with 1 year.
- The median of age for women (26 years) is greater than that for men (24 years) with 2 years.
- The average of age for women (25.96 years) is greater than that for men (24.33 years) with 1.63 years.
- The middle interval (half of cases) for women is bigger than that of men, as follows: 6 years between 23 and 29 years at the women and 5 years between 22 and 27 years at the men.
- We have a low homogeneity both women (16.29%) and men (13.35%).
- Is there a lack of correlation between age and other parameters investigated.

Statistical indicators of height (table 1 and 2; graph 3):

- Compared with older data [8], for best performance, height of women in study is 7 cm higher (171 cm as compared to 164 cm), and in men is 1 cm higher (188 cm as compared to 187 cm).
- The number of cases for women (101) is lower than that of men (152) with 51.
- The amplitude for women (23 cm) is lower

than that for men (30 cm) with 7 cm.
- The mode of height for women is 165 cm and for men 182 cm.
- The median of height for women is 167 cm and for men 182 cm.
- The average of height for women is 168.43 cm and for men 181.02 cm.
- The middle interval (half of cases) for women is lower than that of men, as follows: 7 cm between 165 cm and 172 cm at the women and 11.25 cm between 175 cm and 186.25 cm at the men.
- We have a very good homogeneity both women (2.69%) and men (3.54%).
- Is there a lack of correlation between height and other parameters investigated.

Statistical indicators of weight (table 1 and 2; graph 4):
- Compared with older data [8], for the best female performance, the weight of women in our study is higher with 14 kg (68 kg compared to 54 kg), and in men is lower with 2 kg (71 kg compared to 73 kg).
- The amplitude of weight for women (27 kg) is lower than that for men (39 kg) with 12 kg.
- The mode of weight for women and men is 63 kg.
- The median of weight for women is 57 kg and for men 63 kg.
- The average of weight for women is 57.21 kg and for men 65.52 kg.
- The middle interval (half of cases) for women is lower than that of men, as follows: 6 kg between 54 kg and 60 kg at the women and 11 kg between 60 kg and 71 kg at the men.
- We have a good homogeneity both women (9.30%) and men (10.40%).

This resulted in the following conclusions:
- The average age is 24.33 years for men and 25.96 years for women.
- The average height is 181.02 cm for men and 168.43 cm for women.
- The average weight is 65.52 kg for men and 57.21 kg for women.

References

[1].Puică, I., 2008, Antrenamentul de semifond şi fond la fete, Reeditat de F.R.A. şi Editura Palestra, Bucureşti, p. 4-5

[2]. Nicu Al., 1993, Antrenamentul sportiv modern, Editis Bucureşti p. 203

[3]. CORDUN, M., 2011, Bioenergetică şi Ergometrie în Sport, Editura CD Press, Bucureşti, p. 87-110

[4]. HOLDEVICI, I., EPURAN M., TONIŢA F., 2008, Psihologia sportului de performanţă. Teorie şi practică, Editura FEST, Bucureşti, p. 244-270.

[5]. BOMPA, T.O., 2001, Teoria şi metodologia antrenamentului sportiv. Periodizarea, C.N.F.P.A.,Bucureşti, p. 258

[6]. www.iaaf.org 19.11.2015, 12:40

[7]. www.sports-reference.com 25.10.2015, 17:30

[8]. A.N.E.F.S. Catedra de atletism, F.R.A, 1993, Date statistice privind ultimele 8 ediţii ale Jocurilor Olimpice, f.e., Bucureşti, 42 p.

25

THE IMPACT OF RECOVERY PROCESS ON LOW BACK PAIN

Elena BUHOCIU

Spiru Haret University – Bucharest

Abstract: Background. In physical therapy, the low back pain is a common occurrence, which is why there were proposed over time, numerous scales with which to assess the pain phenomenon that would help both diagnose the initial condition, as well as predict its evolution and the effectiveness of the rehabilitation program.

Method

The study was conducted on the treatment facilities at Hotel Padiş - Felix in July 2015 with the participation of 16 patients of both genders and different age groups, the main criterion for inclusion in the study group being diagnosed back pain - subacute phase with absent or moderate radiculopathy

The patients were evaluated via the Schober Test and two specific methods: VAS for pain assessment and the Roland-Morris questionnaire, assessing perceived disability due to low back pain.

Result

Tracing the evolution of the VAS pain scale reveals that following the consistent application of the kinetic program, there was a significant decrease in pain in 13 patients, representing 81.25%, without regard to gender or age.

In assessing perceived disability (via the Roland-Morris questionnaire), all patients reported improvement of loco-regional and general conditions, although differences in scoring are more than three units in only three cases, representing 18.75%.

Conclusions

1. Studying the perceived disability scores, we find relatively modest decreases in indices, with values of 4 and over being recorded in only 4 cases (25%) and in 1 case the index value reaching 3 – i.e. approaching normality.

2. The degree of disability, which depends on the possibility of accomplishing motor acts specific to daily activities. has a smaller decrease than the pain indices themselves, but is observed among all patients.

Keywords: low back pain, VAS scale, Roland-Morris Disability Questionnaire

Background

In physical therapy, the low back pain is a common occurrence, which is why there were proposed over time, numerous scales with which to assess the pain phenomenon that would help both diagnose the initial condition, as well as predict its evolution and the effectiveness of the rehabilitation program.

Back pain can be found in people of any age, from children to the elderly. 70 -80% of adults [1] report at least one episode of back pain during their lifetime, most being treated at home, through self-medication and rest.

Its etiology varies [1], from disc causes, to inflammation or neoplastic processes. Most often, low back pain has musculoskeletal causes [2] and recovers through kinetic treatment or medical spa means.

The low back pain's evolution can take many clinical forms: acute (onset by a sudden movement or without an identifiable cause) lasting up to six weeks, subacute (persistent six to twelve weeks) or chronic (lasting over twelve weeks) [3].

Essential in recovering a painful lumbar syndrome is evaluating patients and tracking their progress throughout the kinetic treatment. We recommend that the evaluation be conducted both before applying medical treatment, to establish initial parameters and treatment goals during its deployment to assess the effectiveness of treatment, as well as at its end, to quantify the results.

The most common methods to functionally assess low back pain, assessments that are part of the arsenal of physical therapists testing joint and muscle manual. These tests are preferred because they directly assess functional gains in patients during and after kinetic treatment [4]. To study we used the spinal mobility assessment by the Schober Test for flexion and extension movements for spine [5]. According to this test, the distance between a base point at the middle of the sacrum and a point located 10 centimeters above increases up to 15 cm, after serving a maximum flexion of the trunk. The increase in the distance between the two points by less than 4 centimeters indicates a limitaton in the mobility of the lumbar spine. Similarly, one can appreciate the mobility of the spine extension, the distance reducing, normally, by less than 2 cm.

Another simple and effective evaluation method is the use of the VAS (visual analogue scale) for pain assessment - levied by a questionnaire that asks the patient to assess their disconfort level on a scale from 1 (minimal pain) to 10 (maximum pain) [6]. Values above 7 are considered severe pain and require painkiller medication [7].

Throughout the study, the Roland-Morris questionnaire was also used to assess the level of disability experienced by patients. The questionnaire contains a total of 24 items and is used to evaluate patients with low back pain, assessing the degree in which a potentially painful syndrome is affecting the patient's mobility and quality of life. The questions are directly related to current physical activity and movement limitations imposed by pain [8]. Affirmative answers score 1 point, while negative answers score 0. The higher the total score, the more severe the disability associated with a painful phenomenon is. A score of 0 (answered NO to all items of the questionnaire) indicates the absence of disability and a score of 24 (answer YES to all items) indicates that there are severe limitations of movement and activity.

Method

The study was conducted on the treatment facilities at Hotel Padiş - Felix in July 2015 with the participation of 16 patients of both genders and different age groups, the main criterion for inclusion in the study group being diagnosed back pain - subacute phase with absent or moderate radiculopathy

The patients were evaluated via the Schober Test and two specific methods: VAS for pain assessment and the Roland-Morris questionnaire, assessing perceived disability due to low back pain.

After the initial evaluation, patients conducted parallel kinetic treatment based on the Williams programs, neuro-muscular and proprioceptive facilitation techniques (Kabat methods and hold-relax) [9] and analgesic and muscle relaxant physiotherapy [10], as well as hydro-kinetic programs and received daily sessions of regional decontracturant massage.

The recovery program lasted two weeks for each patient.

Results

The study involved 16 patients, the inclusion criteria being the diagnosis of subacute low back pain with absent or moderate radiculopathy and the age between 18 and 60 years.

The patient group was composed of people of both genders, its structure is: 40% men (7) and 60% women (9) (Fig. 1).

Patients from rural areas - 4 people (25%) and urban - 12 people (75%) (Fig. 2).

Patient age ranged from 25 to 60 years, the distribution group are:

- 25-30 years → 2: 10%;
- 31-40 years → 8; 50%;
- 41-50 → 4; 25%;
- 51-60 years → 2, 10% (Figure 3).

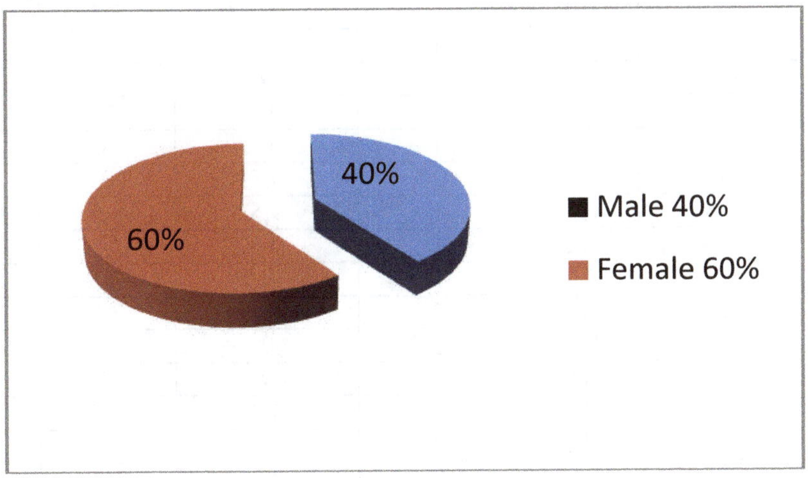

Fig. 1. Group structure by gender

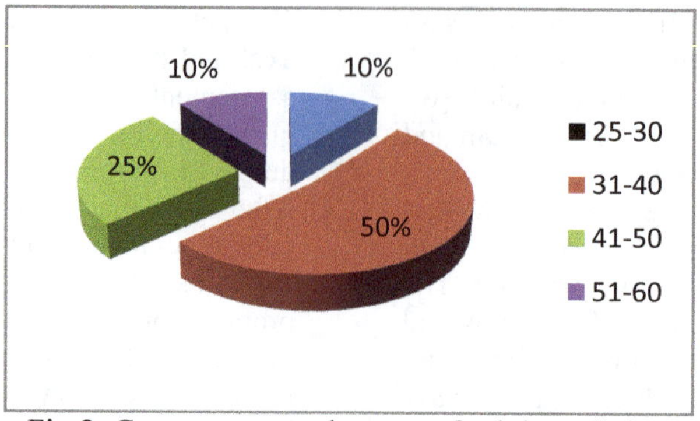

Fig.2. Group structure by area of origin or living

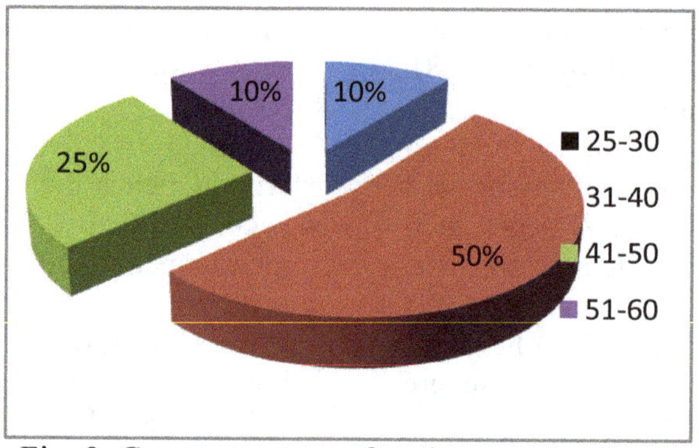

Fig. 3. Group structure after the age of patients

Regarding the evaluation of lumbar mobility in flexion and extension via the Schober test, it can be seen that in all patients, the index has changed after the recovery treatment (Table 1). Values are expressed in centimeters.

Table no. 1. Centralization of data in respect to sheet joint mobility (cm)

No.	FLEXION			EXTENSION		
	Initial	Final	Net Gain	Initial	Final	Net Gain
1.	11,5	13,5	2	9	7,5	1,5
2.	12	14	2	9	8,5	0,5
3.	11,5	12,5	1	9	7	2
4.	12	15	3	9	8	1
5.	12	13	1	9	8	1
6.	12,5	13,5	1	9	8	1
7.	11	13	2	9,5	9	0,5
8.	12,5	13,5	1	9,5	8,5	1
9.	11	12	1	9.5	7,5	2
10.	12	13	1	9	8	1
11.	12	14	2	9	7,5	1,5
12.	11,5	13,5	2	9	7	2
13.	13	15	2	9	7	2
14.	11	12	1	8,5	7,5	1
15.	12	14	2	9	8	1
16.	12,5	14,5	2	8,5	7,5	1

Tracing the evolution of the VAS pain scale reveals that following the consistent application of the kinetic program, there was a significant decrease in pain in 13 patients, representing 81.25%, without regard to gender or age.

In assessing perceived disability (via the Roland-Morris questionnaire), all patients reported improvement of loco-regional and general conditions, although differences in scoring are more than three units in only three cases, representing 18.75%.
Tabulation assess patients through two questionnaires is shown in Table no. 2.

Table no. 2. Evaluation by perceived perception of pain and mobility

No.	VAS Score			Roland-Morris Score		
	Initial	Final	Net Gain	Initial	Final	Net Gain
1.	5	5	0	12	9	3
2.	7	4	3	10	8	2
3.	6	6	0	10	9	1
4.	5	3	2	9	6	3
5.	5	4	1	8	6	2
6.	5	2	3	6	3	3
7.	5	4	1	9	5	4
8.	7	2	5	12	6	6
9.	7	5	2	10	8	2
10.	7	4	3	10	7	3
11.	8	5	3	11	6	5
12.	7	4	3	10	7	3
13.	6	6	0	10	7	3
14.	8	5	3	13	10	3
15.	5	4	1	11	9	3
16.	5	2	3	13	9	4
Average	6	4	2	10	7	3

Discussion

Analyzing the group of patients' parameters, we observed:

- In the studied group, low back pain occurs with higher frequency in female patients (60%);
- The most affected age group is the 31-40 years, followed by the 41-50 years group;
- Environment and lifestyle certainly influence the phenomenon, a painful lumbar spine condition will have a higher incidence in the urban population;
- Limited mobility was observed in all patients, both in flexion and in extension, their condition is improving after treatment, but none has reached the normal values of the Schober test;
- Analysis of VAS scores indicate less pain in 13 cases (81.25%) and 3 cases are being described as having the same intensity;
- From studying the evolution of perceived disability scores, we observed a decrease in median scores (from 6-13 to 3-10).

Conclusions

1. Low back pain is more common in females.
2. Pain greatly influences the mobility and the perceived disability, all study subjects reporting restricted mobility due to the painful musculat contractions.
3. The subjective component of pain is responsible for resistance to treatment - which negatively impacts the effectiveness of the recovery process.
4. Studying the perceived disability scores, we find relatively modest decreases in indices, with values of 4 and over being recorded in only 4 cases (25%) and in 1 case the index value reaching 3 – i.e. approaching normality.
5. The degree of disability, which depends on the possibility of accomplishing motor acts specific to daily activities, has a smaller decrease than the pain indices themselves, but is observed among all patients.

References:

[1]. Cohen SP, Argoff CE, Carragee EJ (2008). *Management of low back pain*. *BMJ* **337**: a2718. PMID 19103627 // in https://ro.wikipedia.org/wiki/Dorsalgie_joas%C4%83 02.10.2016;

[2]. Borczuk, P. (2013). *An Evidence-Based Approach to the Evaluation and Treatment of Low Back Pin in the Emergency Department. Emergency Medicine Practice* in http://

02.10.2016www.ebmedicine.net/topics.php?paction=showTopic&topic_ id=371 //02.10.2016;

[3]. Manusov EG (2012, sept. 1). *Evaluation and diagnosis of low back pain*. Prim. Care 39 (3): 471–9. in https://ro.wikipedia.org/wiki/Dorsalgie_joas%C4%83//02.10.2016;

[4]. Cordun, M. (2009) *Kinantropometrie*. Bucureşti: Editura CD Press;

[5]. Rednic, S., Muntean, L. (2008) *Rheumatic diseases: the unnoticed elephant in the room. Editorial.* The journal of Rheumatology 35:1. Accessed in http://event-consulting.ro/uploads/files/Lombalgia.pdf//02.10.2016;

[6]. Hawker,G.A., Mian, S., Kendzerska, T., French, M. (2011) *Measures of Pathology and Symptoms*. Arthritis Care & Research >Vol 63 Issue Supplement 11. November 2011. Pages S240–S252;

[7].Grant, S., Aitchison, T.,Henderson, E., Christie, J., Zare, Sh., Mc Murray, J. Dargie, H. (1999) *A Comparison of the Reproducibility and the Sensitivity to Change of Visual Analogue Scales, Borg Scales, and Likert Scales in Normal Subjects During Submaximal Exercise.* Elsevier. Volume 116, Issue 5, November 1999, Pages 1208–1217;

[8]. MAPI Research Institute. *Summary of translation method used by*, 27 rue de la Villette, 69003 Lyon, France accessed in http://www.rmdq.org/downloads/Romanian%20MAPI%202004.doc//02.10.2016;

[9]. Drăgan, C.F., Pădure, L. (2015) *Metodologie şi tehnici de kinetoterapie*. Bucureşti: Editura Naţional;

1. Popescu, A. (2009) *Durerea lombară joasă – prima parte*. Articole de specialitate. Accessed in http://dralinpopescu. ro/2009 /durerea-lombara-joasa.html//02.10.2016.

26

SIGNIFICANCE OF EDUCATIVE VALUES OF SPORT IN FORMING PERSONALITY AND HUMAN SOCIALIZATION

Constantin PEHOIU

Valahia University of Târgovişte / Research Centre for Environmental Study, Habitat, Motor Activities and Leisure (Romania)
Corespondence adresse: cpehoiu@yahoo.com

Abstract: Philosophically speaking, the man as element of the natural environment has always related to bonding with the environment. This relation materializes in the nature's supremacy over man, of the one hand, and in what man can do with his own body, of the other hand. We can therefore explain why man, in his evolution, needed and still needs philosophy, the way which allowed him to find or formulate answers to what is fundamental for the meaning of life.
Sociological studies which are centred on the human body consist nowadays in an inventory of the fundamental themes which take into consideration: the way the body was represented, the social and physical space occupied by the body, shapes that the body takes; the manner in which it is socially integrated; body restricting methods; effects of the social changes over the body; its sexuality and experiences which the body goes through.
Components of the educative and formative undertaking, physical education and sports meet, through purpose, objectives, finalities and content, the essential needs of life in community and favour group integration by assimilation of some ethical and aesthetical values such as respect of others, of the law (rules, regulations), discipline (self-discipline), beauty of the physical gesture and implicitly of the sports show. Competition in sports represents a confrontation between two or several personalities mainly conducted on the basis of a physical language doubled by a volitional and emotional background. The competition between two or several athletes represents both a superior expression of their physical capacity and an activity which fully involves their personality.
Key words: personality, socialization, capacity, competition, perspectives

1. Introduction

It is a known fact that the connection between the mental and the physic is biunique and of mutual influence. For the problems approached, this very relation is essential, as the social behaviour of all individuals is mostly conditioned by some of their personality features. Certainly, the individual's socialization is also supported, more or less, by sport – by physical activity in general, considering the fact that social contacts, in their totality, participate to achievement of this process. The causes and maybe even the mechanisms which favour such undertaking are of interest (the movement ensures progress of individual features identified as essential for the society or, more precisely, the social characteristics of sport are the one favouring the evolution of socialization of people who practice a branch of or a sport).

The personality represents a synopsis of the psychological and individual particularities which lead to specific manifestations, from person to person. People are different and education plays in this case a special role, as it influences the dynamic forces, the needs and the motivation. The analysis of the education-motivation relation highlights that the reasons are most times assimilated to some internal causes or impulses, of the one hand, and some behaviours of the individual, of the other hand. In addition, the reasons are associated to emotional psychical processes. They confer satisfactions, contentment, confidence, optimism and personal achievements.

The individual's interest in sport activity is supported by meeting certain needs, interests and ideals such as: staying healthy, need for movement, for walks, for exploration and contemplation of the natural environment, safety or prophylaxis in terms of physiological matters, the need to be with other people, to have personal achievements, to be competent, to receive approval and recognition of the others, the need for beauty, for order, for symmetry, the need for self-achievement along with the need for capitalization of one's own potential and a.s.o. The sociological studies offer interesting ideas on how sport activities may influence the social domain as well as aspects regarding individuals' socialization and forming of their personality. The sociologists define sport activities as activities through which people may experiment new behaviours in sensibly different conditions. These activities are often regarded as means which may prepare successful performance of other future activities.

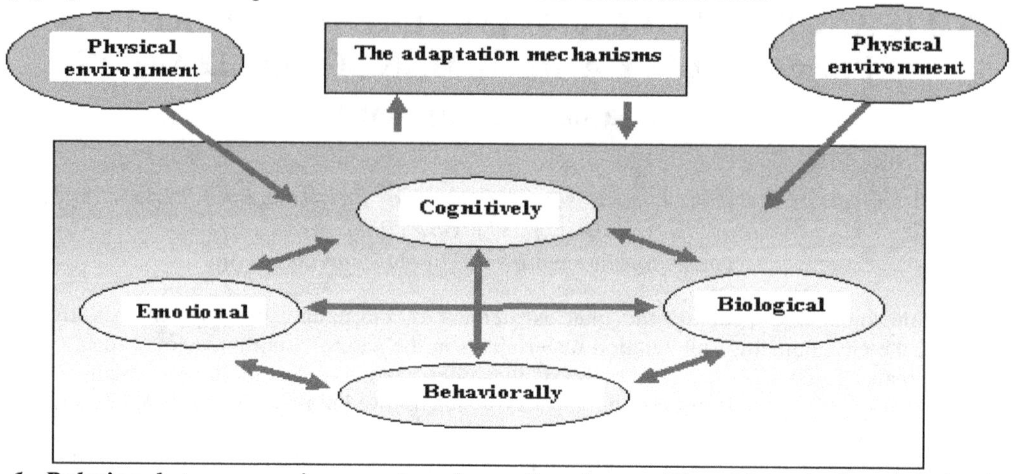

Diagram 1. Relation between environment and emotional, cognitive, biological and behavioural spheres

What seems to be less known and, more importantly, insufficiently substantiated from a scientific, psychological and pedagogical point of view, is the application of the principle of stability and continuity of the human interaction in the diversified environment of the sport activities. The individual becomes aware of the integrator aspect and the ethical valences of the sport activities which trigger new mobilizations in terms of motivation in relation to practice and participation to organizing and performing such activities. These reasons of which range is rather wide may represent the individual's personality, his or her convictions and even passions.

The individual/human subject may be studied and understood cognitively, emotionally, behaviourally and biologically. The personality may therefore be defined as a distinct cognitive, emotional, behavioural and biological pattern of a person which: (a) defines his or her personal style; (b) influences his or her interactions with the environment (diagram 1.).

2. Sport Values

The value represents the dominant norm to which the individual relates in classification of the situations specific to his or her action space which means that it conditions the goal of the person, his or her means to achieve it as well as the strategies to accept the effects triggered by achieving this goal. As a fundamental criterion of socialization, the intrinsic value takes a central place in the structure of the human personality and explicitly orients the sphere of attitudes, judgments and actions of every one of us, because, in a certain way, values manifest themselves in attitudes and attitudes in their turn appear to have instrumental features in relation to values. The closer to the core of the motivational system the values are, the more directly they cause and guarantee defence processes and expressions of ego.

In terms of sport values, the concept of *olympism* expresses, in the most conclusive manner, the existence and development of such values. Seen as life philosophy, *olympism* promotes the fundamental values of mankind – truth, good, beauty, freedom, happiness and justice transposed in fair-play, physical beauty and the beauty of the movement act, tolerance, success in sport, desire to win, self-improvement, perseverance, responsibility, confidence, behavioural balance, fight against vices of modern society, peace promotion, use of knowledge etc. In the light of their diversity, some values specific to sport activity may be interpreted as belonging to the category of vital, moral, aesthetic, economic, political, legal and even religious values. Nevertheless the categories of sport values, irrespective of them including interest, desire to win, to perform well, may be considered the instruments through which the other ones, recognized as values-purpose, may be expressed. Despite the fact that in case of sport values the interpersonal relations no longer represent a purely disinterested act, they should not manifest themselves beyond the categories of values-purpose.

Bănciulescu V. (1986) presents a picture of the

values which may be promoted through sport and sports competition, insisting on their importance in social life and highlighting the athletes' strength of character, their efforts, restrictions and volitive character. "Sportsmen and sportswomen educated in a healthy moral environment, in line with a code of conduct which originates directly in the life principles and norms, have open paths towards a dignified conduct in society" [1].

In a sociological approach, Neacşu I., Ene M. (1987), arguments the psycho-sociological side of the physical education and sport starting from three main functions: the physical education and sport represent "a conviction which raises the sport to the level of art"; the sport is an education, "possibly of the concrete one, more authentic". It forms characters; the sport "is culture as it outlines profound values in space and in time", a culture, it is true, tributary to another set of governing laws. In the authors' opinion, the sport represents "a sui generis synthesis of cultural, moral, aesthetic, social and educational values" [2]. R. Cited by the same authors in 1987, Guillamain believes that the reciprocal actions of aesthetic and ethic values are defining in this area; the sport is the "decisive expression of morality, bearer of the fundamental values of man, of social groups and of society in the global meaning of the term".

Bâtlan I. (2000) approaches the problems of sport values from an axiological point of view and puts together a classification of these issues compared to moral values and unanimously valid values, as follows:

➢ sport values versus moral values – human creations – the former emerge in the specific sphere of competitions whereas the latter characterise the natural, ordinary human relations (moral values such as honesty, correctness, dignity etc. which turn into sport fair play);

➢ sport values versus aesthetic values – the values in the second category come to life and express themselves in large existential environments (these values are active, have a spiritual character, are disinterested, have a unitary purpose and a preponderantly autonomous or heteronomous character), unlike the sport values which are specific to sport school lines of study, of the playful activities, namely agonistic (spiritual – desire to improve; material – physical strength, vitality; they correspond to an interest – the desire to win, to perform well; they are also active; with their help the individual wants to acquire a professional and social statute; therefore, they may be autonomous and heteronomous at the same time).

➢ specific sport values, fair-play representing a high rank value in the axiology of the sport values [3].

Davis E. and collaborators (1991) refer to the following categories of corporal activity values: a) instrumental values, linked to physical performances – development, health/condition, abilities, dexterity; b) economic, the values useful in everyday life and valid for society – preparation for work, free time, ergonomics, sport and leisure, defence, health; c) humanistic values which are the fundament of the complete development of personality, as well as moral personal success, code of conduct, leading possibilities, availability for action and socialization, at emotional level – social feelings, control and expression, insecurity and collaboration, capacity to make the right decisions; d) quality of life which exceeds normality in terms of awareness and commitment in activity: aesthetic taste, vitality, commitment, competition with one's ego, competition with others, creativity [4].

René Maheu (1977) considers that physical education and sport are social activities tightly related to culture and civilisation, capable to enrich the human patrimony and to contribute to a reasonable development of the body and human sensitivity. This is the reason why he pleads that they are more closely linked to the educative process [5]. In his turn, J. Piaget (1970) pinpoints the role of movement in the development of cognitive human mechanisms with children and refers to the unity of action and intelligence in its operational aspect. He concludes that all cognitive mechanisms rely on motility and the process of knowledge is primarily an action on the object, which implies in its roots a permanently motor dimension represented at the highest levels [6]. Similar opinions are expressed by some authors who study social functions of the physical education and sport. In his analysis of the place taken by physical education and sport activities in relation to contemporary culture and the interrelation between these activities and work, Magnane (1964) highlights their importance in terms of means to develop culture for adaptation to work and to influence towards an optimal social behaviour, as well as a manner to form the social and sociability instinct [7]. Other authors, i.e. F.W. Cozens, F.S. Strumpf, G.A. Boucher lay emphasis on the role of the physical education and sport in the influence and development of social relations, stating that the "sport influences relations between classes, interests and connections between them and contribute therefore to the development of integration forces which are important to maintain a democratic way of life" [8].

3. Human Personality in Social Context

The evolution of the human society has seen a succession of waves rolling and changing. It needs an answer to the question ""where does the crest of this wave take us?". The human species would be the result of three waves of changes which each influences and destroys previous cultures and civilisations by propulsion of some new ways of life considered unconceivable by our predecessors in their lifetime [9, 10].

Upon birth man is deprived of personality. Man becomes a personality. Upon birth, man is a candidate to acquisition of this attribute. This acquisition occurs in time, under the influence of many factors [11]. The process of personality forming is not uniform and continuous. It is abrupt and disrupted, with qualitative leaps and potential limitations [12]. Although the process of personality structuring and forming is long, complex, multiphasic and plurifactorial and ranges throughout the individual's lifetime, there are some ages when this process is more heightened. The personality is explained through the multitude of its social determinants, interpreted as various statuses and roles which provide behaviour models. Along these lines, Gordon Allport (1991) appreciates that the interpretation of the social role is a point of the intersection between the personality system (an appanage of psychology) and the social system, as favourite area of sociology and anthropology [13].

The social status represents the position held by an individual in one of the social system dimensions, and is expressed by profession, sex, age etc. It defines the social identity, the explicit role, the rights and obligations of the individual whereas the social role designates a model of conduct associated to a social position. In order to exercise a certain social role, all individuals have to have rights and obligations attached to their position. The system of roles and statuses is constituted as social behaviour learning models [14]. On the other hand, the individual becomes a proper personality which meets several criteria (Table 1).

Table 1. Personality achievement criteria [15]

No	Criteria
1.	becomes aware of the world, of the others and himself/herself;
2.	elaborates a proper personal system of representations, conceptions, reasons, goals, attitudes, convictions, in relation to the world and himself/herself;
3.	carries out socially useful and recognized activities;
4.	makes, affirms and arguments grounded valuable judgments;
5.	creates social values, turns from a consumer into a producer of values and performs an activity in line with his/her creative essence;
6.	has a well-outlined moral noble, coherent profile which enables him/her to devote to some ideas and ideals and to militate for turning them into reality;
7.	has formed a control and self-control capacity in harmony with the significance of the situations, with their permissive and restrictive requirements; has a highly emotional life, mastering what he/she believes and does, consciously taking responsibility and accepting consequences of his/her actions;
8.	integrates harmoniously and proves to be useful in society;
9.	is able to draw attention to himself/herself and get recognition of the others;
10.	may be taken as model in forming other personalities.

Conceived as a system of interactions and progress, all interpersonal relations imply an alternation between the phases of the relative balance and the phases of the improvement balance. Going from one level of balance to the other implies a permanent adaptation, attained through an effort of accepting requirements of this evolution, new attitudes, ideas or feelings of the other. In the self-adjusting process, there emerge three psychological factors which bring about complementary effects, such as:

➢ the first factor, of *to-have* nature, is *self-confidence* which relies on proper competence and positive past experiences of the person;

➢ the second factor, of *to-be* nature, is *self-esteem,* associated with the *self-image* and closely linked to respect for the fundamental social values;

➢ the third factor is of *social* nature and is external to the person as it belongs to the others. This is about his/her appreciation in the meaning of valuable judgment and refers to the interaction between person A and person B, the interpersonal behaviour. The interpersonal relation creates meaning and its functioning is briefly represented in diagram 2.

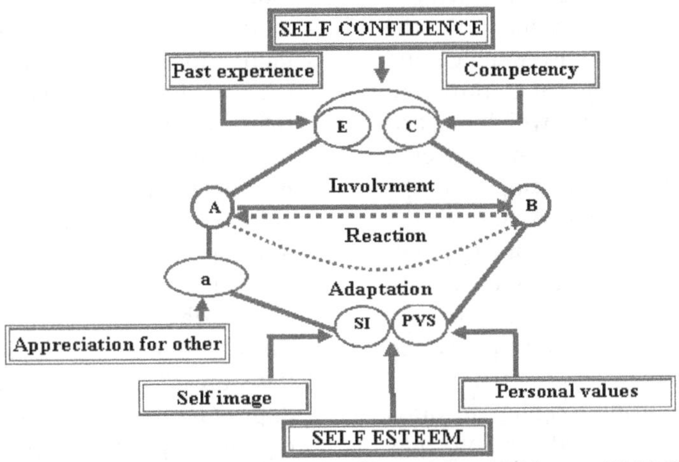

Diagram 2. Adapted from R. Chappuis, 1986, pp. 55 [16]

4. The Sport - socialisation environment

Socialization is the process by which individuals learn skills, attitudes, values and behaviours which make them able to participate as members of the society in which they live. This process is complex and takes a lifetime, which facilitates the transition from one role to the other throughout it.

The sport is deemed to be an environment which contributes to the individuals' socialization process, similar to family, colleagues and friends, school, communities and mass-media. The advantage of the sport is represented by capitalization of the role played by the body and mind. Socialization occurs through movement and the effect of this movement on the development of the personality of the one hand and the nature of the social relations provided by the diversity of the sport branches of the other hand. Thus the sport confers the individual the possibility to assume roles, to understand the necessity of complying with various norms to which he/she should willingly subject, to develop the self-esteem and the identity of his/her ego and to bond with the others. Additionally, one thinks that the cultural values, attitudes and individual and social behaviours learned through physical education are transferred to other spheres of life [17, 18].

Patriksson G. (1995) speaks about sport in terms of a social model establishing contacts, as an institutional reality with social features typical of a modern society, which intertwines with other institutions of this society and thus influences most of its members. This bespeaks the ampleness and the significance of the phenomenon to which we refer in the socialization process, process which widely represents an endeavour by which the members of a society become active participants inside it, throughout their lives. The popularization of the sport as means of the individual's formation, particularly among children and young people, emphasizes the substantiation of the goal, its contents of many norms and values specific to a certain society. Therefore, sport specifically contributes to spatial and temporal propagation of these values without excluding, evidently, the development of skills, knowledge, norms and values typical of this area [19].

The phenomenon to which we refer in this study has seen, in its long evolution, a continuous development, although, in some stages of society development, the manner of understanding its effects on the body has not surfaced pointedly, as a theoretic and practical ensemble. The physical exercise has however spread and we find it in various areas of manifestations of human activities. For instance, it exists in medical recovery, in institutionalized forming of children and teenagers, as a means of military training, not to mention its permanent use in sport training, in sport competitions, in leisure activities a.s.o. This wide conceptualization has led in the same stages of human society development, to new landmarks in understanding the phenomenon of physical exercise practice and has spread in most human and profound human activities, up to the ones which most of us know today as a starting point in the social, economic and technological development. As a specific form of man's action in general, the physical exercise goes beyond a starting point, it designates a social process, a concrete reality in the process of becoming, marked by the evolution of each social and economic formation [20].

The man's aspirations and longings towards a model of behaviour and action has determined keeping in the sphere of human values the ones which have proven priceless and durable in all areas, with a view to social integration under all aspects – physical, intellectual, moral, aesthetical, where the sport activity forms part of such aspects. It is actually known that every society projects a certain type of personality, as expression of the integrality of the social relation existing at a specific and well determined historic moment. As one may conclude, sport activities, conceived as a *sine qua-non* condition of the individual's formation, always developed by practice and theory throughout society development, are nowadays considered as integrants of permanent education. In this context, considered even global, it is necessary that the modern individual becomes the *sports man* permanently concerned with quality and performance, as a result of the desiderata on his/her physical development at all moments of his/her activities, for personal hygiene and implicitly on increasing his/her life expectancy.

In Epuran M.'s opinion (2005), the functions of the body activity (Tab.2) and all relating aspects are fully compliant with the ideal of the *modern man*'s development and formation, the integrating psychological and social aspects harmonising with the ones regarding provision and development of health, of psychological and motility development, of conveying values and traditions, improvement of social performance in order to reach a superior level of life quality [21, 22]. By the sphere of influence and behaviour targeted, the functions above are in line with objectives on structural development of the body, some at motility level, others at psychological and motility level, cognitive, or objectives at motivational and emotional and volitive level.

In a document published in 1992, the International Society of Sport Psychology tackles from a psychological point of view the beneficial effects produced by physical activity throughout times of growth and development of the individual by fruition of the unity between body and mind, which means favouring formation of personality. These effects are highlighted by positive transformations in terms of forming and improving self-esteem, development of thinking, positive approach of situations, elimination of stress and anxiety, increase of confidence in own power, self-appreciation, reduction of energy consumption and implicitly increase of performance, positive emotions and feelings a.s.o. [23]

The importance of movement, of playing, in relation to learning to socially cohabit as a child, is incontestable, all its forms give the children the possibility to accept various social roles and to learn important functions in a large social context. Cited by Sage G.H. (1986), Mead G.H. (1934) asserts that playing may be considered a powerful factor with a supporting role in the child's socialization throughout evolution in his/her life towards maturity, aspect which may undoubtedly be seen in real life. The child "*takes over and plays roles existing both in the immediate world and in the large social world, and, while embodying such roles, he or she learns to come out of himself or herself, and to therefore develop a reflection of his or her own as a social object different from the others and yet connected to them (...)* along with other factors, playing represents the form, the method and the means necessary "*to socially adapt during childhood and serves as a basis for the adult's manifestation inside society*" [18].

Table 2. Functions of education and sport – acc. to Dragnea A. and collab., 2000, p. 123 [22]

No	Sphere of Influence	Functions of Physical Education	Functions of Sport
1.	biological and sanogenetic	function to optimise the biological potential and the potential of improving health;	function to maximize the biological potential, in line with requirements of sport branch and to reduce the effects of unilateral or excessive effort;
2.	capacity of movement	function to develop psychological and motility capacity;	function to develop performance capacity
3.	psychosocial	function to develop intellectual, moral, volitive quality; socialization function;	function to outline (improve) the mental profile of a test, sport branch; agonistic function; function of excellence;
4.	cultural	function to convey spiritual and material values, function to reflect physical activities as cultural acts; function to develop aesthetical qualities (body and movement);	function to convey traditions, rituals, moral values (fair-play); function to capitalise result of science in this area; function of show of sport branches; function of symbol of the sport Olympic ideal;
5.	economic and leisure	function to improve professional and school performance; function to spend free time in an organized pleasant manner; function to support professional integration;	Functions relating to the following aspects: investments, creation of jobs, development of a sport industry;

Compared to the childhood age, when the socialization process through sport is conducted rather automatically and sometimes instinctively, through playing, and the teenage time under the impulse of the desire to stand out and impress the people of the same age, the adults' interest in the physical activity is more complex and various; the distinction is now made between the professional sport activity and the leisure sport activity, specific to ordinary people. In harmony with such approach, one thinks that even the results are much more various, they target the respect to oneself, the body concept and the image, self-control, self-evaluation, discipline, responsibility, a better physical training, better communication and relations with other people, professional success, better free time management, abandonment of some habits, all these being reflected in a higher quality of life. With regards to issues involving elderly, the discussion may be adapted in two directions: the first refers to elimination of the quality of vital functions and increase of exposure to becoming sick whereas the second relates to change in the social status – retirement, sometimes very difficult to accept and which may trigger various dysfunctions, from partial isolation to depression, anxiety, abuse of alcohol and medication etc. The sport activity may have an important role and contribute to slowing down functional degradation of the body in favour to an optimal health, to keeping the concept of oneself and self-awareness, may positively and directly influence the social contacts of the elderly people, increasing their high spirits and decreasing their depressive condition, etc. In addition, sport represents an important environment of the socialization process which aims people with special needs and supports social integration of different categories of delinquents.

Attitudes are most times the consequence of one person's manifestation to another, manifestation which may be emotionally appreciated. In case of performance athletes, as a result of their autonomously conducted training, one may speak of a reduced negative attitude and an increased positive attitude in relation to their coach, manager, other athletes, public etc. By analogy, one may consider that the people who practice sport regularly, in an organized or disorganized manner, have the possibility to change their negative behaviour in favour of the positive behaviour, namely to become self-confident and to easily, independently detach from certain adverse pressures coming from other people, be such pressures real or imaginary.

Relying on the tradition manifested in the research of the sport socialization, Patriksson G. (1995) affirms that one may make the difference between *socialization through sport* and *socialization through* or *supported by sport*. The distinction emerges upon analysis of the socialization support by sport, because the usefulness of practising a sport is usually pinpointed in terms of the effects on the other areas of life – the degree of transferability of attitudes, skills, rules and norms learned in sport to other domains of activity. *Socialization in sport*, as asserted by the author cited, refers to what is acquired in sport by each person who practises sport, without targeting precisely the usefulness beyond its area. Due to the analytical characteristics, such differentiations are not accessible at any time, socialization is characterized in reality by a permanent dynamism, in the sense that the feelings, experiences, skills and habits assimilated in a specific time of one's life tend to influence what will happen later, in a new stage. Consequently, the anticipative socialization in family, in playing groups and groups of friends, may confer a partial answer on the causes determining certain children to start practising a sport branch, while others do not, and similarly on why there are differences between active and non-active people in relation to practising a sport [19].

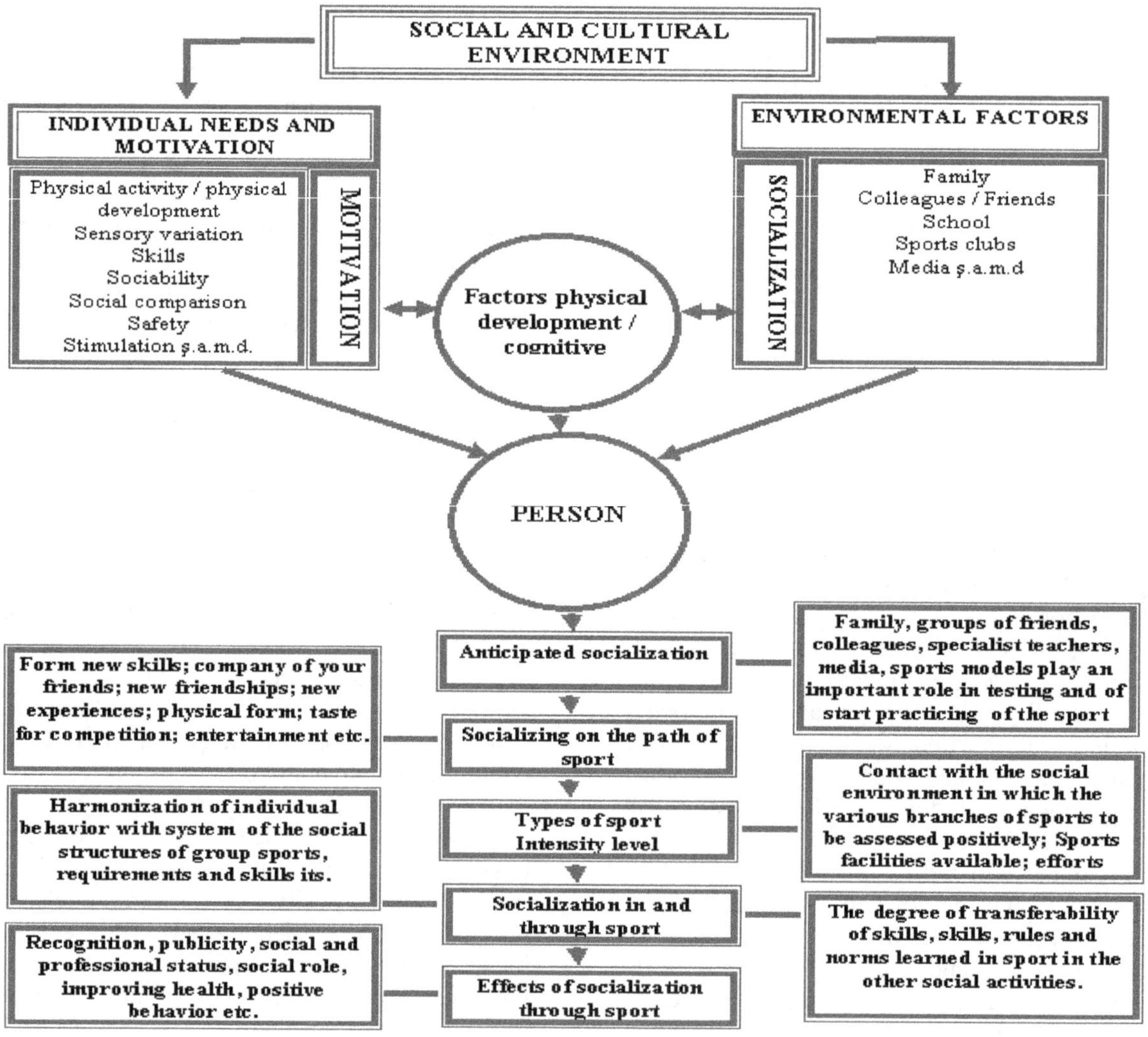

Diagram 3. Schematic model of the socialization process through sport by Patriksson G., 1995 [19], improved by us

The existence of the human being is primarily corporal and it is a component of a society with the same characteristics, affected by its experiences, values and norms of the culture to which it belongs. This is the explanation for the multitude of ideas which seek to render the body meaningful, from one society to another. The body has nowadays ceased to be perceived as a normal fact of life, a biological entity. It represents now what we must *model* instead of simply accepting. The appearance, form and dimensions of the body are open to most various reconstructions, depending on what every person desires in line with the cultural requirements of the time and the place.

The sociological researches focused on the human body comprise today an inventory of fundamental themes which consider among others: the manner in which it was represented; social and physical space it occupies; forms under which it expresses itself; manner in which it is socially integrated; restricting methods; effects of social changes; sexuality and own experiences. Reading literature takes us to the definition of a fundamental concept, i.e. body image – "the representation which the subject makes about his or her body, the manner in which the body appears to the subject, more or less consciously, in a social and cultural context particularized by personal history" [24]. From this point of view, one may see that at present many individuals of both sexes, who belong to societies considered developed, are dissatisfied with their physical appearance, especially the dimensions and the shape of their body. Therefore, the women are the ones who stand out as they are more interested in changing their physical appearance. Most times, women try to achieve this objective through diets or extreme methods of weight control, including starvation, voluntary elimination of ingested food, abuse of laxatives and diuretics or extreme physical exercises which sometimes lead to nutrition dysfunctions recorded much more often in case of women than of men. Therefore, it is useful to situate the body image issues as well as the nutrition issues, depending on their gravity, on a continuum. The desideratum is to find a good body image and self-esteem at one end of this continuum and an inventory of the nutrition diseases at the other end.

The development of a body image in different manners has determined increased interest to detect the factors which contribute to their formation and which continue with appropriate body modelling. Some of these factors are judgments and comments from the other people, sexual and racial harassment, stigmatization, *gender* stereotypes and socialization, social and cultural values which are predominant yet not permissive, physical changes during puberty, menopause, pregnancy, violence, certain life and work conditions, diseases and disabilities a.s.o. Among these factors, one must remember the social and cultural factors relating to the body image, namely the cultural pressure to relate to the ideal of socially-accepted physical beauty; sex and socialization stereotypes; exposure to messages conveyed by mass-media.

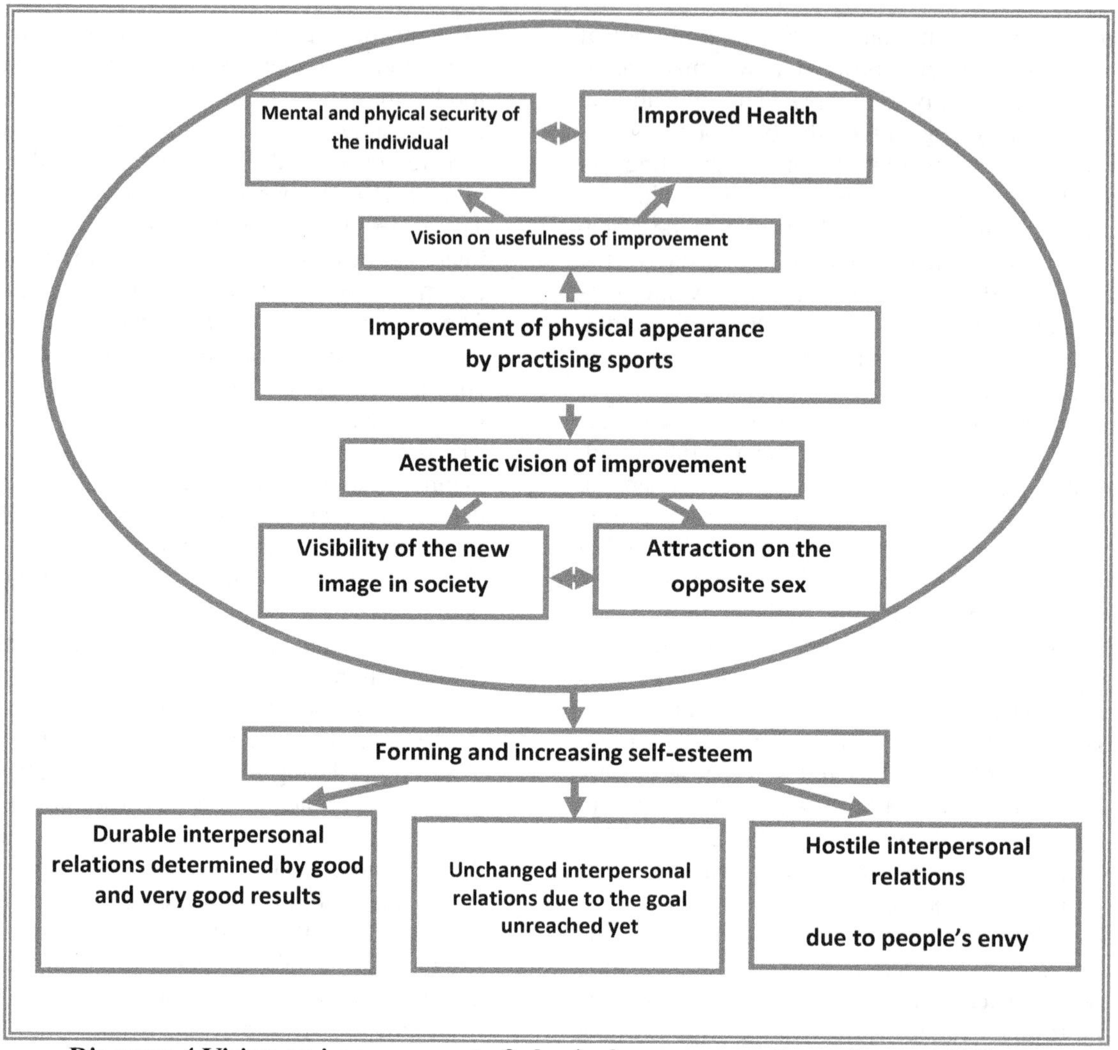

Diagram 4 Vision on improvement of physical appearance through sport [25]

4. Conclusions

Benefiting of a well structured network in contemporary civil society, the sport confirms its social importance, which is also obvious if we look at the increasingly number of people who practice sport, the public support and the economic impact manifested. Component of the educational endeavour, the sport promotes both respect for moral values, through the concept of *Olympism*, and essential values of life in collectivity, favouring social integration through assimilation of such values by the members of whichever human community. Through its current dimension, the sport offers the man a unique opportunity to meet and socialize with the other people, to achieve different roles, to assimilate some social habits, such as tolerance, respect for others, compliance with legislation, self-education, self-assessment etc., to agree in relation to the behaviour connected to a specific type of activity which influences personality development.

Additionally, the sport activity involves and ensures new experiences, less encountered in other domains of activity, acceptance of a new life style which includes, among others, a rational nourishment, controlled movement and breaks, to the detriment of the sedentarism and obesity, working in a team and consolidating the patriotic feeling, as a consequence of the performances achieved by athletes who have the same citizenship or nationality as us, irrespective of the geographic space where they live.

Although we have the tendency to consider that the main goal of sport practice is promotion of a free association of individuals in order to establish new social contacts, communication and understanding between them are not sufficient as they represent only means to achieve socialization and not direct effects. This is the reason why monitoring and management of sport activities are extremely important, especially among the young people, socialization in and through sport means to highlight the moral qualities and not to promote harmful temptations and habits specific to modern life.

The behaviour, the skills and rules learned through practice of physical exercises may be transferred and adapted to all and any social domains, irrespective of their specificity. Sport activities fructify formation and development of personality, improvement of health ratios and increase of life quality, effects of such activities being obvious in time, in the direction of forming and improving self-esteem, elimination of stress, anxiety, increase of confidence in own forces, self-appreciation, reduction of energy consumption and implicitly, increase of performance, of positive emotions and feelings a.s.o.

References

[1] Bănciulescu, V., (1986) *More than a Victory,* Bucureşti, Albatros Publishing House;

[2] Neacşu, I., Ene, M., (1987) *Education and Self-Education in Forming Sports Personality şi autoeducaţie în formarea personalităţii sportive*, Bucharest, Sport Turism Publishing House, pp 19-21;

[3] Bâtlan, I., (2000) *Sports Values. An Attempt to Establish a Sports Axiology*, Bucharest, Semne Publishing House, pp. 24-41;

[4] Davies Elwood, Craig & Miller, Donna Mae. The Philosophic Process in *Physical Education. Second edition*, Philadelphia: Lea & Febinger, 1967; Somerset. England, Wolfe Publishing Ltd., 1991;

[5] Maheu R., (1977) Sport and Culture, in *Sport Abroad*, nr. 75/1977, CNEFS;

[6] Piaget, J., Inhelder, B., (1970) Psihologia copilului, Bucureşti, Editura Didactică şi Pedagogică ;

[7] Magnane, G., (1964) *Sociologie du sport,* Paris, Gallimard ;

[8] Ceauşescu, N.N., Mitra, Gh., (1982) Physical Education in Todoran, D., coord., (1982) *Fundamental Issues of Pedagogy*, EDP, Bucharest, 1982, Cap. V, p. 118-126;

[9] Toffler, A, şi Toffler, Heidi., (1995) *Creating a New Civilization*, Bucharest, Antet Publishing House;

[10] Toffler A. (1995) *Power in Movement*, Bucharest, Antet Publishing House;

[11] Zlate. M., (1972) *Social Psychology of School Groups,* Bucharest, Didactică şi Pedagogică Publishing House; no.1/1996, Routledge, Taylor & Francis Groups;

[12] Golu, M., (1993) *Dynamics of Personality,* Bucharest, Geneze Publishing House, pp 23-29;

[13] Allport, G., (1991) *Structure and Development of Personality,* Bucharest, Didactică şi Pedagogică Publishing House, pp 57 -59;

[14] Zamfir, C., Vlăsceanu, L., et al., (1993) *Dictionary of Sociology*. Bucharest, Babel Publishing House, pp. 517-518;

[15] Zlate. M., (1988) *Man Facing the World,* Bucharest, Albatros Publishing House;

[16] Chappuis, R., (1986) *La psychologie des relations humaines,* Paris, PUF, Paris, pp.55;

[17] Anshel, M.H., editor, (1991) *Dictionary of the Sport Exercise Sciences.* Champaign, Human Kinetics Books;

[18] Sage, G.H., (1986) The Effects of Physical Activity on the Social Development of Children, in G.A. Stull, H.M. Eckert (Eds.), *Effects of Physical Activity on Children* (p. 22-29), Champaign, Human Kinetics Publ;

[19] Council of Europe Committee for Development of Sport (CDDS), (1995) *The Impact of Sport on Socialization. Significance of Sport for Society,* translation Vol. II/1996, Bucharest, CCPS, pp 7-75;

[20] Pehoiu, C., (2004) *Continuity of Physical Education Activity in Pre-elementary, Elementary and Secondary Education,* Târgovişte - Cetatea de Scaun, pp 5 -7;

[21] Epuran, M., (2005) *Methodology of the Body Activity Research* (second edition). Bucharest, FEST Publishing House;

[22] Dragnea, A., & collab (2000) *Theory of Physical Education and Sport,* Bucharest, Cartea Şcolii Publishing House, pp. 123;

[23] ***International Society of Sport Psychology, (1992) Physical Activity and Psychological Benefits: a position statement, in *International Journal of Sport Psychology,* 23, 86-91;

[24] David Le Breton, (2009) *Anthropology of the Body and Modernity*, Timişoara, Amacord Publishing House, pp. 144 ;

[25] Savu C., Pehoiu C., Pehoiu, Andra, Georgiana, (2009) Fitness, an efficient of building your physical image, in *Sports Medicine Journal,* supplement 2 - October 2009, pp 369-372, Craiova, Universitaria Editure.

27

PASSES CONTRIBUTION TO THE ACHIEVEMENT OF AN EFFECTIVE POSSESSION OF THE BALL IN THE GAME OF FOOTBALL IN JUNIOR FOOTBALL PLAYERS

Dumitru BARBU, Doru STOICA

University of Craiova, Faculty of Physical Education and Sport, Craiova, Romania

Abstract: In this paper we aim to highlight the importance of the possession of the ball in the game of football teams, which must comply with the terms of theory and methodical training and especially with the procedure of taking over and passing the ball - important aspects of the art of the game in order to improve efficiency completion. In the training both possession and position specific exercises were used, exercises aimed at improving the technique and specific exercises to develop motor skills involved in achieving effective possessions through progression in order to lead the ball on the shortest way to the goal. This has allowed the establishment of a proper dynamics of the game, the ball movement and the corresponding requirements of modern football players. The experiment demonstrates what level of time ranges the possession of the ball and how effective it is according to the exercises presented in the paper and used in training juniors, an urgent need to find new ways of working which take into account the increased speed of the game, choosing the effective ways and means to be exploited for the players.

The results show that research hypotheses were confirmed and they constitute benchmarks to achieve results consistent with the requirements in the game of football.

Keywords: football, training, technical, possession, effective passing of the ball.

Introduction

Starting from the idea that the first rule of education and instruction is not to ease too much the exercise whose purpose is overcoming the difficulty (beyond a certain degree of effort), we pursue tenaciously the aim that the trainings do not lose their lesson character, learning, so, whenever and however, they should not replicate the seniors training structure and much less to have seniors training finality. In full agreement and permanent conception from which we started, the whole process of training and education must have a dominant technical-tactical character, built on a high and stable fund of general physical training and capitalizing the psycho-intellectual resources of talented children selected for the great performance.

Since the attack phase is the crucial moment of the game, the means of collaboration have a more active relationship with the other game. Relations between players in offensive phases have a constructive character, achieved by the joint and direct participation of players to build the defensive actions and interventions needed to overcome teh proximity target. Cooperation established between the players has a conscious character is resilient and creative and results from the continuing struggle and sometimes from quite aggressive actions taken by the defense. When recovering the ball (positive transition), it is essential to consider [1]:

- where in the field the ball was recovered;
- who and how many players participate in recovery;
- how many and which players should or may participate in the attack;
- free areas that to be decided whether to play by short or long step;
- how to organize the attack team in the new situation;
- What is the fastest way to reach completion;
- Who balances the defense of loss of possession.

On the cooperation of players in their attacks, the specific features of the organization and completion of a team's tactical actions, confers to the team its personal style in attack, style that is apparent even in the conception of the game. Collective tactical actions are performed using technical procedures in the field of motion: heading the ball, feints, taking over and shooting at the goal,, the execution of which should follow the principles and rules of individual tactical actions.

By finding new ways and means of physical, technical and tactical training, the players have learned and mastered in game-like conditions (speed of execution, simple and straightforward processes but executed in maximum speed, interference between posts) relations between the players taking part in the attack phase have acquired new dimensions by the appearance of ball movement and players, to support and aid the player with the ball and the group around him.

Research Purpose

It is represented by the contribution to the improvement of the football training process by lifting the indices on sports training factors, such as the physical, technical, tactical, especially the technical to a higher level:, using the appropriate physical development methods and specific means to be closer to the aim pursued in the educational process - effective possession of the ball for team performance objectives.

Research Hypotheses

1. Adding to the hours of training a number of additional technical elements through appropriate exercises that exhibit a high degree of complexity and increasing the number of repetitions in procedures execution higher indices on specific skill or capacity to control the ball, and on the speed of the game, shall be recorded, allowing an effective possession of the game.

2. Making specific training focusing on learning to connect the technical element to other elements appropriated separately in the themed game, in the school game, learning basic technical element, hitting the ball particularly in the process of completion - shot on goal, will record superior indices on accuracy, efficiency, boosting the "refresh" quick different situations.

Material and method

In view of the collection, processing and interpretation of the findings and the analysis we had a permanent observation on the receptivity of players to the targeted exercises and games used at different times of the lessons and training periods. There was a continuous dialogue with the athletes to address weaknesses, but also on individual and collective technical elements that have been successful in training and games.

The experiment conducted for the elaboration of the paper has an ascertaining character, of verification of the hypotheses proposed and created by developing a methodology for using the exercises, movement games with and without the ball head to achieving effective possessions of the game. Tests have allowed an assessment as close possible to the real possibilities of the athletes, but also an assessment of the correctness character of this period mainly training preparedness of future athletes.

We watched in the training that the workload for technical and tactical training meet the organization towards the increasing of efficiency in phase possession game in particular by improving the quality of passes. So, we used specific exercises that focused on developing skill, speed of reaction and execution, strength, endurance and targets under speed, but also exercises and games to acquire the main elements and techniques: improvement of takeovers, ball heading, perfecting misleading movements. The strategy involves teaching situations for lining contexts, for the construction game, situations on starting the game from the goalkeeper, primarily exercises without adversity. [2]

Regarding the organization of the game for positioning exercises, working knowledge of the specific role of each player in its region of operations were used. In games positioning we can use more players (9-16), whose role is to assist the player with the ball on the outer sides of the playing space and freedom of movement against players who are trying to recover. They will use passes until they will reach the situation of numerical superiority, thus avoiding 1vs1 situations because they assume the appearance of fatigue and get away from the proposed objective[3].

The collective research subjects are a sufficiently homogeneous mass, consisting of 20 junior players born in 1998 and 1999, from the Centre for Children and Juniors from Universitatea Craiova active in the Championship elite League Organized by the Romanian Football Federation.

Results

To see whether the team performed an efficient ball possession we realized time recordings on how effective each player has been in the possession of the ball, whether the continuation of the rally was a success or a failure. Thus we was conducted two tests of this kind, with the same team in both the tour and in return (F.C. Braşov).

After the initial testing in team training we introduced specific exercises to improve the playing technique as well as specific exercises for possession from 2vs1 to 11 vs 11. This situation is repeated several times, with different recovery times, with average duration and intensity on large ample space. The length of games will be split into several parts in order to achieve greater capacity of concentration of players and greater intensity. We shall not use the whole field to a greater density of actions and will avoid prolonged outages to ensure continuity [4].

Each player was registered with a timer based on the position held in the team system, and in case of replacement, the new entrants were taken over.

To achieve records in good condition, both games were scheduled on the same type of pitch (artificial), which allowed a smooth ongoing actions within the game. The recordings were made only on field players and not for goalkeeper's own or opposing players. The time difference was materialized in ball out of play out or for the execution of various set pieces etc.

Table on players' recorded times - ball possession

Nr Crt.	Team Position	Registered time (sec)			
		Tour	**Return**	**Mean**	**Dif. 2-1**
1	Right back	114	142	**128**	**28**
2	Center right midfield	120	145	**132.5**	**25**
3	Center left midfield	132	157	**144.5**	**35**
4	Left back	111	154	**132.5**	**43**
5	right midfield	117	160	**138.5**	**43**
6	defensive midfield	150	170	**160**	**20**
7	ofensive midfield	137	163	**150**	**26**
8	left midfield	119	164	**141.5**	**43**
9	striker1	102	109	**105.5**	**7**
10	striker 2	110	123	**116.5**	**13**
Total team		**1212**	**1487**	**1349.5**	**273**

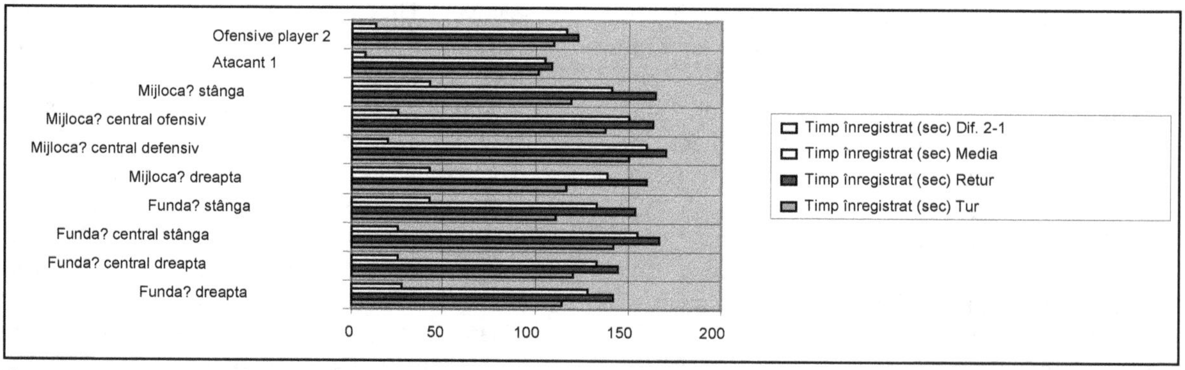

Fig. 1. players on the positions' possession of the ball, round-trip time and average time realized

Analyzing the times registered by players on positions, we observed as was only natural that due to labor and position in the team, midfielders recorded the highest values in time: 160 minutes / game central defensive midfielder and 150 sec / game central offensive midfielder. Next, the left defender the possession of 144.5 sec / game due to his involvement in the construction phase of the game, the last one striker 1 standing with a clear sec./joc 105.5

Table total time of possession realized by the team per game and the differences between return and tour

Position in the game	Registered time (sec)			
	Tour	**Return**	**Mean**	**Dif. 2-1**
Total team	**1212**	**1487**	**1349.5**	**273**

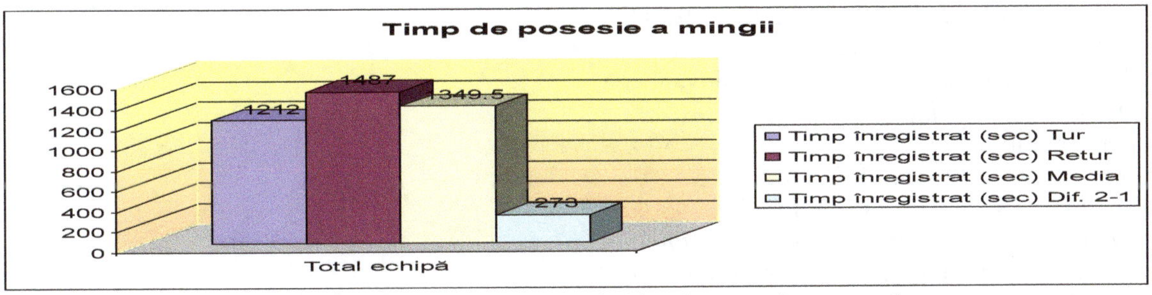

Fig. 2. Graph for the total time recorded by the team in tour and return

Discussions

After applying specific training programs for achieving effective possessions of the game, there is a clear increase in the time between tour and return 273 seconds (4.55 minutes), the team having possession of 1,212 sec / game tour and 1487 sec / game in return.

This aspect had effects on the team efficiency on the scoreboard. Thus, if the teams finished tied in the tour game - 1-1 in the return the score has risen the team winning 5-1, due in particular to work extended for the possession that put the team in multiple situations to score.

Future football must have a special dynamic design and player technique should refer to this dynamic expressed in the athletes stimulated by addressing all stakeholders. So players will have to move constantly in order to create spaces and not narrowing the field (low technical teams with prefer this priority objective in the defense). The support for the player with the ball will hold defender intervention.

Therefore, the team should think about how to work together to impose themselves despite the opposition side. This requires the building of patience, thinking appeared in every space defense that can be speculated, thinking of the concept of space-time, tactical concept of wide field (wide) with games from side to side [5].

When performing passes they will take into account the following aspects of training [6]:

- the Quality of the pass is imperative;
- many technical executions;
- Accuracy and execution need to pass in the right time;
- Head up for documentation on reception and transmission vision;
- Keeping possession of the ball on the ground;
- Use both feet to pass and receive the ball,
- Choosing the best directions for passes.

Conclusion

1. The technical factor is one of the basic factors of the game of football and is considered to support the others. We must emphasize the importance of this factor in the juniors of all categories, it remains one of the means of selection, following that during the preparation to adopt appropriate forms and methods so that juniors grow in value with age and experience.

2. In modern football, the midfielders are "the engine team," channeling attacks. They must ensure change the pace of the game in attack and acceleration of completion. For those players they must have some technical and tactical, mental, qualities, which stand out from the others. Players from the middle compartment must be counted in the current context of football those who can overcome on one or more chapters the duties of other players.

3. The cooperation established between the players has a conscious character is resilient and creative and results from the continuing struggle and sometimes quite aggressive actions taken by the defense.

4. By finding new ways and means of physical, technical and tactical training, which players have learned and mastered in game like conditions (speed of execution, but simple and straightforward procedures performed in maximum speed, interference between posts), the relations between the players taking part in the attack phase have acquired new dimensions by the appearance of ball movement and players, of support and aid for the player with the ball, and the group around the player with the ball.

5. The assumptions of the work were confirmed, which means that the exercises used in training can be a model of training to increase efficiency in the possession game.

References

[1]. PASQUALE USSIA (*03 - 0 7- 2012*) - *Le transizioni nel calcio moderno*, Corso Master

2011-12, Coverciano, TESI di FINE CORSO, Relatore : Renzo Ulivieri, p. 6.

[2]. FC Internazionale, Settore Giovanile, (2011) - *"La fase offensiva"*, stefano.bellinzaghi@inter.it, *Sito: intercampus.inter.it/cgi-bin/res/login,* f.p.

[3]. [4]. JAVIER LOPEZ LOPEZ – *La preparacion del futbolista basada en el futbol* – bases teorico-practicas del entrenamiento especifico del futbol – volumen 1, p. 146, p. 150.

[5]. SANTIAGO VÁZQUEZ FOLGUEIRA (2001) - 1.022 EJERCICIOS DE ATAQUE EN FÚTBOL, Barcelona. Editorial Paidotribo Consejo de Ciento, p. 103.

[6]. *Basic passing and cooperation* (2012) - Pro-SoccerDrills.com, p. 7.

THE INFLUENCE OF PHYSICAL EXERCISE ON SOME ANTHROPOMETRIC PARAMETERS

Florin NEFERU
University C-tin Brâncuşi, Tg.Jiu

Abstract
Physical education and sport are identified by many experts, as indispensable for affirming the individual's personality. The development of motor, intellectual and moral skills through physical education and sport is a right and should be mandatory within the educational systems. The study has proposed the validation of fitness programs in order to remodel the body of 50 students (aged 20 ± 1,5years). For 6 months, the subjects have participated in work programs that included specific means of fitness. At the end of the experiment an improvedbodymass, bodymass index and chest-hip ratio was highlighted.Thus, fitness exercises can be successfully used in physical education lesson, giving it attractiveness and efficiency.
Keywords: fitness, bodymass, students

Introduction
Physical shape is considered an indicator of vitality and youth and, as such, it is desired and appreciated both in professional and everyday life. A body modeled after existing templates, specific to a certain period of evolution of society is desirable for most individuals. This can be achieved through Physical exercise, one that can interfere with objective stimuli on certain body segments or on the entire body. The effect of movement on the individual is manifested through a substantial contribution to developing and maintaining functional capacity, keeping body structures and limiting their deterioration due to age and lack of stimulation. Analyzing the effects of Physical exercise on students body, Tremblay and Chiasson [1] state that these are much higher on the adiposity of those who practice fitness, than are perceived generally by specialists and health agencies.
Physical development of young people is a matter of strict actuality, our interest particularizing especially on students in the first years of college, on the biological significance of indices and parameters determinant of good health, reason for which we intend to demonstrate the need for specific means using bodybuilding as a form of maintenance and selective influence of the musculoskeletal system, but also as an effective body reshaping.
Proscribing sports exercise is a fact in our country, putting this to a lack of culture for movement, which should be cultivated since childhood. [2]
Placing the movement of human activity in an educational context, holds as an argumentative foundation the close ties it can develop, along with those of major biological functions with mental processes and especially with the cognitiveones [3]

Methods
For 6 months, 50 subjects (20 ± 1,5years) participated in fitness and bodybuilding lessons 2 times a week, each session lasting 60 minutes.
The programs were individualized based on the weight of the need and the driving experience prior to each subject, aiming at two major goals based on constitutional type ie decreasing body fat and / or muscle tissue mass growth.
The exercises were generally loaded (with many repetitions), aiming at muscular hypertrophy, the workload being high. Each subject was given at each meeting a worksheet where weight and exercises dosage was different, depending on the objective (to increase muscle mass and / or decreasing body fat).
The research subjects were tested before the implementation of work programs and at the end of the experiment, monitoring their progress.
The evaluation consisted in the measurement of weight and waist, according to which the body mass index was performed and the waist-to-hip ratio was calculated. Waist-hip ratio is used increasingly particularly in health, for predicting the risk of cardiovascular or metabolic diseases.

Inclusion criteria were established for the experimental research as follows:
- age 18-20 years
- BMI <30,
- TA and FC age appropriate limits,
- Without neuromuscular disorders,
- Participating in the exercise program,
- Participants who follow the rules imposed by the appropriate conditions, thus limiting errors.

Exclusion criteria established for the experimental research were:
- Metabolic syndrome
- Diabetes,
- Neurological pathology,
- hypertension,
- Orthopedic disorders,
- Subjects participating in specific sports workouts.

Results

Tabel 1. Descriptive statistics for body mass T1

	N	Min	Max	Mean	Stdv	Cv
weight	50	58.70	97.3	70.112	10.23	14.60
Valid N	50					

50 of the analyzed students, recorded an average body weight of 70.11 (± 10,23kg). The coefficient of variation indicates a relatively homogeneous group (14.60%), the body weight is one of the indicators that provide information on health status, this indicator values ranging between 58.70 kg and 97.3kg, reporting the ideal weight (weight- 100), with 16 subjects and 10 exceeding these values falling below this threshold.

Tabel 2. Descriptive statistics for body mass T2

	N	Min	Max	Mean	Stdv	Cv
weight	50	58.00	94.6	68.92	9.42	9.60
Valid N	50					

On the second test, the body mass was 68.92 (±9,42 kg), only 8 students surpassing the ideal values and 5 being under the recommended scale, the latter improving muscle mass and have won in what body mass is concerned.

The body mass index has an average value of 23.36 (± 2.10) to values which lie between 20 to 32 (Table 3). This parameter is within the normal range recommended by the World Health Organization, though there are 10 subjects that exceed the maximum (25) and 2 which are categorized as obese (values greater than 30), according to data given by this higher forum. The coefficient of variation indicates a homogenous group.

Tabel 3. Descriptive statistics for BMI T1

	N	Min	Max	Mean	Stdv	Cv
BMI	50	20	32	23.51	2.50	10.64
Valid N	50					

Tabel 4. Descriptive statistics for BMI T2

	N	Min	Max	Mean	Stdv	Cv
BMI	50	20	32	22.93	2.06	9.01
Valid N	50					

Waist-hip ratio (WHR), a parameter that I followed in selecting subjects for the final experiment showed an average of 0.86, this parameter fitting in the normal range indicated by WHO but there are 12 subjects that exceed the maximum of 0.90. The group is homogeneous, the coefficient of variation being 9.73. At the final testing, this aspect has improved, WHR ratio being 0,86

WHR ratiowas reported at values below:

- Excellent acceptable- under 0.85;
- Well 0.85-0,90;
- Inacceptable- average from 0.90 to 0.95;
- Large 0.95 to 1;
- extreme is 1

Tabel 4. Descriptive statistics for WHR T1

	N	Min	Max	Mean	Stdv	Cv
WHR	50	0.78	0.97	0.86	4.93	9.73
Valid N	50					

Tabel 5. Descriptive statistics for WHR T2

	N	Min	Max	Mean	Stdv	Cv
WHR	50	0.82	0.96	0.84	4.22	5.92
Valid N	50					

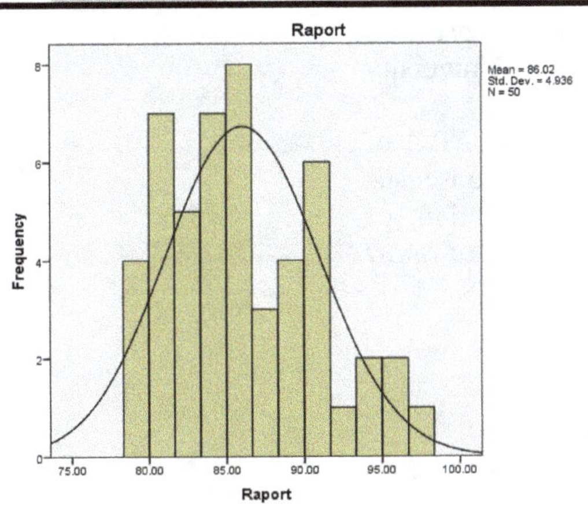

Graph 1 WHR T1

Conclusions

O'Donoven G. & authors [4] recommends for a healthy adult to perform at least 150 minutes of moderate aerobic physical activity with effort every week or at least 75 minutes of high intensity. Weight training, circuit and other complementary exercises aerobic activity are preferred. Also to support their physical condition, people who have crossed the threshold of initiation and doing sports at least 6 months can get benefits on health line by performing physical activity for 300 minutes per week at a moderate intensity

. They recommended exercises with weights 2 times / week as they can improve muscle elasticity.

Regardless of the number and complexity of daily problems, good physical condition gives an increased satisfaction to sports activities, develops muscle strength, can positively influence both the aesthetic appearance of youth and the functional one, many experts saying that the highest increases in force development are recorded at the age of 20-30 years, fitness being one of the subjects acting in this direction. The work programs applied have proved their efficiency, the indices monitored being positively influenced by the means used. Thus, the proposed fitness program can be extended to a larger group.

References

[1].Tremblay A., Chiasson L., (2002), Physical fitness in young college men and women, Canadian Journal of Applied Physiology, vol.27, nr.6, pp.563-574

[2]. Marcu V., Ciobanu D., (2009), *Exercițiul fizic şi calitatea vieții*, Universitatea din Oradea, pag 137

[3]. Neagu N., (2010), *Teoria şi practica activității motrice umane*, Ed. University Press, Tg. Mureş, pg.19

[4]. O'Donoven G.&all, (2010), The ABC of Physical Activity for Helth: A consensus statement from the British Association of Sport and Exercice Science, *Journal of Sport Sciences, 28:6, 573-591.*

STUDY OF ELECTROENCEPHALOGRAPHIC ACTIVITY AT DIFFERENT CATEGORIES OF PROFESSIONAL SPORTSMEN

Denisa ENESCU BIERU, Mihaela ZĂVĂLEANU, Luminiţa BRĂBIESCU CĂLINESCU, Cătălin FORŢAN

Faculty of Physical Education and Sport, University of Craiova, Romania
Correspondence author address: Denisa Enescu Bieru, E-mail: alunis_dendeni@yahoo.com

Abstract: Our purpose was to emphasize a neurophysiologic pattern associated to different categories of professional sportsmen, handball and volleyball players, by assessing their electroencephalographic classic rhythms waves (theta, alpha).
The study was performed on a group of 17 professional sportsmen, with average ages, heights and weights, 9 handball players and 8 volleyball players, characterized by different stress degrees of the upper members, active for between 5 and 12 years in one of the sportive activity.
The EEG response was recorded with surface electrodes, placed on the scalp according to the electroencephalography 10-20 system and the EEG waves obtained during some activities (successive relaxation and contraction of both fists), were measured using the Nihon-Kohden EEG-9200 device.
By processing the results recorded at handball group, was remarked the presence of classic rhythms specific to wakeful state at adult, both during relaxation and contraction moments, with a diminution reaction characteristic to each rhythm, depending on relaxation-activity moment.
Volleyball players, unlike handball players, presented during both, relaxation and contractions periods, a theta band activity, aspect mentioned in literature as accompanying the motor memory process, which dominates at volleyball players.
EEG complex testing of professional sportsmen, as well as the outlining of an EEG pattern specific to studied sportive disciplines, represent an original aspect of this study.
Key words: professional sportsmen, electroencephalograph.y, neurophysiologic pattern.

Introduction

The technique of cerebral electrical activity acquisition during a period time, through electrodes placed on the scalp, is named electroencephalography (EEG) and offers only partial information about the functional state of the central nervous system. According to frequency, one of the EEG specific parameters, were identified four types of waves (rhythms): alpha 8-13 Hz, beta 14-30 Hz, theta 4-7 Hz and delta 0,5-3,5 Hz.

Our purpose was to emphasize a neurophysiologic pattern associated to different categories of professional sportsmen, handball and volleyball players, by assessing their electroencephalographic classic rhythms waves (theta, alpha).

Material and methods

The study was performed on a group of 17 professional sportsmen, with average ages, heights and weights, 9 handball players and 8 volleyball players, characterized by different stress degrees of the upper members, active for between 5 and 12 years in one of the sportive activity.

The studied sports were chosed, taking into account the more extensive representation of the upper limbs in the motor cortex, thus, a higher number of plastic changes are possible to appear as a result of repeated complex movements performed during specific training [1].

The testing was performed under current ethical rules, each participant being informed of the experimental processes.

All the investigated sportsmen have been subjected to electric-neuro-physiological investigations by measuring the EEG waves, using Nihon-Kohden EEG-9200 device. The EEG response was registered with surface electrodes which have a letter to identify the lobe (F frontal, T temporal, P parietal, C central, O occipital) and a number to identify the hemisphere location (even numbers refer to electrode positions on the right hemisphere, odd numbers to those on left hemisphere), placed on the scalp according to the electroencephalography 10-20 system (Figure 1), bipolar acquisition, 16 channels, the reference being the two ears (A1, A2), using a time constant of 0,3 seconds and a filter below 50 Hz. In consideration of the study objective, we recorded the EEG line during some activities which can emphasize the possible characteristic cerebral patterns.

So, the activities followed during EEG recording were: first relaxation time ((R1), right fist contraction (A), left fist contraction (B), right fist contraction order without performing the move (C), left fist contraction order without performing the move (D), after every mentioned moment was recorded a relaxation time (R1-R5) (Figure 2)..

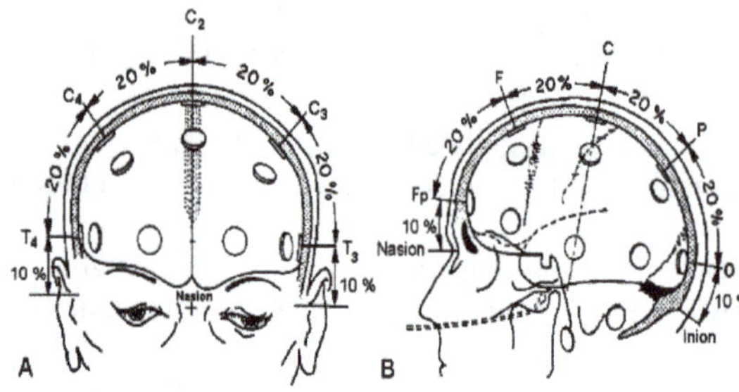

Figure 1. 10-20 electrode placement system

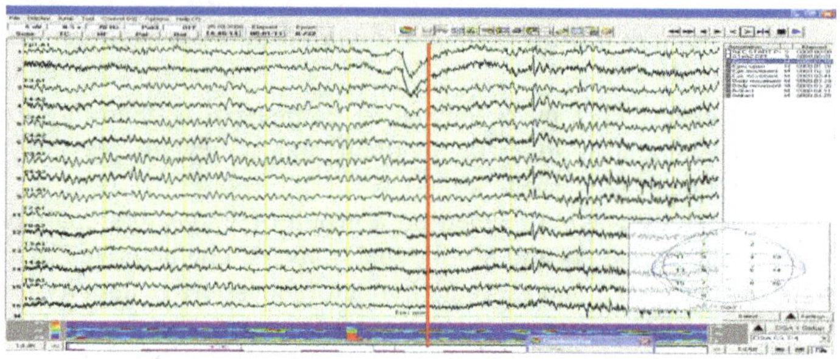

Figure 2. Modification of EEG line by changing an

The EEG analyze was made by assessing the classic rhythms: Theta [4-8Hz], Alpha1 [8-10Hz], Alpha2 [10-13Hz].

Results

For handball group, was remarked a slight increase of the theta wave values, during entire recording, as showed in Table 1.

Table 1. Theta values at handball group for every studied moments

channel	R1	A	R2	B	R3	C	R4	D	R5
T5-A1	0.275	0.582	0.511	0.597	0.263	0.189	0.330	0.252	0.504
T3-A1	0.787	0.681	0.786	1.334	1.259	1.119	0.665	0.739	0.602
F7-A1	0.328	0.237	0.261	0.359	0.285	0.232	0.329	0.254	0.281
O1-A1	0.789	0.700	0.869	1.014	1.263	0.974	0.731	0.670	0.627
P3-A1	0.446	0.445	2.652	0.478	0.531	0.420	0.505	0.444	0.475
C3-A1	0.549	0.546	0.581	1.271	0.736	0.663	0.527	0.641	0.533
F3-A1	0.477	0.373	0.540	0.414	0.654	0.394	0.500	0.489	0.475
Fp1-A1	0.585	0.629	0.912	1.104	0.981	0.748	0.533	0.583	0.619
Fp2-A2	0.428	0.365	0.790	0.576	0.700	0.426	0.445	0.425	0.396
F4-A2	0.512	0.391	0.514	0.423	0.630	0.403	0.520	0.440	0.485
C4-A2	0.391	0.449	0.486	0.523	0.447	0.387	0.399	0.400	0.449
P4-A2	0.362	0.355	0.380	0.349	0.318	0.266	0.345	0.320	0.311
O2-A2	0.273	0.207	0.332	0.261	0.300	0.235	0.262	0.266	0.204
F8-A2	0.452	0.359	0.406	0.376	0.498	0.415	0.488	0.407	0.359
T4-A2	0.216	0.157	0.258	0.187	0.278	0.202	0.229	0.181	0.194
T6-A2	0.551	1.165	0.741	1.142	0.506	0.555	0.607	0.520	0.675

At volleyball players our study emphasized the biggest values for theta waves, in comparison with the handball ones, as in Table 2.

Table 2. Theta values at volleyball group for every studied moments

channel	R1	A	R2	B	R3	C	R4	D	R5
T5-A1	0.325	0.293	0.35	0.565	0.3	0.24	0.29	0.412	0.453
T3-A1	0.748	0.721	1.23	3.696	0.84	2.126	0.87	0.939	1.6
F7-A1	0.188	0.206	0.17	0.534	0.16	0.152	0.15	0.148	0.151
O1-A1	0.845	1.696	2.87	2.379	0.81	1.332	1.91	1.127	1.3
P3-A1	0.57	0.554	2.74	0.634	0.74	0.624	0.62	0.589	0.761
C3-A1	0.716	0.775	0.85	1.373	0.7	2.008	0.78	0.841	1.553
F3-A1	0.559	0.487	0.46	0.439	0.5	0.511	0.53	0.457	0.643
Fp1-A1	0.75	1.731	1.54	1.721	0.74	1.228	0.84	0.974	1.048
Fp2-A2	0.39	0.425	0.88	0.537	0.39	0.313	0.37	0.349	0.424
F4-A2	1.491	1.186	1.52	1.496	1.38	1.329	1.6	1.1	1.569
C4-A2	0.352	0.372	2.49	0.424	0.34	0.315	0.42	0.357	0.45
P4-A2	1.208	0.845	1.55	0.997	0.96	1.006	1.27	0.994	1.255
O2-A2	0.268	0.268	0.24	0.665	0.23	0.263	0.27	0.251	0.329
F8-A2	0.577	0.568	0.53	0.667	0.56	0.572	0.57	0.608	0.569
T4-A2	0.264	0.316	0.31	0.772	0.28	0.236	0.25	0.254	0.415
T6-A2	1.012	0.809	0.9	1.049	1.01	1.086	1.07	0.889	1.129

Handball athletes' alpha1 activity was proved to be more homogenous and with classic reactivity, being lower during any active moment and higher during repose moments, regarding alpha1 EEG activity for volleyball players, that one was lower in the dominant hemisphere, as presented in Table 3 and Table 4.

Table 3. Alpha1 values at handball group for every studied moments

channel	R1	A	R2	B	R3	C	R4	D	R5
T5-A1	0.934	0.711	0.97	1.031	1	0.345	0.91	0.520	1.01
T3-A1	0.792	0.519	0.94	0.887	1.39	0.806	0.8	0.595	0.813
F7-A1	0.661	0.407	0.74	0.675	0.72	0.409	0.91	0.338	0.695
O1-A1	1.085	0.934	1.26	0.865	1.58	0.912	1.44	0.677	1.366
P3-A1	1.717	1.057	2.65	1.293	2.54	1.087	2.5	1.340	1.915
C3-A1	0.313	0.314	0.33	0.609	0.48	0.408	0.35	0.320	0.347
F3-A1	2.093	2.209	4.68	2.174	3.09	1.858	3.45	2.260	1.931
Fp1-A1	0.334	0.323	0.4	0.586	0.45	0.429	0.31	0.312	0.366
Fp2-A2	0.685	0.309	1.11	0.489	1.09	0.447	1.06	0.451	1.054
F4-A2	2.681	2.348	2.46	2.082	2.12	1.706	2.6	1.568	1.793
C4-A2	0.57	0.275	0.71	0.404	0.93	0.414	0.76	0.601	0.664
P4-A2	1.505	1.213	1.61	1.385	1.38	0.854	1.5	0.976	1.159
O2-A2	1.803	2.685	3	1.478	2.24	1.805	2.34	1.836	1.467

F8-A2	1.304	0.979	1.03	0.932	0.94	1.024	1.07	0.906	0.699
T4-A2	1.067	0.757	1.88	0.783	1.66	0.69	1.58	0.893	1.251
T6-A2	2.282	4.076	0.74	1.876	1.68	1.711	1.61	1.581	1.034

Table 4. Alpha1 values at volleyball group for every studied moments

channel	R1	A	R2	B	R3	C	R4	D	R5
T5-A1	2.298	2.210	1.72	1.765	1.46	1.321	1.47	1.504	2.67
T3-A1	1.412	1.166	0.88	1.492	0.9	1.564	1.1	0.963	1.54
F7-A1	0.34	0.353	0.33	0.445	0.36	0.363	0.36	0.358	0.436
O1-A1	0.641	0.568	1.18	0.867	0.57	0.992	1.89	0.858	0.855
P3-A1	5.043	5.418	2.74	3.812	4.14	3.818	4.17	3.302	5.034
C3-A1	0.542	0.540	0.5	0.591	0.58	1.399	0.63	0.55	0.968
F3-A1	1.817	1.411	1.66	1.289	2.24	1.752	1.78	1.716	2.221
Fp1-A1	0.486	0.562	0.71	0.638	0.51	1.129	0.65	0.58	0.729
Fp2-A2	0.41	0.271	0.63	0.362	0.35	0.291	0.37	0.271	0.441
F4-A2	11.92	10.668	10.6	5.542	16	24.13	17.4	8.718	16.61
C4-A2	0.381	0.324	1.14	0.380	0.34	0.328	0.42	0.311	0.452
P4-A2	7.878	8.182	6.49	4.316	7.58	9.223	9	5.108	9.865
O2-A2	0.67	0.514	0.89	0.814	0.98	0.616	0.95	0.658	1.04
F8-A2	5.035	4.832	4.23	4.971	4.76	3.54	4.36	3.509	4.232
T4-A2	1.983	1.484	0.85	0.704	1.29	1.593	1.77	0.935	1.669
T6-A2	4.535	5.823	4.2	2.764	5.04	5.429	6.08	3.871	7.207

Alpha2 values are lower for handball players in comparison with the volleyballs' ones, that are also characterised by a small activity of the left hemisphere, reflecting a ″quiet″ conduct, aspect revealed in Table 5 and 6.

Table 5. Alpha2 values at handball group for every studied moments

channel	**R1**	**A**	**R2**	**B**	**R3**	**C**	**R4**	**D**	**R5**
T5-A1	0.522	0.401	0.7	0.618	0.61	0.469	0.52	0.393	0.577
T3-A1	0.732	0.413	0.75	0.747	1.24	0.616	0.69	0.494	1.202
F7-A1	0.608	0.458	0.73	0.692	0.78	0.613	0.68	0.548	0.736
O1-A1	0.62	0.328	0.9	0.511	1.37	0.719	0.82	0.532	1.412
P3-A1	1.767	0.913	2.52	1.829	2.43	1.881	2.42	1.457	1.973
C3-A1	0.255	0.218	0.35	0.454	0.42	0.425	0.37	0.341	0.429
F3-A1	2.114	1.460	3.64	2.967	2.77	1.783	2.63	2.037	3.363
Fp1-A1	0.232	0.229	0.37	0.381	0.41	0.354	0.25	0.224	0.37
Fp2-A2	0.625	0.243	0.95	0.846	1.33	0.594	0.81	0.490	1.216
F4-A2	2.402	1.679	3.08	2.799	3.02	2.798	2.7	1.860	2.597
C4-A2	0.667	0.394	0.87	0.961	1.13	0.691	0.78	0.498	1.152
P4-A2	1.086	0.752	1.52	1.637	1.3	1.101	1.19	0.883	1.382
O2-A2	0.749	0.527	1.38	0.868	0.85	0.52	1.04	0.827	1.263
F8-A2	2.233	1.531	2.55	2.128	2.62	3.046	2.9	1.629	2.046
T4-A2	0.404	0.216	0.78	0.510	0.59	0.339	0.71	0.419	0.807
T6-A2	1.778	1.814	2.6	2.171	2.4	2.26	2.18	1.354	1.459

Table 6. Alpha2 values at volleyball group for every studied moments

channel	**R1**	**A**	**R2**	**B**	**R3**	**C**	**R4**	**D**	**R5**
T5-A1	1.381	1.585	1.79	1.518	1.96	2.178	2.05	2.254	1.67
T3-A1	0.788	0.731	1.01	1.121	1.11	1.357	1.04	1.121	1.206
F7-A1	0.447	0.490	0.53	0.597	0.62	0.558	0.65	0.57	0.66

O1-A1	0.678	0.667	0.91	0.739	0.78	0.813	1.13	0.971	1.016
P3-A1	1.875	1.454	2.41	1.724	4.45	4.502	3.87	3.406	2.717
C3-A1	0.333	0.300	0.29	0.335	0.4	0.692	0.43	0.431	0.652
F3-A1	1.279	1.087	1.59	1.086	2.31	2.102	2.32	1.74	1.938
Fp1-A1	0.317	0.427	0.41	0.385	0.33	0.423	0.41	0.465	0.456
Fp2-A2	0.414	0.251	0.51	0.337	0.46	0.432	0.52	0.337	0.577
F4-A2	6.534	5.684	5.89	5.505	8.16	9.659	7.96	8.247	7.353
C4-A2	0.341	0.238	0.62	0.324	0.41	0.46	0.44	0.385	0.482
P4-A2	5.629	5.701	5.81	4.705	6.44	7.759	7.36	6.811	7.326
O2-A2	0.568	0.556	0.71	0.631	0.72	0.59	1.14	0.743	0.818
F8-A2	4.206	4.408	4.52	3.970	5.99	6.184	5.59	4.931	4.346
T4-A2	0.817	0.704	0.85	0.729	1.03	0.971	1.11	0.965	1.011
T6-A2	4.317	3.899	4.61	3.161	5.08	6.43	4.79	4.458	5.167

Discussions

Because our study aimed the identification of neurophysiologic patterns specific to a long sportive activity, the attention was directed towards athletes of whom the initial cerebral plasticity process stopped and the morphologic differences are born especially in M1 (primary motor) area.

Was suggested the importance of theta wave, in order to understand, evaluate and measure the motor memory processes, but especially, for improving the motor performances, in our case, the sportive ones [2], [3].

Thus, is considered that a decrease of alpha activity (non-synchronization) and an increase of theta one (synchronization), reflects a high capacity of memorization [4]. Following during our study, the electroencephalographic activity of each studied sportive discipline, we observed different response patterns, but constant for the same group of athletes, specific changes being reported by Pearce in 2000, by using magnetic stimulation [5]. At the beginning of the recordings, neither of the studied sportive disciplines presented theta power spectrum activity. The same moment of recording showed for handball group an alpha frontal-occipital activity, with a larger spreading but a smaller power, as for volleyball players, is recorded a frontal-occipital activity for alpha wave, but only for the non-dominant hemisphere, aspect described by Andrew and Pfurtscheller in 1997 [6]. The dominant hemisphere presented only an occipital activity at handball group, aspect reported by Klimesch in 1998 [7] and Babiloni in 2009 [3]. The right fist contraction moment produces spectacular EEG modifications in comparison with initial moment ones.

Volleyball players presented an increase of the theta band activity, so the theta band was very well represented in left frontal, parietal and occipital-temporal, well outline areas, while the theta band for the right hemisphere was not systematized, as was in the dominant hemisphere.

The handball group did not show the same theta activity during right fist contraction.

Group of volleyball athletes presented minor right frontal modifications for alpha2 bands. Is sustained the affirmation that for volleyball players, the changes during right fist contraction were mostly in theta band, having a long duration motor memory for the performed move [7].

For handball alpha1 and 2 decreases were obvious during this action, showing a high attention [7], so another EEG feature was outlined, that emphasize the difference between the two sports.

During relaxation moment R2, theta activity is constant or increases at volleyball group and alpha2 activity presents a slightly increase in parietal area, for handball, the frequencies bands had an increased activity in the areas where these frequencies already existed, characteristic for these is an alpha2 increase, more difficult to explain. The left fist contraction determined the same changes for alpha frequency bands as the right one, additionally appearing little left frontal-temporal-occipital areas that presented minimum increase of theta spectrum at handball players.

The changes find until now at the two sportive disciplines can not be totally explain by the literature, there are maybe the final result of an intermediary processes pointed out by other authors.

From this moment, the EEG characteristic patterns of the two sports, remain constant, being a small theta increase for handball in the left hemisphere and a alpha majority for both hemispheres at the same sport.

Alpha 1 activity is not higher in the right hemisphere at volleyball athletes, instead, alpha2 activity is higher in the left parietal area. The last recording moments are not so different from the initial moments at handball players, but for volleyball athletes the theta activity remains dominant for temporal and central areas.

Because of the particularities of each sportive discipline, is outlining the idea of some sportsmen presenting a performed movement imagination bigger than the one of other tested sport, which is produced by structural changes, signaled by Pearce in 2000 [5].

The whole EEG testing aimed to emphasize the classic rhythms power spectrums modifications, produced by different orders (fists successively contractions, movement thinking without perform it), in comparison with the relaxation moments between actions. The literature describes many observations regarding the motor memory, our objective study was to emphasize the differences inter-sports, an original aspect enough conspicuous outlined by the previous affirmations.

Conclusions

Emphasizing some neurophysiologic patterns specific to long period sportive activities through electrophysiological tests is imposed as a viable method and easy to use for cerebral electrogenesis appreciation, in presence of functional plastic changes determined by the training.

By processing the results recorded at handball group, was remarked the presence of classic rhythms specific to wakeful state at adult, both during relaxation moments and activity, with a diminution reaction characteristic to each rhythm, depending on relaxation-activity moment.

Volleyball players, unlike handball players, presented both during relaxation and movement thinking, theta band activity, aspect mentioned in literature as accompanying the motor memory process, which dominates at volleyball players.

EEG complex testing of professional sportsmen, as well as the outlining of an EEG pattern specific to studied sportive disciplines, handball and volleyball, represent an original aspect of this study.

Acknowledgement

All authors have equal contributions.

References

[1]. Fattapposta, F., G., Amabile, M. V., Cordischi, D., Di Venanzio, A., Foti, F., Pierelli, C., D'Alessio, F., Pigozzi, A., Parisi and C., Morrocutti, 1996, Long-term practice effects on a new skilled motor learning: an electrophysiological study, *Electroencephalography and Clinical Neurophysiology*, Volume 99, Issue 6, pp. 495-507

[2]. Aglioti, S.M., Cesari, P., Romani, M., Urgesi C., 2008, Action anticipation and motor resonance in elite basketball players, *Nature Neuroscience,* Volume 11, pp. 1109-1116

[3]. Babiloni, C., Del Percio, C., Paolo, M., Rossinib, D.F., Marzanog, N., Iacobonig, M., Infarinatoc, F., Lizioc, R., Piazzah, M., Pirritano, M., Berlutti, G., Cibelli, G., Eusebi, F., 2009, Judgment of actions in experts: A high-resolution EEG study in elite athletes, *NeuroImage,*Volume 45, Issue 2, pp. 512-521

[4]. Tianbao, Z., Hong, Z., Zheng, T., 2008, Revelations of the new developments of brain science on early education, Computer and Inormation Science, No. 3, Vol. 1

[5]. Pearce, A.J., et al., 2000, Functional reorganisation of the corticomotor projection to the hand in skilled racquet players, *Exp Brain Res* 130, pp. 238-243

[6]. Andrew, C. and Pfurtscheller, G., 1997, On the existence of different alpha band rhythms in the hand area of man, *Neurosci Lett* 222, pp. 103-106

[7]. Klimesch, W.M., Doppelmayr, H., Russegger, T., Schwaiger, J., 1998, Induced alpha band power changes in the Human EEG and attention, *Neuroscience Letters*, Volume 244, Issue 2, pp. 73-76

30

RECOVERY OF THE HIP-FEMORAL JOINT DISEASES THROUGH SPECIFIC MEANS FOOTBALL

Georgeta Ioana GHEORGHE[1] , Dan Gheorghe PĂUN[1], Ioan Laurian PĂUN[2], Mihai Cristian NEGOESCU[3]

[1] *Spiru Haret University, Faculty of Physical Education and Sport*

[2] *Str. Barbu Lăutaru No.10, Brasov School No.1*

[3] *Moldova State University, Faculty of Psychology and Educational Sciences*

Abstract: Etiopathology adepistarea hip leads to the following conditions at the hip joint femoral: Bursitis Meralgia iliopsoasă and paraesthesia. Other causes pain, primary or secondary osteoarthritis of the hip, femoral neck fracture, bone metastases at the proximal end of the femur, rheumatoid arthritis, ankylosing spondylitis, psoriatic arthritis, lumbar discopathy.

Static standing hip hip supposed to be extended and indifferent position rotations and abduction - adduction. The extension is limited pressing iliofemoral ligament femoral head in acetabulum and is called "ligament standing position".

Static methods: progressive relaxation after Jacobson, autogenous training after Schultz

Dynamic Methods: eutonia after Gerda Alexander, Biofeed-back

Football specific means used in the recovery of the hip-femoral joint mobility

Treatment is done only after evaluating patient.

Recovery through physiotherapy include affected limb posture, Musculoskeletal the hip joint manipulation, mobilizations passive, active and active resistance.

The recovery program should begin immediately after mobilization exercises being amplified gradually, depending on the degree of the condition.

Medical rehabilitation is aimed to increase joint mobility and tone, she made through physical therapy exercises, physiotherapy and therapeutic massage.

Keywords: the hip-femoral joint, illness, recovery, specific means football

Introduction

The hip joint - is a joint synovial femoral, spheroidal, with three axes of movement, locomotion very important state and comprising the following articular surfaces: the means of connection.

Joint stability is ensured by three factors [1]:

- bone factors represented by:
- coaptation of the articular surfaces;
- articular axis obliquity;
- factors ligament;
- muscle factors:
- anterior-posterior stability (large gluteal muscle);
- lateral stability (gluteal muscle medium);
- participates in the stability:

pelvitrohanterienii (fixed femoral head in acetabular cup) and longitudinal muscles - adducts balanced with abductorii (tend to luxeze femoral head);

Biomechanics is a enartroză hip and has three degrees of freedom allowing flexion-extension movements, abduction-adduction, internal-external rotation and the combination of movement circumducţie. Femoral neck length and angle cervical-diaphyseal make the movements of flexion, extension, abduction and adduction to associate with rotation.

Treatment is done only after evaluating patient. The drug involves NSAIDs, painkillers, cortisone with systemic or topical administration (infiltrations). They are useful and Physiotherapy and remedial gymnastics. If infectious arthritis, patients benefit from antibiotic treatment for several months. In systemic rheumatic diseases, immune system therapy will address and will treat all affected joints. Bone metastases in bone antiresorptive therapy can be done and / or cytostatic, after identifying the primary tumor. In some cases, treatment is interdisciplinary, with physiotherapist, orthopedics, oncology and infectious disease.

There are other local causes hip pain less common in medical practice. For example, septic arthritis (infection after an invasive procedure intraarticular often local) or tuberculous arthritis.

Hip disease can occur in patients who have a beginning necrosis of the femoral head or those with Duchenne hip that evolution is towards osteoarthritis.

Methodes and materiales

Overall recovery objectives and means hip affected [2]:

1. Relaxation

It's paramount objective in the recovering hip. Relaxation addresses both the stress, muscle tension and mental condition because the hospital atmosphere. Relaxation exercises can be obtained by muscle relaxation and overall divided into two groups:

Static methods: Progressive Relaxation by Jacobson - involves learning proper muscle tone control, from muscle contractions caused by a scheme targeting specific body parts in the following order: upper extremities, lower abdomen, paravertebral region, thorax and facies.

Autogen training, after Schultz - aims to reduce tonic and motor stimuli to induce a state of self-delusion by sustained concentration. It includes acknowledging the weight and heat (muscles) focus on respiratory rate (breathing) sensation of heat in the abdomen, focusing on heart rate, feeling cold frontal region.

Dynamic Methods: Eutonia after Gerda Alexander - the dynamic plan involves body awareness and static and dynamic knowledge of the body in space. Muscle relaxation after Bio Feed-back method is performed using an electromyography to record muscle tension and transmit information in the form of virtual or acoustic signal allowing his patient tone recognition, thus facilitating muscle relaxation.

2. Fight Pain

Hip pain may originate in any of the components of articular and periarticular pain relief is important in the recovery plan, it could cause neofuncţie. Pain can be treated using: frecvenţă- low currents diadynamic currents, currents Trobert, galvanic current; Local heat-paraffin; Shortwave; massage-smoothing; reflex massage

3. Fight joint inflammation - is sometimes present, forming a continuous source of pain. In the paper, the main means used in this direction were: Sleep and thrust the ax-articular pressure drop; Local massage with anti-inflammatory drugs (NSAIDs). It insisted on the groin and buttocks; vibromassage

4. Develop stability - This objective was achieved by isotonic exercises and izometonice. They will be presented in the personal experiment. Primary objective is the development of stability in recovering leg. Avoid force development adductors and psoas.

5. Develop mobility şoldului- traction in the shaft, passive mobilization, mobilization autopasive, mobilization activo-passive, active mobilization, hydrokinetotherapy

6. Re-education gait - This is achieved using fixed braces. Is used both for physical therapy for the passive and active. In the first case mechano facilitates passive movement to its execution and in the second, loading resistance opposes the effort to be stretched muscle power.

Massage - is another means necessary. It is one of the oldest therapeutic means - improves blood circulation and lymphatic helping to eliminate passive hyperemia and catabolite; stimulates contraction of muscle fibers increasing their excitability. The massage is recommended before physical therapy sessions.

Hydrokinetotherapy - is another means used in treatment. Water temperature: 35-37 ° C. Action hydrotherapy refers not only to the changes on skin temperature and peripheral circulation but also on metabolism in general. Hydrokinetotherapy was used both in individual tubs and collective hidrokinetoterapie Basin. Here runs passive physical therapy, active, and active resistance.

Discussions

The recovery program should begin immediately after mobilization exercises being amplified gradually, depending on the degree condition ..

Medical rehabilitation is aimed to increase joint mobility and tone, she made through medical gymnastics exercises (physical therapy), physiotherapy and therapeutic massage.

Medical rehabilitation gives patients several benefits:

• Prevention of possible complications due to prolonged immobilization
• Restoring stability joints and muscle tone
• recovery and improvement in joint mobility / eliminate pain in mobilizing
• Recovery of muscular strength and improve blood circulation locally
• Increased resistance joints by progressive loading
• Regaining amplitude moving
• Resume driving

Recovery through physiotherapy include affected limb posture, Musculoskeletal the hip joint manipulation, mobilizations passive, active and active resistance [3].

Earlier recovery practice various exercises assisted maintenance limb affected, preventing

edema, and the installation of movement disorders.
The exercises, performed properly, increase the degree of stability of the balance (through muscle toning), while increasing mobility and hip, to obtain functional movement ideal angles.
Electrotherapy sessions also help to relieve pain, various forms of effects with current pain relievers, muscle relaxants, and anti-inflammatory decontracturante.
Also, laser therapy stimulates circulation locally, increasing metabolism and accelerating the healing process.
Massage can increase joint mobility and muscle tone, being allowed only focus away from the fracture.
Made by special techniques, aimed at favoring the return veno-lymphatic specialist combat muscular contractions responsible for the appearance of pain.

Specific means football game used in recovering the hip-femoral joint mobility [4]

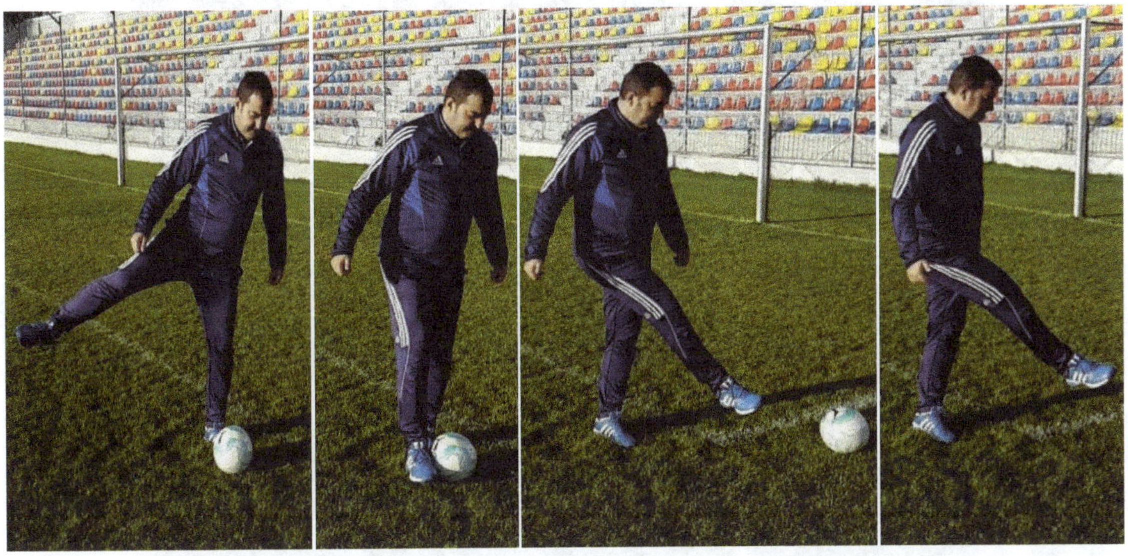

Fig. 1. Hitting the ball with the flat ground level

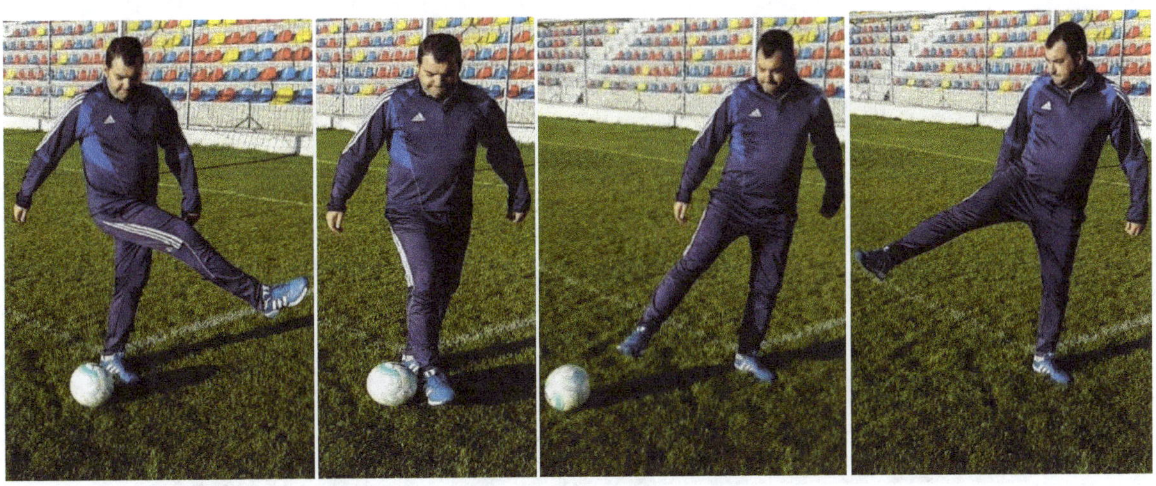

Fig. 2. Hitting the ball with the flat top

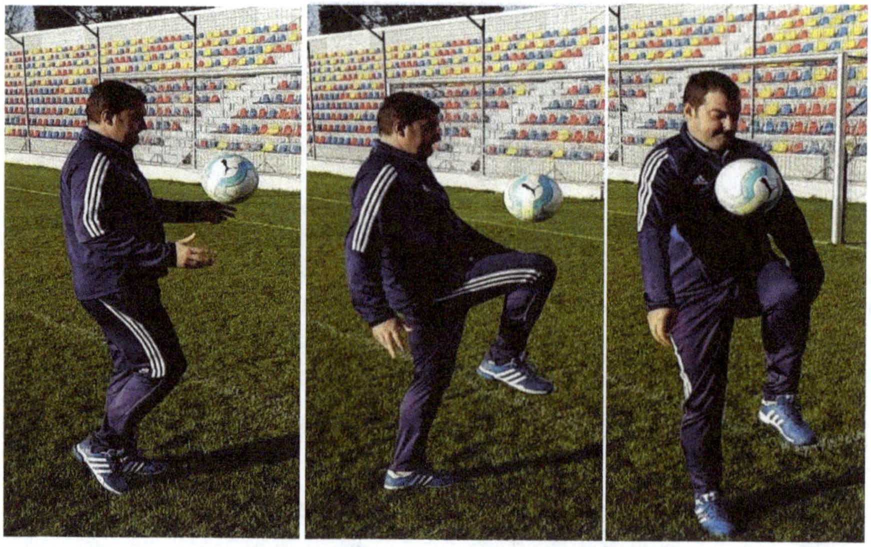

Fig. 3. Hitting the ball with the thigh

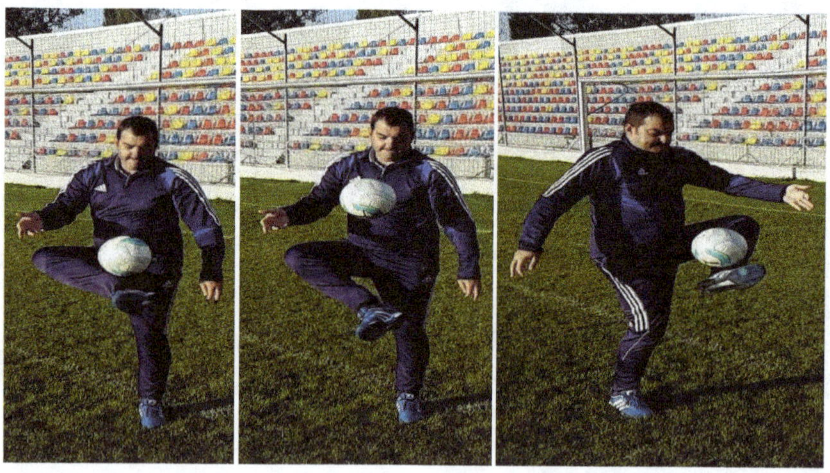

Fig. 4. Hitting the ball with the flat of sagittal position both inwardly and externally

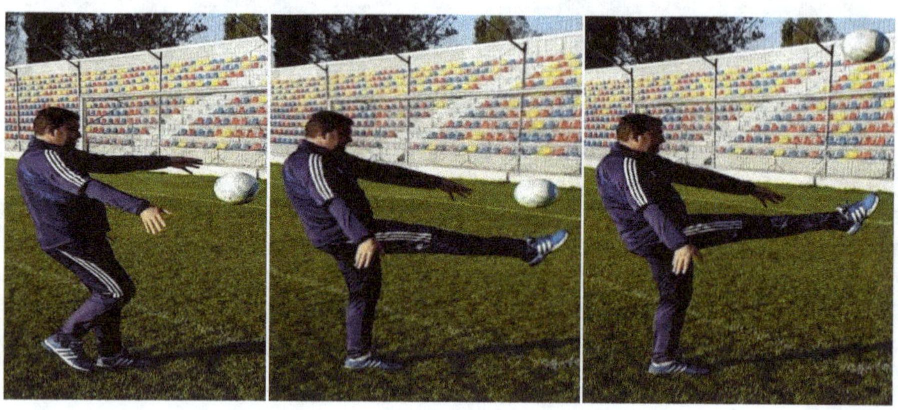

Fig. 5. Hitting the ball with shoe full height

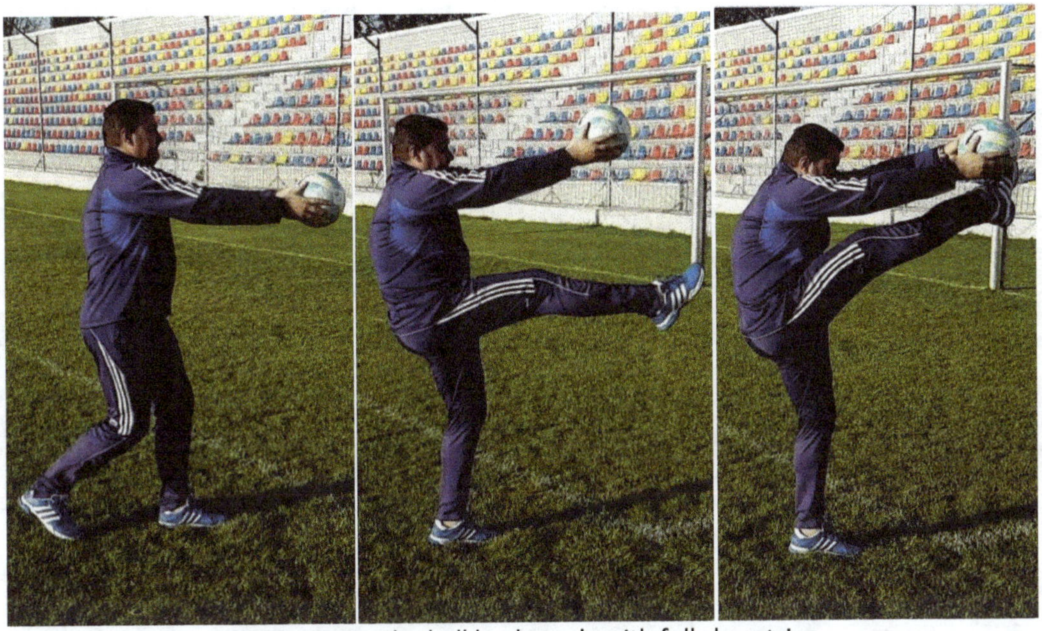

Fig. 6. Hitting the ball backwards with full shoestring

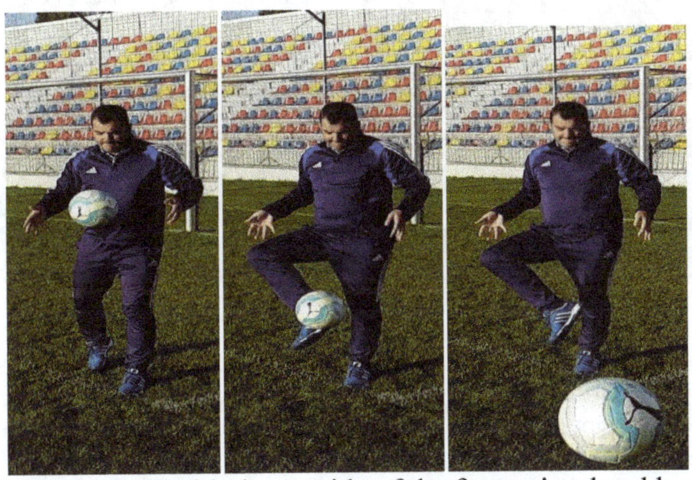

Fig. 7. Hitting the ball with the outside of the foot twisted and bent inward

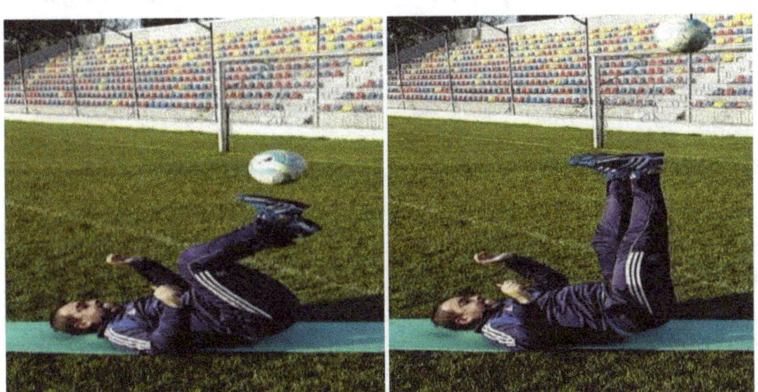

Fig. 8. Lying back, hitting the ball with the sole path High

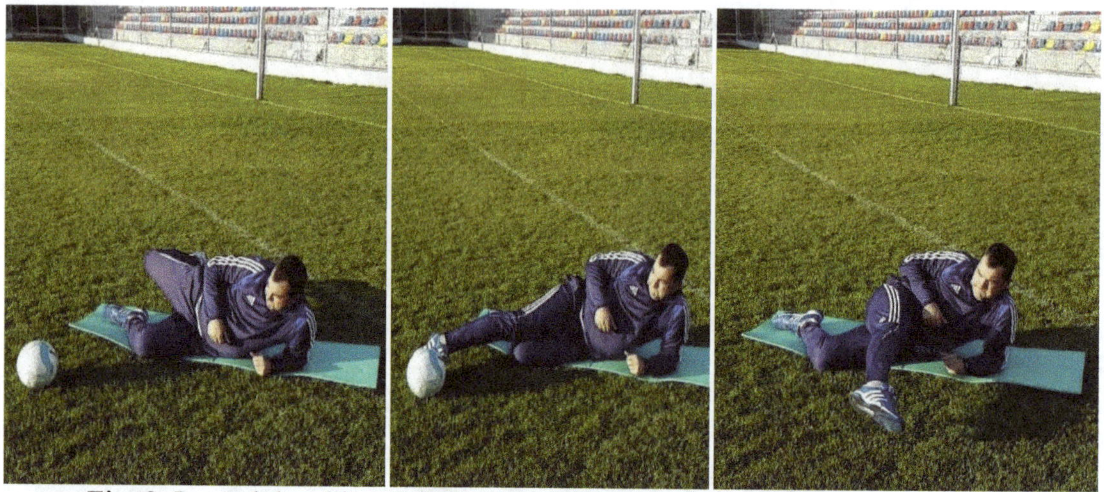

Fig. 9. Lateral decubitus full shoelace hitting the ball with the back forward

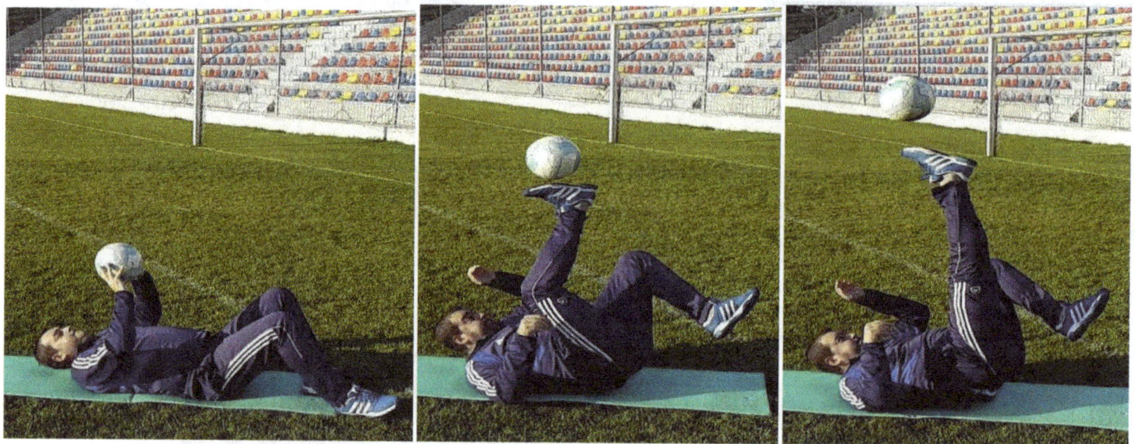

Fig. 10. Throwing leg

Conclusions:

1. Recovery of the affected limb posture include physical therapy, Musculoskeletal manipulations in the hip joint, passive mobilization, active and active resistance [5].
2. Recovery Program must begin immediately after mobilization exercises being amplified gradually, depending on the degree of affection.
3. Medical rehabilitation is aimed to increase joint mobility and tone, she made through physical therapy exercises, physiotherapy and therapeutic massage.

References

[1]. Cioroiu, S. G. (2006). *Esenţial în anatomie şi biomecanică*. Braşov: Editura Universităţii Transilvania, pp. 56

[2]. Creţu, A., coautor Bratu, M., (2003). *Refacere în sport*, Bucureşti: Editura Alexandru 27, pp.98

[3]. Cernăianu, C., (1997). *Teoria şi practica jocului şi antrenamentului modern*, Bucureşti: Editura Fundaţiei România de Mâine pp118

[4]. Păun, D., (2011). *Fotbal – tehnică şi tactică*, Bucureşti: Editura Bren, pp105

[5]. Untea, Gh., (1984). *Aspecte metodico-biologice în fotbal*, Bucureşti: Editura Sport-Turism, pp79

31

STUDY ON DEVELOPMENT OF JOINT MOBILITY TO MIDDLE SCHOOL STUDENTS

Ioana Maria BUȚU, Simona Anemari TEODORESCU, George Cristian CĂTUNĂ

Faculty of Physical Education, Sport and Physical Therapy, Spiru Haret University, Berceni Road, nr. 24, sector 4, Bucharest

Abstract: ***Introduction.*** The ability to easily execute a broad movement is known as a mobility and sometimes flexibility is especially important in training. It is a prerequisite execution skills and develops with amplitude greater ease with which the athlete can perform fast movements. The success of the execution of such movements depends on the amplitude of the joint (or the extent of movement), which must be larger than that required by the respective movement. Therefore it requires a reserve of mobility, that person must develop in order to be safe.

Material and methods

Methods for the development of mobility are three in number, namely the method of activating technique to obtain a maximum mobility of the joint, only by activation of the muscle; liability method to acquire a maximum mobility with the help of exercises with a partner or by using weights and combined method (FPN) require the person to flex active segment up to the joint, then execute a contraction isometric maximum resistance from a partner.

Results

Small schooling stage, the ability flexion of the joints pelvis, shoulder, spine continue to grow, reaching maximum values to 8-9 years.

Discussions and conclusions

In step 10-14, mobility training should be continued because improvements are achieved harder; belt spine mobility and scapular-humeral do not increase, unless action is taken in this regard.

Keywords: mobility, middle school, students.

Introduction

Mobility determines the correct performance of technical procedures and other preparatory exercises from different branches of sport, or for the acquisition of basic motor skills correctly and applied. Usually, mobility is associated with better physical performance, with coordinated movements and associated with a well developed musculoskeletal system. Good mobility is required in all driving documents. Mobility is a quality motor, as with other parameters determine the characteristics and movements [1].

Mobility is man's ability to perform the movements of the body segments with different amplitude.

It is expressed in degrees, given that locomotor movements segments are different angles between them. The structure determines the nature and type of joint movements to be performed in them, and the amplitude is mainly dependent on the impression quality ligaments, tendons and muşchiurilor. Within their muscle elasticity may change to a large extent by neuropsychological processes influence muscle relaxation and stretching exercises stretching type. It considers that the reduction in elasticity antagonists movements amplitude is determined by reflex action defense, reducing the extent of the contraction, the resistance movement.

As you increase the mobility (muscle elasticity is increased through practice, without negatively impacting the return to the original position) simultaneously with exercises to increase flexibility as is recommended exercises of force, which in turn causes joint mobility.

Suppleness is defined as the body's ability to perform large amplitude driving actions. In our case we prefer the term flexibility to define greater or less than the magnitude with which a movement - mobility (joint) and elasticity (tendons, ligaments and muscles), the terms used by some authors to name this capacity It is subordinate body suppleness, highlighting particular aspects of it [2].

Suppleness low creates numerous drawbacks, namely:

- Lengthens driving properties and improvement activities;
- Favors injuries;
- Reduce development indices other driving skills (speed, skill, strength and endurance) and limits their use with maximum efficiency;
- Decreases efficiency in carrying out the driving actions, lack suppleness being supplemented by further efforts by large energy expenditure;

- Decreases execution quality, expressive movements could no longer be enforced, offhand, breezy and easily;
- Suppleness levels peak around age 15-16 years, and at the joints and movements even later. After this age, especially in the neexersării, flexibility decreases gradually. The assertion that there is a suppleness in children (joint mobility) higher however is not fully justified. The fact is that childhood is the most effective for developing this quality [3].

Joint mobility within the natural manifestation is a characteristic feature resulting from the very existence of the joint system of the body. It can be said that an individual has a sufficiently developed motor quality in relation to the requirements of a particular activity if sports nostrum. This quality must be so developed and perfected as to integrate smoothly into gear entire body in that activity and to support easily the role that it has a role that he can not only do amid other qualities dead which is filled permanently.

The naturalness of joint mobility is subject to a number of general factors such as age and gender, especially by a number of specific factors: the nature joints, atructura capsule, ligaments, tendons, and muscles that directly concerned. It is known that motor activity evolves inversely with age. Throughout its evolution, the joint undergoes a series of changes in the degree of mobility. We therefore witness a biological process of gradual loss of a deadly qualities result in limiting the amplitude in carrying out movements.

Experiments conducted proved that the loss of these qualities may be delayed by special physical practice of exercises that maintain, develop joint mobility and muscle elasticity degree higher natural motion [3].

Exercise by tension, pressure or torsion exerted on the joints, activates them, thanked them maintain a degree of mobility year delay and, if possible, aging, deosificare premature, so squeeze their functions.

Given that joint mobility and muscle elasticity are influenced by other qualities dead and they in turn influence appears as a necessity concern for increasing and improving the mobility and eleasticitate [4].

The purpose of the paper is to observe the development of joint mobility to students participating in the experiment by participating in physical education classes, namely those aimed at developing the driving attributes.

Materials and methods

The active method is a technique that yields a maximum joint mobility, muscle activation exclusively. This method refers to the degree of flexion of the agonist muscle and to relax and releasing of such a force to the antagonist muscles. If using a static method, the athlete flexes two segments of a member to the point of extreme mobility while maintaining the position for 6-12 seconds. Athlete ballistic method achieved by balancing the assets of a segment's membership is mobile segment to another building [5].

Passive method to acquire maximum mobility with the help of partner exercises or using weights. In the first case, the partner keeps or pushes a member to peak mobility without active involvement of the subject. This method can be applied to the following joints: ankle, pelvis, spine, shoulder, wrist. It is recommended to use weights (barbells, gantele) for the development of mobility ankle, knee and shoulder. But I do not recommend the pelvis or spine joints because the weight may exceed the tolerance Athlete can press on two segments of a joint bending them over limits, cee needles can lead to possible muscle tears. In any case, the weight must be reduced, carefully applied and gradually increased. Such training should be performed always under strict surveillance [6].

Combined method (FPN) requires the athlete to actively flex segment up to the joint, then perform a maximum isometric contraction to resistance from a partner. Athlete voluntarily flex segment to an angle exceeding previous limits. Runs same isometric contraction through a broader and stronger resistance against opposite a partner. To meet the needs methodological isometric contraction is maintained for 4-6 seconds and carried out series of repetitions to limit the athlete's physical tolerance.

Scale joint mobility comprises 3 levels of Cartage and 3 hypermobility:
0 - joint ankylosis;
1 - severe limitation;
2 - slight limitation;
3 - normal mobility;
4 - slightly higher than normal;
5 - steep increase over normal;
6 - joint instability.

The experiment was conducted at elementary school no. 169, Bucharest students of class V-C during September 2015 - June 2016. The group of students included 16 girls, 12 boys and underwent initial testing and final.

Results:

The tests were as follows:

1. Evaluation of scapulo-humeral joint mobility. The initial position: standing off, raising and lowering their arms stretched above his back. We measure the distance between the hands (in cm).

2. Evaluation of complex mobility of trunk muscles (spine) and legs (hamstrings, hamstrings, triceps sural). One of the evaluation tests of mobility part coarse trunk - hip - standing torso forward bend test. The initial position: sitting on the edge of a bank, bend the trunk forwards (knees straight), measure the distance from toes to fingertips.

To assess the scapulo-humeral mobility we obtained the following results of the two tests (see Figures 1 and 2).

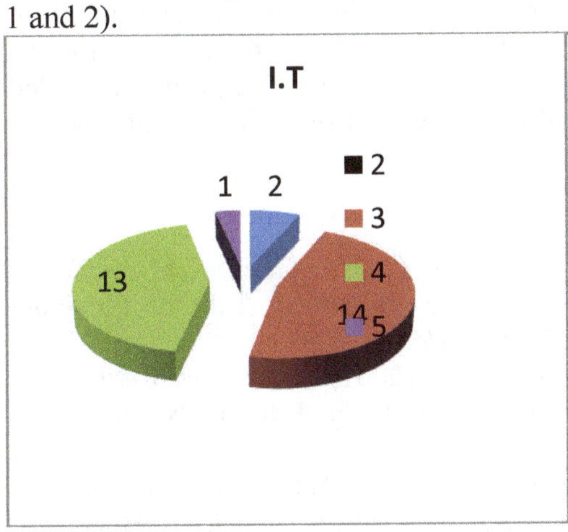

Fig. 1. The results of initial testing for scapulo-humeral joint mobility assessment

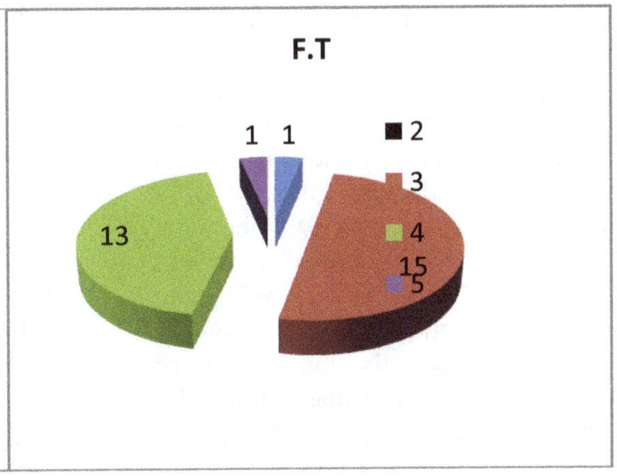

Fig. 2. The results of the final testing scapulo-humeral joint mobility assessment

Figures 3 and 4 are the results obtained in evaluating the mobility of the trunk and legs.

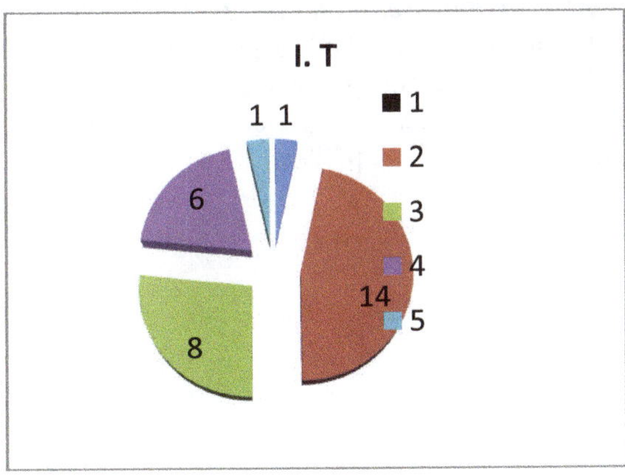

Fig. 3. The results of initial testing for mobility assessment torso and legs

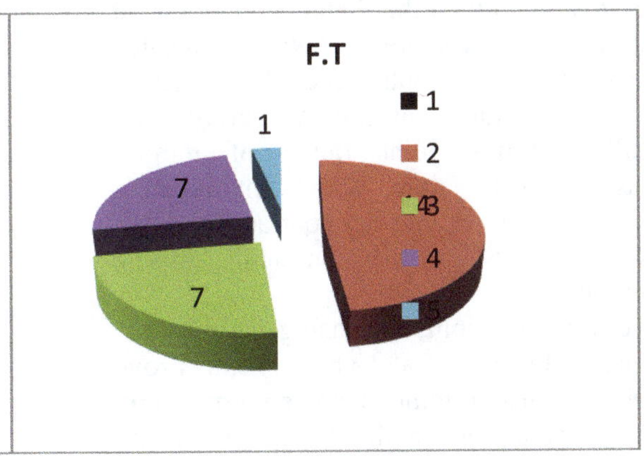

Fig. 4. The results of the final testing mobility assessment torso and legs

Discussion and conclusions

Mobility deficit may be due to soft tissue or damage (contractile and / or uncommitted) crossing a hinge or joint damage through proper mechanism lesion times due to both cases.

Loss of normal motion amplitude meets:

- Prolonged immobilization segments (hip spica cast posts subject imposed by pathology);

- Restrictions to mobilize all normal spring due to pain, bone deformation stations or vicious;
- Loss of flexibility that determines the non-use of areas of joint mobility;
- Neurological disorders that cause muscle imbalances (paralysis, spasticity);
- Connective tissue disease (as in rheumatic diseases) or the existence of joint superjacent skin disorders (eg - cellulitis);
- Tisulo-articular trauma (direct trauma to the articular structures - such as the rupture of the meniscus, local inflammation, plaque, burns).

In appreciation of deficiency joint mobility must differentiate true deficit limiting active mobility due to insufficient muscle strength, a limitation of mobility due to pain (which has no correspondence in place or intensity of joint damage), or a joint stiffness (absence of a pathological substrate - spasticity, rheumatic stiffness) because stiffness, defined as weight (embarrassment) to mobilize the joint can occur due to the thixotropic phenomenon. In humans, the thixotropy is the cause of prolonged rest, resulting in a macromolecular arrangement in such a manner that it prevents the movement.

Limiting mobility impairment that is based on is called soft tissue contracture. The soft tissue is represented on the one hand muscles composed of muscle tissue (the tissue contractile par excellence) and the fibrous skeleton, and on the other hand necontractil of uncommitted structures (skin, capsule, ligament, tendon). Contracture of muscles is called contracture miostatică nature and logically limiting joint range of motion because muscle may only Involvement substrate tissue or muscle contractile tissue Involvement Co and the contractile muscle necontractil.

Above a certain limit, increasing mobility (as evidenced by the scale above) can prove negative as tension joints become permanently active. Passive joint stability by compromising or appliance capsuloligamentar (elongation, breaking it) remains the only active component stability ensured by periarticular muscle tonic contraction. In case of fatigue or muscle relaxation increases the risk of these dislocations or sprains. Hipermobilitatea, which allow for normal physiological movement outside amplitudes in time will cause a premature wear of the cartilage of these joints.

Thus, glenohumeral joint assessment by the two tests, shows an improvement in mobility to students participating in the experiment. The fact that the top two values on the scale that expresses the degree of mobility has not been assigned any of the students demonstrate that they have no severe limitation or joint ankylosis. Also, no child has joint instability.

When evaluating mobility torso and legs, students have achieved an improvement in values obtained in final testing, from baseline. Here is observed, due to the results recorded that the students did not stiffen joints, but no joint instability.

References

[1]. Buțu I.M. (2015), *Gimnastică ritmică – baze generale*. Bucureşti: Editura Fundației *România de Mâine*, p. 56.

[2]. Bompa T. (2001), *Dezvoltarea calităților biomotrice,* Constanța: Editura Ex. Pronto, p. 67.

[3]. Dragnea A, (1991), *Teoria* şi *metodica dezvoltării calităților motrice,* Bucureşti: Compendiu, p.98.

[4]. Dragnea, A., (1996), *Antrenamentul sportiv*. Bucureşti: Editura Didactică şi Pedagogică, p.23.

[5]. Hidi, I.L., (2007), *Fitness programe pentru optimizarea condiției fizice*. Bucureşti: Editura Didactică şi Pedagogică, p.51.

[6]. Şerbanoiu, S., Tudor V., (2007), *Teoria şi metodica educației fizice şi sportului*, Bucureşti: ANEFS, p. 29.

32

REHABILITATION FOR THE POSTSURGICAL ACUTE ACHILLES TENDON RUPTURE - A CASE STUDY

Ilona ILINCA[1,2], Eugenia ROSULESCU[1,2], Mircea DANOIU[1]

[1]*University of Craiova, Faculty of Physical Education and Sport, Craiova*

[2]*Neuromotor Adults Rehabilitation Center St. Maria, Craiova*

Abstract: Background & Purpose. Treatment options for an Achilles tendon rupture include surgical repair and conservative non surgical rehabilitation. Surgical repair is typically recommended for patients who expect to return to relatively high functional activities required of recreational athletics. Surgical repairs allow quicker mobilization and return to activity. The purpose of this case study is to apply postoperative rehabilitation protocol after an Achilles tendon total rupture and to assess the results on heel pain and function, joint mobility, strength and balance.

Case Description. Our subject was a 33-year-old male recreational athlete diagnosed with complete Achilles tendon rupture and subsequent repair. One week after removed plaster cast he presented to physical therapy with pain, muscle trophic modifications, calf atrophy, joint block and extreme compensation strategies during ambulation.

Outcome Measures. The subject underwent a functional evaluation that included: the heel pain intensity (VAS scale) articular testing (goniometric measurements), manual muscle test, static balance (The Unilateral Forefoot Balance Test), girth measurements and functional scale (LEFS). The rehabilitation treatment included the information and education of the patient, physical therapy, electrotherapy, criotherapy and assistive gait devices. Measurements were repeated at 1-month, 2-month and 4-month follow-up.

Results. The data shows an important difference in all parameters measured (VAS, ankle ROM, muscle strength, girth measurements, balance and functional abilities) comparing four stages of evaluation, where the intermediates and final evaluation provided a better results compared with the initial one.

Key words: Achilles tendon , rupture, rehabilitation

Introduction

The Achilles tendon also called the calcaneal tendon is a tough band of fibrous tissue that connects the calf muscles to calcaneus and is essential for walking, running and postural control. It is the largest, toughest and strongest tendon in the human body. The Achilles tendon originates from the two tendon portions formed by the extension of the gastrocnemius, with its medial and lateral head originating from the condyles of the femur, and the soleus muscle, and inserts into the calcaneal bone. The goal of the tendon is to transmit force of these muscles to the calcaneal bone. The calcaneal insertion is specialised to assist the dissipation of stress from the tendon to the heel bone.

Achilles tendon ***ruptures*** are ***partial*** or ***comple te.*** While a partial rupture can be completely asymptomatic or may cause a mild symptomatology, in the complete rupture the patient experience intense pain and sudden loss of strength and mobility of the affected leg. Ruptures can also be divided into acute traumatic ruptures and chronic or neglected ruptures when the injury has been left untreated for 4 weeks or more. Most Achilles tendon ruptures occur in male, recreational athletes between the ages of 30 and 40 years[1]. Ruptures not attributed to sports activity are usually caused by falls or stumbles that also require sudden acceleration or deceleration movements.

The pathogenesis is debated but it is commonly thought that ruptures are due to sudden overloading of the musculotendinous unit in a poorly conditioned individual.

The physiologic capacity of the Achilles tendon may be compromised by intrinsic or extrinsic factors. Extrinsic, mechanical forces may exceed the physiologic capacity of the Achilles when: a forcefully push off the forefoot while the knee is extending, a sudden dorsiflexion with full weightbearing, a sudden and intense dorsiflexion when jump from a height and landing on a plantar-flexed foot. Intrinsic risk factors include: hypovascularity, repetitive microtrauma and the associated inflammation and degeneration, endocrine function and nutrition.

Several studies demonstrate that the middle-portion of the tendon, approximately located 4-5 cm proximal to the calcaneal insertion is a relatively hypovascular area. This hypovascularity may account for the fact that most of the ruptures occur in this area[2]. Age is also considered an important risk factor associated with Achilles tendon rupture; blood flow diminishing significantly with age.

Treatment options for an Achilles tendon rupture include surgical repair and conservative non surgical rehabilitation. Patients who have a neglected rupture and a functional deficit are managed optimally with surgery[3]. Decision making is based on age, past medical history, and desired level of functional return. Surgical repair is typically recommended for patients who expect to return to relatively high functional activities required of recreational athletics. Surgical repairs allow quicker mobilization and return to activity.

The purpose of this case study is to apply postoperative rehabilitation protocol after an Achilles tendon total rupture and to assess the results on heel pain and function, joint mobility, strength and balance.

CASE REPORT

History of Presenting Condition

Our subject was a 33-year-old male recreational athlete diagnosed with complete Achilles tendon rupture and subsequent repair. The surgery was performed 5 days after the injury. Following the repair, the patient was immobilized in a below-knee plaster cast with the ankle at a 90 degree angle for 6 weeks. Full weight bearing was allowed after 3 weeks. One week after removed plaster cast he presented to physical therapy with pain, muscle trophic modifications, calf atrophy, joint block and extreme compensation strategies during ambulation. Due to pain, swelling, associated with mobility impairments and indications for partial weight bearing the patient uses axillary crutches for ambulation. At the initial evaluation the patient presents the following: ankle AROM plantarflexion 18^0, dorsiflexion 5°, inversion 20^0 and eversion 14^0. Strength ankle DF: 3-/5, PF 3/5, INV 4/5, EV 4/5. Atrophy of the left quadriceps and gastrocnemius muscle. He ambulates with canes and antalgic gait pattern with decreased push-off on the left foot. The incision is clean and dry, with mild redness and warmth to palpation.

Physical therapy intervention

Physical therapy interventions were chosen according to the patient's function impairments, activity limitations, and participation restrictions. The rehabilitation treatment includes the information and education of the patient, physical therapy, electrotherapy, criotherapy and assistive gait devices. Therapeutic ultrasound and laser therapy have been used to shorten the time needed for correct lesion cicatrisation. The patient received physical therapy for 60 minutes, 3-4 times per week for 12 week and periodic visits for up to 24 weeks.

The physical therapy intervention based on Manual therapy (soft tissue mobilization, passive range of motion, joint mobilizations), Neuromuscular Reeducation to retrain lower extremity postural awareness, recruitment patterns, and balance, Gait training to decrease compensation and restore normal gait pattern and Therapeutic exercise to restore strength, range of motion and to reinforce proper movement patterns. A home exercise protocol was given the patient to supplement therapy on days.

The goals of therapy intervention:

- The management of pain and swelling with physiotherapy, criotherapy and elevation
- Improvement Range of motion through scar and soft tissue mobilization- triceps surae complex, plantar fascia and the Achilles tendon
- Improvement joint mobility restrictions utilized joint mobilizations to the talocrural and subtalar joint and the first metatarsophalangeal joint.
- Improvement strength of the muscle groups that have been damaged by immobilisation after surgical treatment.
- Strengthen ankle plantarflexors through full ROM and the gastrocnemius/soleus complex
- Restore normal walking ability
- Restore the dorsiflexion and plantar flexion of the ankle joints

6-8 WEEK AFTER SURGERY	
Joint mobilization Scar tissue mobilization Soft tissue mobilization -gastrocnemius/soleus, Achilles tendon	
Active ROM exercises for knee (flexion/extension), hip (flexion/extension, abduction/adduction), and toes	2-3 sets of 8-12 repetitions
Hip strength: gluteus medius/ abduction (Straight Leg Raises, Clam-	2-3 sets of 8-12 repetitions

shells)	
Isometric quadriceps contractions	10x6sec
Isometric knee extensions	10x6sec
Stretching of the hamstrings, gastrognemius, and quadriceps – straight leg lifts, hip abduction	2x30sec
Begin active dorsiflexion to neutral with passive plantar flexion	1-2 sets of 8-10 repetitions
Supine ankle Alphabet	1 set
Seated calf raises	2-3 sets of 8-12 repetitions
BAPS board in sitting	20x each direction
Progressive weight-bearing, using axillary crutches	

8-12 WEEK AFTER SURGERY	
Same exercises as last 2 week	
Joint mobilizations of the talocrural joint, both anterior and posterior, if needed	
Stretching Gluteus Maximus, Medius, Piriformis, Rectus Femoris	2x30sec
Gentle Gastroc/soleus stretching	3x15sec
Continue knee and hip range of motion exercises from phase 1	3 sets of 8-12 repetitions
Continue to strengthen all other area of the body	3 sets of 8-12 repetitions
Initiate active plantar flexion	2x8
Advance active dorsiflexion to neutral	2x8
Inversion/eversion ROM	2x10
Active range of motion exercises, isometric exercises, progressing to light resisted	2-3 sets of 8-12 repetitions
Exercises using tubing or manual resistance – to all weakened ankle and foot musculature	2 sets of 8-12 repetitions
Bridges bilateral (10 week)	3x8
Minisquats (bilateral)	3x8
Double leg standing	5x30sec
Bilateral concentric heel raises	2x10
Begin stationary bike with heel push only	10 min
Gait training – used the appropriate height heel lift, if necessary, to attain normal loading	

12- 20 WEEK AFTER SURGERY	
Same exercises as last 2 week	
Continue with active exercises, isometric and isotonic	
Calf muscles stretching, isotonic exercises with elastic bands.	2x30sec
Begin single leg stance on uninjured leg	5x10sec
Bridges unilateral	3 x8
Heel-raise exercises	3 x10
Functional movements: minisquats unilateral,lunges/ reverse lunges	3x10
Knee straight - gastrocnemius drop	3x8
Knee Bent- soleus drop	3x8
Balance exercises on balance board and one-leg exercises	2 sets of 10 repetitions
Single leg stance on half foam roler	5x10sec
Steps ups, steps downs	3x8
Sidestepping	theraband, 3x20 feet
Stationary bike	5 min
Elliptical (week 12)	5 min
Waking at the treadmill (week 14)	5 min
Jogging may start at week 16	

Outcome Measures

The design for this study was a pre-test post-test design. The subject underwent a functional evaluation that included: the heel pain intensity (VAS scale) articular testing (goniometric measurements), manual muscle test, static balance (The Unilateral Forefoot Balance Test), girth measurements and functional scale (LEFS).

Visual analogue scale (VAS) Pain was assessed using a visual analogical scale (VAS) [4]. The VAS consists of a 10-cm line, with the left extremity indicating "no pain" and the right extremity indicating "unbearable pain." The subjects were asked to mark the intensity of the heel pain that he felt at rest and level of heel pain following activity. Higher values suggest more intense pain.

The active range of motion (AROM) for talocrural and subtalar joint was measured and recorded in degrees using a goniometer which has been demonstrated to be a sufficiently reliable tool for measuring lower limb ROM [5].

The strength of the ankle was measured, recorded and graded by manual muscle testing on a five-point scale. (grade 5 - movement against gravity with full resistance; grade 4 - movement against gravity with some resistance; grade 3 - movement against gravity only; grade 2 - movement with gravity eliminated; grade 1 - visible and palpable muscle contraction but no movement and; grade 0 - no contraction). Manual Muscle Testing is an easily accessible and reliable method of determining the strength of individual muscles [6].

The static balance of the patient was measured with The Unilateral Forefoot Balance Test. This test is based on the single leg stance test but uses a reduced base of support. At this test the subject balances on the forefoot by placing the weight on the ball on the foot and lifting the heel just off the ground without raising it up high. The subject should not elevate the non-supporting leg beyond mid shin and it must not rest on the other leg. We recorded the time covered between the moment the person's heel cleared the ground and the moment when the elevated foot touched the ground[7].

Circumference of the superior medial malleolus and calcaneus was measured with a non-stretchable 150cm measuring tape. Circumferential girth measurements are commonly used to document atrophy or swelling in an extremity[8].

The Lower Extremity Functional Scale (LEFS) is a self-report, 20-item, uni-dimensional, region-specific measure that quantify the perceived difficulty of a variety of activities. Each item is scored on a 5-point scale (0-4). Item scores are summed to yield a total score ranging from 0 to 80, with higher scores representing better functional status [9].

Results

The evolution of the subject had a positive trajectory registered noticeable improvements in almost all measured parameters, in the period between assessments.

The initial intensity of heel pain rest and following activity, assessed by VAS scale was moderate at rest (5/10) and severe after activity (8/10). Ten weeks after surgery the intensity decreases reaching 4/10 (VAS following activity) and 2/10, two months follow up as shown in table 1.

After the rehabilitation strategy significant increases were observed in ankle range of motion (plantar flexion, dorsiflexion, inversion and eversion). Total active motion angles of the ankle joint were increased progressively over time from 5^0 to 19^0 for dorsiflexion, (10^0 being sufficient for walking activity) from 18^0 to 42^0 for plantarflexion and for inversion/eversion from $20^0/14^0$ to $37^0/25^0$ (table2).

Table 1. Evaluation of VAS score

VAS Scale	8 weeks after surgery	10 weeks after surgery	2 months after surgery
VAS at rest	5/10	2/10	-
VAS **following activity**	8/10	4/10	2/10

Table 2. The measurements of ankle ROM

Ankle ROM	Pre-treatment	After 1month of treatment	After 2 months of treatment	After 4 months of treatment
Plantarflexion	18^0	25^0	38^0	42^0
Dorsiflexion	5^0	15^0	17^0	19^0
Inversion	20^0	26^0	32^0	37^0
Eversion	14^0	18^0	22^0	25^0

Gradually over the next four months, ankle strength improved considerable when comparing with initial moment. Re-evaluation of dorsiflexion, plantarflexion, inversion and eversion muscle performance revealed increased strength of the previously tested. After four month of rehabilitation, manual muscle test grades of 4+/5 and 5/5 were given for both ankle dorsi- and plantar-flexor. For ankle inversion and eversion, strength had improved to 5/5.
Girth measurements were also used to assess how much edema was still in the affected ankle. At first evaluation the value of difference between superior medial malleolus circumference of the affected leg and the normal leg was 3,4 cm. After one month of rehabilitation the difference between medial malleolus circumferences improved with 2 cm. The next evaluation showed an improvement of 1cm in the difference of medial malleolus circumference. After 3 months of rehabilitation treatment there was no difference between circumferences measured. Initially the calcaneus circumference of the uninvolved ankle was smaller than the involved ankle by 1,3 cm (table3).

Table 3. Evaluation of the girth measurements (cm)

Girth measurements(cm)*	Pre-treatment	After 1month of treatment	After 2 months of treatment
superior medial malleolus	3,4	1,4	0,4
calcaneus	1,3	0,7	0,2

* the value of difference between affected leg and the normal leg

After 2 weeks of rehabilitation we assessed static balance and we noticed that the patient was able to single-leg-balance only for 5 seconds. Satisfactory improvements were obtained at all evaluation moments as shown in table 4.
The LEFS score showed a better improvement after four months (table4). The LEFS score was 38 points after 1 month of rehabilitation therapy, which is 47% of maximal function if compared to 20

points (25%) before any rehabilitation treatment. After two months of rehabilitation the LEFS score showed 56 points (70% of maximal function) growing after 4 months at 74 points (92%).

Table 4. Evaluation of Unilateral Forefoot Balance Test and LEFS score

	Pre-treatment	After 1month of treatment	After 2 months of treatment	After 4 months of treatment
Unilateral Forefoot Balance Test(sec)	5`	15`	30`	90`
LEFS score	20/80	38/80	56/80	74/80

Discussion

Acute Achilles tendon rupture is a frequent and potentially disabling injury. Variations in functional treatment protocols are large and the efficacies of different rehabilitation protocols are unclear[9].Our patient was treated surgical repair with postoperative immobilization (6 weeks). After surgery, the important outcomes refer to recovery of full function and the ability to return to previous activities including sports without an increased risk of re-rupture and of developing other overuse injuries.

The patient completed the rehabilitation program consisting of exercises therapy and electrotherapy with no complications and there were no adverse events registered after our rehabilitation. Physical therapy intervention described in this case report focused on manual therapy, exercise therapy and gait training aimed to reduce pain and inflammation, restore strength, joint mobility, balance, to increase functioning and improve levels of activity.

The subject made steady progress in terms of regaining ROM and strength once he began physical therapy. Plantarflexion ROM returned more quickly than dorsiflexion ROM, perhaps suggesting that his Achilles tendon had slowly lengthened. Ankle ROM is usually used as an indirect measure of tendon elongation. Increased dorsiflexion after an Achilles tendon rupture is assumed to result from tendon lengthening. Plantarflexion and dorsiflexion strength was significantly impaired but made dramatic improvements toward the end of this bout of therapy. There were important differences for intensity of the heel pain and girth measurements in the different moments of evaluation during the therapeutic intervention. Between 2 months and 4 months post-surgery, the patient achieved a significant functional improvement compared with the first period of evaluation.

In addition, the patient improved his compliance with a home exercise program, which also may have factored into his enhanced.

Conclusion

The outcomes of this case report indicate that electrotherapy combined with a therapeutic exercise programs appears to be an effective means to improve functional capabilities following Achilles tendon repair. Furthermore, strong compliance with a home exercise program is favorable to enhance rehabilitation outcomes. The correlation of orthopedic-surgical intervention and rehabilitation measures, the earliness recovery measures enforcement can create the necessary support for obtaining a proper ant complete rehabilitation of the patient.

References

[1]. Soma C.A:, Mandelbaum B.R. Achilles tendon disorders. Clinics in Sport Medicine. (1994).13(4):812-23.

[2]. Pierre-Jerome C, Moncayo V, Terk MR.(2010). MRI of the Achilles tendon: A comprehensive review of the anatomy, biomechanics, and imaging of overuse tendinopathies. Acta Radiol. May;51(4):438-54.

[3]. Porter D., Mannarino, F. Snead D., Gabel S., Ostrowski M. (1997) Primary repaire without augmentation for early neglected Achilles tendon ruptures in the recreational athlete. Foot and

Ankle International, 18(9):557–64.
[4]. Downie WW, Leatham PA, Rhind VM, Wright V, Branco JA, Anderson JA. (1978) Studies with pain rating scales. Ann Rheum Dis. 1978;37:378 – 81.
[5]. Norkin CC, White DJ. (1995) Measurement of Joint Motion: A Guide to Goniometry. Philadelphia: FA Davis Company.
[6]. Mendell J.R., Florence J., (1990) Manual Muscle Testing. Muscle nerve. (Supll):S16-20. PubMed.
[7]. Clark M.S. (2007) The Unilateral Forefoot Balance Test: Reliability and validity for measuring balance in late midlife women. New Zealand Journal of Physiotherapy 35(3): 110-118.
[8]. Whitney S.L., Mattocks L., Irrgang J.J., Gentile P.A., Pezzullo D., Kamkar A. (1995) Reliability of Lower Extremity Girth Measurements and Wight- and Left-Side Differences. Journal of Sport Rehabilitation. pp. 108-115, Human Kinetics Publishers. Inc.
[9]. Binkley JM, Stratford PW, Lott SA, Riddle DL. (1999) The Lower Extremity Functional Scale (LEFS): scale development, measurement properties, and clinical application. North American Orthopaedic Rehabilitation Research Network. Phys Ther. 79:371-383.
[10]. Kearney RS, Achten J, Lamb SE, Plant C & Costa ML (2012) A systematic review of patient-reported outcome measures used to assess Achilles tendon rupture management: what's being used and should we be using it? Br J Sports Med 46(16): 1102–1109.

33

THE ROLE OF IN OPTIMIZING PROFESSIONAL PREPARATORY GAMES PROFESSIONALLY APPLIED OF PHYSICAL TRAINING

Dănut STOICA[1], Valeriu JURAT[2]

[1]University of Physical Education and Sport, Chişinău, Republica Moldova
[2] University of Physical Education and Sport, Chişinău,Republica Moldova

Abstract: Professional preparatory games are the easiest model to boost loved professional actions of the operators from order and public security system in active breaks, substantiating professional activity, together with professional progress, evolving liked in the physical and psychical plan. To this form of practical activity is observed from the beginning two distinct structures (education and occupation) during the process instructions which efficiently complement each other. After a longer time professional preparatory games evolve in mentally and motor plan acquiring complex and varied characteristics , approaching as much as they can teh operators profession. With the passing to the step of creativity of the game takes shape and content clearly for the operator by developing the psyche and its motility, thus participating relaxed, conscious and active physique and psyche to the real professional actions that areto fulfill in their daily duties.
Keywords: games, training, professional, practical.

Introduction

Professional preparatory games have an important role in the physical training professional content applications and are useful and effective in the educational process with a dynamic character development major functions of the body, establishing a clear harmony between them, providing an active psychic and motor.Here by the content, structure and application adapts and complements creating permanent professional content accessibility implementation games for different ages.Between these two types of exercises (physical and mental) that are in the contents of games, it needs to make a clear distinction between the foundation, which is designed as a means to actively instruct and as guidance psychomotor in the evolution and progress of people arrived at an high level of professional psychomotor maturity to reset psychomotor intense effort to solve practical professional duties.[1,2,3].

Professional preparatory games strengthen physique and psyche of the human being, developing thinking, imagination, creativity rapidly, exerting an important influence on the character of conduct of such business and pleasure.The Permanence of improvement of moral-volitional qualities plays a key role in the development of muscle which in turn indirectly influences breathing, circulation and psyche of that person.[4,5].Most experts in the field made permanently linked impossible to distinguish between play and work, showing the important role it plays in development adding that "therefore can not fix an absolute border between play and work.Play and work are not only the same line poles, along passing imperceptibly from game to work"[6].

Materials and methods

The definition of game is made easiest and targeted by "The terminology of physical education and sport" (1973), which states that "the game is a complex activity, predominantly motor and emotional, which occurs spontaneously established rules having previously recreational, sporting and while adapting to social reality "[7]. (professional).The game is a psychomotor activity practice, running natural, spontaneous, pleasant, leisure, recreational activity primarily aimed at restoring the body after intense physical and mental effort. This is the fast, safe, pleasant and efficient working method as a means of acquiring and consolidating the contents psychomotor and professional staff policy and public security system.[1,4, 7].

Preparatory professional game has a key role in the continued development of psychomotor qualities having a formative influence in the training process by deepening knowledge previously acquired professional execution.Throughout working life, man is a being active practice and professional preparatory games you can engage in activities without any previous specialized training, requiring only a strong personality and well-developed driving skills.[2,8] Multilateral contribution to preparing creates an active influence on the human body, only if properly designed, organized, led and coordinated permanent instructors. In the course of preparatory games professionally requested maximum of physical attributes and specific professional skills, moral-volitional qualities, while strengthening the confidence and the know-how.

Specific professional driving skills are improving rapidly consolidating and especially through the game, creating new and complex professional connections here by harmonizing practical interests of professional activities.Using games preparatory professional operators develops rapidly in a pleasant work environment, initiative, rapid adaptation, group work, tolerance, responsibility for execution, accepting mistakes, group cohesion, independence movement, self-confidence itself, etc ..[2,6,9].

Choosing the most efficient requirements in games preparatory professional are based on a number of criteria such as purpose, content, objectives, motivation, equipment and technical means, working time, the degree of effort used by health, venue, weather conditions, develop physical fitness, volitional qualities, etc ..The influence of psychomotor and professional preparatory training games on the operator determines the purpose, content and structure of their overall participating intensively and effectively to the training objectives that are essential implication on future operational content. They require time, precision, coordination, speed, strength, flexibility, mental mobility that much work is done only by rational and objective that required intense observation, attention, will, imagination, motivation, etc ..

It was observed that, lately, the Interior Ministry granted increasingly less time professional preparatory games and sports specialist. But back to the original idea: is it an important professional preparatory game in applied professional physical preparation? It's worth it to pay this special attention and support as? It requires specialists in applied professional physical preparation? Does our efforts are doomed from the start? To acknowledge and clear answers to these questions need to look a little more closely professional preparatory games.[9, 10]

Playground is varied (sporting grounds, parks, housing, etc.) which increases the possibility of practical concern to human movement, which can be as varied; and the joy and pleasure of victory or defeat clearly affects psychomotor skills, quickly triggering mechanism moral-volitional qualities especially self-control and strengthen the will.Therefore, in a short time professional preparatory games helps to counteract the effects of sedentary satisfying their urge to move them. Most games require a multilateral body, which develops the final effects of physical attributes (speed, coordination, endurance, strength) with perfect perseverance and desire to prepare physically and professionally.[2,5,8]

Professional preparatory games energises and mobilizes all forces and psychic driving, keeping up the interest and practical progress, which we maintain by using motivation, the desire to reach the final maximum efficiency. The motivation is stronger, the operator will be stronger in confidence, instructor assisting him with compliments positive during the action.Will try as much as possible as compliments to strengthen its self-confidence and practical knowledge, the will and desire to do more and better. Any process psycho-pedagogy of learning the professional knowledge to be executed to start the game pregătitore professional because the pleasure of practicing "gives them wings", encourages and motivates, allowing people that they can choose for themselves the most effective, after desire and purpose. It would otherwise have underlined the importance of professional preparatory games disconnection from mental stress, the most effective method of active rest, enabling the use within leisure in the educational process.[3,9,10]

Preparatory professional games, if learned correctly during the action will develop the spirit of fair play, which is needed because of the freedom of action and that actually is the basic principle that all games are built to move. The game itself properly during continuous learning process influences individual behavior during social and professional life.Through it man is customary to bear with dignity and externalize defeats during victory. Those who depend on it during the competition and acquire him permanently translating it into social and professional activity.

One could mention a lot of qualities moral-volitional which is cultivated through games preparatory professional that intelligence has an important role by repeating permanent movements, coordinating them precise content and quick creation of environmental conditions favorable that can enable effective cultivation of the thinking capacity of each operator, developing the spirit of sacrifice, professional perseverance, courage, that can develop even using the most simple and fast motion gaming.[7,10]

Another feature of the game is to develop professional preparatory personality traits, characterized by dynamism and speed of thought, which developing practical and logical memory in short time and effectively. These positive influence multilateral development operator, combativeness, discipline, spirit of trust and responsibility of what is running. It should be stressed also that the game manifest liked not only positive traits of character, but while negative ones, such as lack of interest in coexistence with selfishness, pride immeasurable modesty, honesty cunning, etc .. The game itself does not cultivate negative qualities, but sometimes they emerge and are enhanced excessive unintentional. A feeling of belonging to a certain group is the one that gives priority positive traits. Each operator is aware that the spirit of sacrifice is a professional quality. Of affirmation and manifestation of an operator to dominate others and must be combated at all times because behavior between ideal and practical contradictions positive behavior can occur. But the presence of the instructor provides prevention and resolution of conflicts. Because of this preparatory games professionally designed have organized a stronger effect than spontaneously, provided that the instructor be familiar with the basic rules of the game, running technique and his professional order. Word, gesture, instructor's personal example, can have a key influence, can mitigate and avoid negative traits effectively developing basic motor skills and specific training.[2,6,7,9].

Discussion and conclusions

At a deeper analysis of professional preparatory games emerges the importance and role in educating the will and self-restraint in tense situations professionally, that is needed to have the ability to coordinate movements psychomotor work safer and more efficient.Once it develops visual acuity, hearing, intelligence, observation, etc., that the variety of their content is an effective means of development and improvement of the physical and psychic operator.Clearly shown by I. Moraru that "between play and work is still an essential difference: the game only produce pleasure and enjoyment, but does not produce objects (goods) necessary to society" [6]. This clearly shows the essence of each key role which plays in civil society and professional activity daily.

Just proving something you can reach the initial allegation, that applied professional games are one of the most efficient, enjoyable and important means of instruction. Any instructor, once convinced of this, it realizes that it is necessary to know as many different games with professional content, to be able to analyze and select adapting their professional activity on the right to execute.[3, 9]

The games are challenging and professional preparatory multilateral body in a pleasant environment, with the highest efficiency if performed under the guidance and observation instructor to the following specific features games:

- lack of fatigue or lack of interest in play;
- attractive and fun of the game;
- spontaneous movements;
- mobilize all mental and motor skills;
- psychomotor maximum effort;
- maintain continuous desire to move;
- power mobilization of all forces in a short time;
- psychomotor quick disconnect;
- of affirmation;
- observation during the game lack of interest (selfishness, envy, wickedness, malice, etc.);

The true professional is not limited to the content of the game, leaving him to proceed to chance. If a teacher take people then retreats to perform another task will fail to capitalize on a series of educational resources and professional game. An effective multilateral exercises influence the game organized and coordinated closely followed the instructor intervening and directly influencing the content and purpose of professional preparatory games.[2,5,10].

Those who want to call themselves specialists in applied professional physical preparation need not identify during work on game play free, but know this game previously deployment. The game is entertaining from start activity, then the trainer to treat it consciously as an occupation full responsibility.

References

[1]. Mitrea, Gh., Mogoş, Al.(1980). *School Physical Education Methodology.* Bucureşti: Ed. Sports -Tourism.

[2]. Simister, C.J. (2011).*Games for the development of intelligence and creativity of children.* Bucureşti: Ed. Polirom.

[3]. Simion. Z.M.(2000). *The game in physical education in primary teaching* - degree project.Târgovişte: University of„Valahia"Târgovişte

[4]. Epuran, M.(1974). *Psychology and sport in present.* Bucureşti: Ed.Stadion.

[5]. Chiriţă, G. (1983). *Education through movement games.* Bucureşti: Ed. Sports - Tourism.

[6]. Moraru, I. (1992). *Interdisciplinarycreative strategies*. p. 22-25, Bucureşti: Ed. Romanian Academy

[7]. *** *The terminology of Physical Education and Sport.* (1974). Bucureşti: Ed. Stadion

[8]. Verza, E. (1978). *Man, play and fun.* Bucureşti. Ed. Scientific and Encyclopedic.

[9]. Şchiopu, U.(1970). *Psychological problems of the game and entertainment.* Bucureşti: Ed. Didactic and Pedagogic.

[10]. Cârstea, Gh.(1997). *Theory and methodology bases.* Bucureşti: Ed. A.N.E.F.S.

WAYS TO ENHANCE THE SPEED IN TABLE TENNIS SPORT TRAINING AT THE LEVEL OF THE SECOND FORMATIVE PHASE

Dragoş DIACONESCU, Eliana LICĂ, Marian DRAGOMIR, Laurenţiu LICĂ

University of Craiova

Corresponding adress: dragosdiaconescu31@yahoo.com

Abstract: Introduction. The process of preparing performance in table tennis requires the training of table tennis players and keeping the performance to a level as high as possible. Training begins with the selection of players and continues with an educational process of formation of sportsmen personality consistent with the requirements of specific sports performance in modern table tennis. Methods. Thus, this paper aims to identify the best strategies that lead to optimizing speed training in junior tennis players. For 5 months, 12 subjects (male, aged 8-11) had in their workouts means directed mostly to speed development. Results. At the end of training significant progress was identified in all tests, thus speed emerged as significantly enhanced.

Key words: tennis table, speed training, junior.

Introduction

Table tennis competition has become very fierce, competitors trying to surprise and overcome their opponents, always looking to find new ways and solutions that contribute to improving the game and training process. The modern table tennis requires very good motor abilities like speed, agility, strength, endurance, balance and good reflexes and sense of touch [1]. Speed of movement is along with the coordination and movement touch, the important feature of many tennis specific movements [2].

Acceleration speed is the individual's ability to cover a given space in a short time [3] V. Tudor, 2005, p. 108) and is regarded as a complex form of manifestation of speed (A. Demeter 1981, p. 38) [4] expressed by the relation between space and time [1] (V. Tudor, 2005, p. 108). Acceleration speed is thus a complex form of manifestation of speed with maximum quickness, rapidly completing a distance, which is in a relative interdependence with other manifestations of speed and influenced by other motor quantities - power, agility, endurance.

The aim of our work was to identify experimentally the most effective teaching strategies to improve speed in table tennis sport training at the level of the second formative phase.

Method

For 5 months, work programs which had musical media in its structure intended to interfere with the development of speed , among which: Running with active knees lifting; speed Running on 20 m in groups of 4-8 students on auditory stimuli in competition; Running with different tasks to auditory signals (shouts a name, answer a question, etc) were applied 2 times per week to a total of 12 athletes (aged between 8-11), working at CSS Craiova, Dynamic games; defense of the entire table with frontal light, an opponent which will direct the balls mainly to the sides of the table; counter forehand on 3 quarters of table, forehand directed only towards the opponent; combined counter alternatively forehand and backhand directed from the backhand corner, on the left half of the table, directed at the opponent's backhand; counter from all mass freely routed with permanent change of distance from the table, combining counters next to the table with the remote ones, were implemented.

The subjects were tested before and after implementing the work programs, the tests were:

speed Running - 50m. Technical specifications. Horizontal running color ground. standing Start, timing the motion without shoes with nails. Results are recorded in seconds, tenths and hundredths. We give two attempts with a 15 minute- break. We record the best.

10 x 4m lateral displacement. Description: we mark a 4 m wide lane; we place a pole that can be hit without falling 30cm outside the lines elastic aisle. Execution: lateral movement with footsteps add up until the sole of the foot on the direction of displacement touches the aisle, followed by the line change in the opposite direction. When the direction of the game changes, the game hand touches the pole through a similar movement of the ball hitting racket, either backhand shot or forehand or, if applicable. We are timing the required interval for 10 lateral displacements, displacement being a 4m displacement.

10 x 4m forward-backward displacement. Description: we mark a 4m aisle with two lines; 50cm outside the front line, outside the aisle we place an elastic pole. Execution: forward and backward *displacement* with added steps. Every *forward displacement* they have to touch the pole with the game hand. The sole of the foot on the direction of displacement must touch the marking line.

In this research, we used a 4 motor control tests. For each of the proofing tools we have done the following determinations for each of the two tests, initial and final.

1. arithmetic mean of data string;
2. the deviations from the arithmetic mean of each value and their sum;
3. variance or dispersion of data string;
4. standard deviation;
5. coefficient of variation;
6. „ t "- value student test;

In this way, through specific methods and techniques of scientific research we can support assertions concerning the homogeneity of the group and veracity of data and information.

Table 1. The value of determined parameters - 50 m sample

Nr. crt.	determined parameter	Initial test	Final test
1	arithmetic mean	8,51"	8,35"
2	The Sum of deviations from the arithmetic mean	6,7"	6,0"
3	Variance	0,61	0,55
4	standard deviation	0,78	0,74
5	Coeficient of variation	9,16	8,86
6	Student test	2,60	2,47

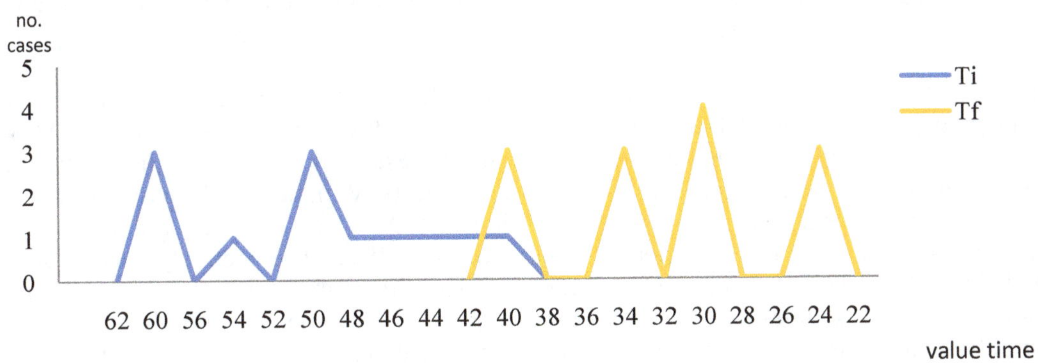

Figure 1. Representation of the distribution of the results according to the values from initial testing to final testing

In the speed running test - 50 m with standing start, the arithmetic mean between two test results achieved by the experimental group shows an increase of 1.6 tenths of a second, in six cases the progress being 2 tenths. The coefficient of variation / variability has values of 9.16 and 8.86 is below 10, suggesting a lower dispersion and a high homogeneity of the group. „ T test "has a calculated value of 2.60, 2.47 respectively. At a significance level of 0.05 and a confidence level of 95%, the value of„ t "critical, according to student test while the group of 12 people is 2.20. „ T test calculated values "means that there are more than 95% chance that the effect is the consequence of the underlying causes and not accidental. In this case the null hypothesis is rejected and the working hypothesis admitted.

Table 2. Value of parameters determined in the test of 10 x 4 m lateral displacement

Nr. crt.	determined parameter	Initial Test	Final Test
1	arithmetic mean	15,9”	15,6”
2	The Sum of deviations from the arithmetic mean	12	12
3	Variance	1,09	1,09
4	standard deviation	1,04	1,04
5	Coeficient of variation	6,54	6,67
6	student test	3,48	3,48

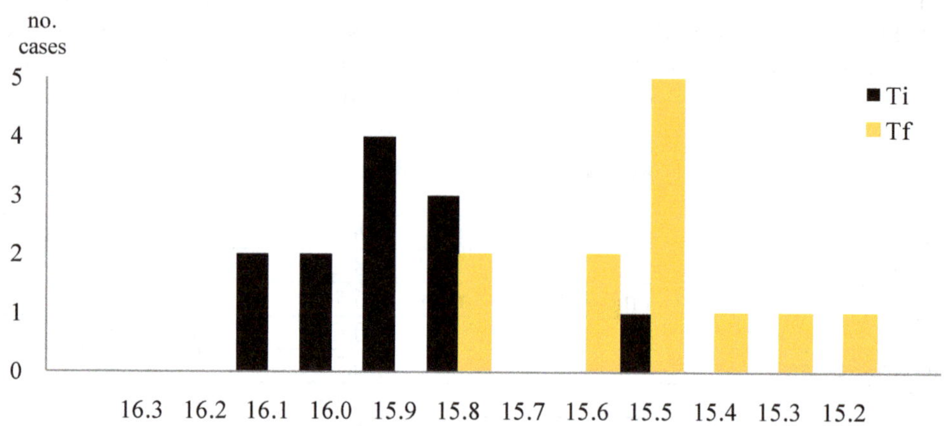

Figure 2. Representation of the distribution of the results from the experimental group initial testing and final test 10 x 4 m lateral shift

In the test of 10 x 4 m lateral displacement, of specific speed, the average of the results of the experimental group increased between the two tests with three-tenths, respectively 1.92% (Table 10.2). There is an increase in the block data seen in the results as the sum of the difference of the arithmetic mean is maintained the same through the two tests. Variation of the experimental group is 1.09 in the initial testing, being maintained in the final one. As a result the standard deviation is equal in the two tests of 1.04 and the coefficient of variation is 6.54% and respectively 6.67%. Both values being below 10% indicates a small dispersion of homogeneity of the large group. „ T "calculated has a value of 3.48 and is larger than „ t" critical for a group of 12 subjects, while the materiality / trust threshold of 0.01% is 3.11. In these circumstances, t "calculated is higher than„ t" critical for a significance threshold of 0.01% , the probability that the test results be the consequence of other variables, unchecked, is less than 1%. Therefore, the null hypothesis, considering that the results are the effect of experimental interventions as in the alleged assumptions. The curve distribution of values in the two tests is relatively normal for each test, with the mention that in the final testing it is shifted to the right, as a consequence of the results changes.

Table 3. Value of determined parameters in the test 10 x 4 m displacement Forward - backward

Nr. crt.	Parameter	Initial Test	Final Test
1	arithmetic mean	16,4”	16,1”
2	The Sum of deviations from the arithmetic mean	12”	12”
3	Variance	1,09	1,09
4	standard deviation	1,04	1,04
5	Coeficient of variation	6,09	6,45
6	student test	3,52	3,52

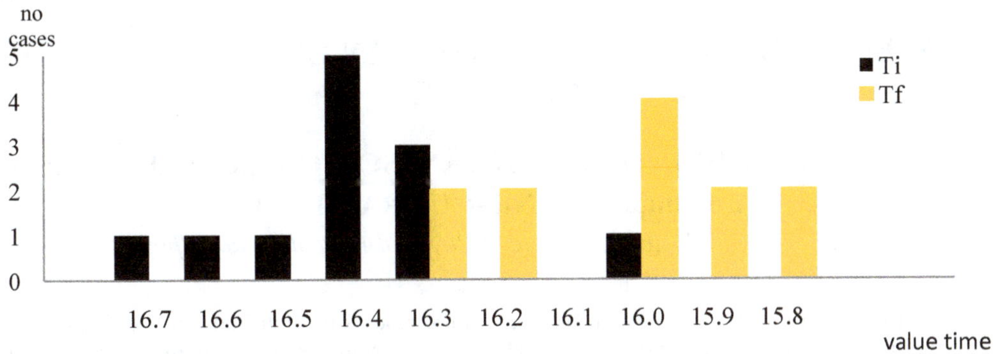

Figure 3. Representation of the results distribution from the experimental group initial and final test 10 x 4 m Forward - backward

Table 10.3 and 10.10 chart are given parameter values statistics in the test of 10 x 4 m Forward - backward and the distribution of results obtained by each member of the experimental group is plotted. We found the same trends as in the test described above: the arithmetic mean is growing from a test to another - 16.4 / 16.1 – the difference of individual values from the average is constant from a test to another - 1.2 / 1.2 sec., an aspect that makes a variation of 1.09 and standard deviation equal to a 1.04.

The coefficient of variation of 6.09 and 6.45 in the two trials indicate a low dispersion of values and a high homogeneity of the experimental group. Test,, t "calculated is 3.52, higher than,, t" critical for a significance threshold of 0.01%, which is 3.11. This means that the probability that the effect is due to other causes is less than 0.01%, which results in statistical confidence. This provides the basis for rejection of the null hypothesis and the admission of the assumptions as valid. The distribution of the values is normal for a selected group of athletes and shows at the same a trend shift to the right of the curve values as a result of growth in performance.

Conclusion

The developments in modern society in general and especially in sports performance lead to a general conclusion that continuous improvement is a requirement, a social and performance one. This involves development, upgrades and adaptations in multiple ways, including the promotion of scientific research in support of performance. The role of physical training was considered significant in recent years in many sports, especially team sports in the area, including the table tennis. This guidance was generated by changes in regulations and training of systemic vision on the training factors according to which, the expression of superior technical and tactical indices was not possible without motor qualities to sustain technical expression at the targeted performance levels.

Acknowledgement

All authors have equal contributions.

References

[1]. Grosser M., Kraft H., Schonborn R.,(2000), Speed training for tennis, Meyer&Meyer Sport, p.10

[2]. Kondric M., Milic R., Mandic G., 2007, Physiological anaerobic characteristics of slovenian elite table tennis players, Acta Univ. Palacki.Olomuc., Gymn., vol.37, no.3.

[3]. Tudor V., (2005), Măsurare şi evaluare în cultură fizică şi sport, edit. Alpha MDN, Buzău, p.108

[4]. Demeter A. (1981), Bazele fiziologice şi biochimice ale calităţilor fizice, Editura Sport–Turism, Bucureşti,p. 38

35

THE ROLE OF ASSOCIATED FACTORS IN LEARNING HANDBALL TECHNIQUE

Roberta Georgiana GHEŢU, Dorina ORŢĂNESCU, George Bogdan BURCEA, Luminiţa CĂLINESCU BRABIESCU

University of Craiova, Faculty of Physical Education and Sport.

Abstract: Performance in general, but also in handball is the result of a multitude of variables,with a highly degree of conditioning and mutual determination. The research starts from the premise that detecting and actuating correctly on progress or limiting factors, with a particular impact on learning is a viable solution to learning and perfecting technique. We appreciated that studying and assessing the level of expression of attention, memory and thought in the process of learning the technique in handball, is an enlightening approach of their effectiveness on learning.

Methods - Applying a set of attention tests, memory and thought on a group of junior children III, which followed a learning program, we aim to highlight the correlations between the level of learning the technique and the quality of investigated factors.

Results - Data analysis reveals significant differences obtained by the experiment group in appropriation of the concerned techniques after the program run. Direct correlations can be made between the investigated factors and the quality properties of the technique, sometimes with significant differences on groups of stations.

Keywords: learning, program, technique, factors.

Introduction

Competitions highlight certain aspects that characterize the conduct of handball. One can appreciate that handball exhibits dynamic, influenced and defined by the level of expression posed at a certain time given by some conditionings that can be likely methodical, organizational or regulation.

Sports performance dynamics of the game of handball require knowledge of development trends, design features of the game but also the elements of progress or limiting. All these are essential requirements underlying conception, orientation and training of sporting achievement.

Choosing this theme is primarily due to my professional concerns, to understand and effectively address the problems encountered, however, and based on accumulated scientific and methodical knowledge.

The performance athlete is a complex entity, with strong psychomotor peculiarities and often contradictory. It is necessary to outline the idea that there is a difference between athletes, in terms of ability to execute proper technique and specific efficiency especially during the game.

The necessity of finding solutions to streamline the work of athletes in order to increase the efficiency in preparation aiming the qualitative and the temporal component of learning, motivated me to conceive and realize this approach, willing to make our contribution to optimize the conceptual and practical technical training in handball the junior level III.

We believe that the investigation that we propose assumes importance in the context of the discussion the level of the handball player (with psychical abilities and driving records through evaluative criteria) comparable with a model internationally expressed.

Being aware of determinations between theoretical research and practical work, by addressing to the topic of handball performances, we wanted to highlight the importance of operation based on a concept of training, accessing knowledge from the biological sciences, pedagogical, psychological and health representing an inspirational source, but also a guarantee of a stingent election of means and methods to be applied.

It is known that the demands of training and competition can only be coped by athletes who have the ability to accumulate technical and tactical knowledge, corresponding to its level of use and efficiency. They pose a higher bio-motric potential developed and a proper motivation an applicant going through the process of preparing . The major concern in developing variable preparation and in particular the technical one was to realize a project of scientifically based training, where the instructional objectives to be realistic and in accordance with the level of players applying a methodology for adequate training of this level, assessment and reassessment of one of the regulating factors of the activity.

Regardless of the content, learning process involves a chain of mechanisms which are included in two categories: instrumental-operators and motivational. The first category includes attention, cognitive system which is consisting of perceptions, representations, imagination, memory, understanding and thinking and also creativity. In the second category are the needs, the aspirations, the emotional provisions, the inclinations and the desires. In the process of learning and training handball technique is recommended that the means which are used to be such as to require the greatest enrollment of tasks with a great coverage of attention. [1]

The role of memory and thinking and attention in learning the art handball:

Memory

As a process, the memory is considered a prerequisite,being a premise but aloso a product of other mental processes, being involved in all major human behavior: knowledgement, understanding, motor intelligence, creativity.[2] The study addresses the issue of memory from this perspective, trying to establish some parameters of subjects endowment concerning the manifestation of the memory based on learning technical process program.

Thinking

Thinking is a defining process for humankind because, as individuality it allows him to consciously act in solving the problems of adaptation to the environment and society. [3]Consequently, the learning and training process, in our case, handball, must comply the thinking development stages, by selecting the appropriate ways and means.

Attention

The role of attention in learning handball specific techniques:

In sports, attention is regarded as the most significant indicator of mental state since it is proved that attentin reflects cerebral energy levels, mental strength, tension characteristics, fatigue.[4]

In the process of learning and training handball technique is recommended that the means used to be such as to require the enrollment tasks with a great coverage of attention.

Material and methods

Casuistry research is consisted of two groups (experiment and control), their composition is as follows:

- experiment group, consisting of 16 players from C.S.Ș.Craiova Club, which fall in the category of juniors III and are activating in the National Junior and Schoolchildren Championships. In terms of age, subjects fall within juniors III, 12 to 14 years.
- control group, that followed its training program as the established schedule, was made up of athletes from C.S.M Craiova, working in the National Junior and Schoolchildren Championships, with age within the limits of 12- 14 years.

The working method consisted in establishing the level of acquiring the handball technique based on a compex assessment, control tasks, of on the one hand and the level of factors expression associated with learning (attention, memory, thinking) based on enlightening tests on the other hand.

Test "Focusing the attention" after G. Arădăvoaice

Test evaluation of memory "Attention to detail" adapted from Philip Carter

Test (adapted) for kinesthetic sensibility and motor memory

PORTEUS Maze

Establishing correlations between technical and drive ability and quality benchmarks of attention, memory and thinking of subjects.

Scientific nature of designing methodology of actuation means derives from using evaluative parameters and conditional factors of technique learning, taking into account both the physical development, motor ability, level of acquiring the handball technique and the qualitative benchmarks of attention, memory and thinking. In this regard, preliminary research aims identifying those factors in order to design a training program ment to interfere with objective stimuli on possible discrepancies found. Using the results of testing indicators a training program has being designed in order to positively affect attention, memory, thinking.

Means to optimize attention

Mean	Dosage
arranged in groups of three forwards at every semicircle, they pass the ball in high speed three times until the opposite semicircle, they pass the ball and they come back as defenders; the exercise is repeated by another group.	2x15 x,15 sec.rep.30 sec.series.
running 10 m with an opponent, achieving the steps that lead up throwing the ball, on a trail;	3x 3min, 1min break.
2x1, strikers, defender, sits striker support series. They are positioned to receive the ball;	2x15x,30 sec. break active defender
three forwards, two of them positioned to 9m with the ball, one player at semicircle. At signal, one passes to the player without the ball and catches, than passes again.	2x10x, 20sec break
the same exercise, a defender is inserted	2x15x,30 sec. break
1x1the players pass the ball with 2 hands from traveling the length of the field	1x10x
two players arranged at a distance of 3m from a wall perform passes by recoil.	2x15 x,20 sec.break
two players seated on 6m semicircle facing his own goal	2x10x,15 sec.p
at 9 m are two different color balls, the coach always changes their place. At signal the players run to recover their own ball.	

Means to optimize driving memory

Mean	Dosage
the players execute 2-3 structures of jumping variations, successive on 1 or 2 feet. At the order they must execute the structure.	5-6x
3 methods of throwing are demonstrated. The player shots on goal with an indicated process and the athlete evaluates the fairness.	5x3 p
the execution of individual actions on a trail 5-6x. Resuming execution on an unmarked trail in the same conditions.	2x8x
The players execute 2 technical processes of throwing proceeds (preceded by the cross and leap jump) encodes (A, B) preceding the indicated code execution the player must execute the process.	

Means for optimizing tactical thinking
all individual and collective tactical actions carried out opponents with varying degrees of adversity

Results

Analysis of the results obtained in these tests of attention, memory and thinking

Analysis of results from tests of attention

Table no.1

"Attention to detail" test values

Subjects	1	2	3	4	5	6	7	8	9	10	11	12	13	14	15	16
Experiment Gr.	5	4	5	5	5	5	7	5	6	7	4	4	6	5	6	7
Control Gr.	6	6	4	7	6	7	8	6	6	5	6	4	8	5	6	8

Table no.2

The analysis of the results of benchmark tests of memory

Subjects	1	2	3	4	5	6	7	8	9	10	11	12	13	14	15	16
Experiment Gr.	5	4	5	5	5	5	7	5	6	7	4	4	6	5	6	7
Control Gr.	6	6	4	7	6	7	8	6	6	5	6	4	8	5	6	8

Table nr.3

Motor memory and kinesthetic sensibility

Subjects	S1	S2	S3	S4	S5	S6	S7	S8	S9	S10	S11	S12	S13	S14	S15	S16
Exp. Gr.	41	40	39	35	44	40	35	37	43	44	46	37	49	45	43	40
Contr.Gr.	49	51	47	43	40	46	41	45	42	40	37	45	47	49	52	44

A. **Fairness tactical and technical execution test**

The following game structures have been consisted and denoted with a mark from 1-10 :

Evaluating procedures of throwing:

- thrust throw with a hand over the shoulder in jump;
- shot on goal from side angles from jump, with increasing the angle of throwing;

Passing processes evaluating:

- thrust pass with one hand above the shoulder;
-bounced pass;

B. Test for accuracy determination

The Handball Gate was bounded by adhesive tape in 9 areas, making each each subject to throw 6 times in each area and percentagely recording the achievements of each subject.

1	2	3
4	5	6
7	8	9

Test regarding motric memory

There have been developed 3 technical-tactical structures for attack and defense phase, the players have to play only the actions, at first execution.

Discussions

Results achieved by evaluation of precision and driving memory

Test accuracy - 1-5 zones Ti, Tf

Table no.4

	Zone 1 Ti	Zone 1 Tf	Zone 2 Ti	Zone 2 Tf	Zone 3 Ti	Zone 3 Tf	Zone 4 Ti	Zone 4 Tf	Zone 5 Ti	Zone 5 Tf
Arithmetic average	47.86	72.87	47.85	75.99	48.90	81.21	46.81	77.04	50.98	74.96
Standard deviation	13.36	11.99	14.69	12.15	12.80	13.46	13.83	13.45	12.80	13.62
CV	27.92	16.46	30.69	15.99	26.17	9.58	29.54	17.46	25.10	18.17
Ttest	-9.51*		-11.267*		-12.11*		-8.720*		-11.264*	

*p<0.05

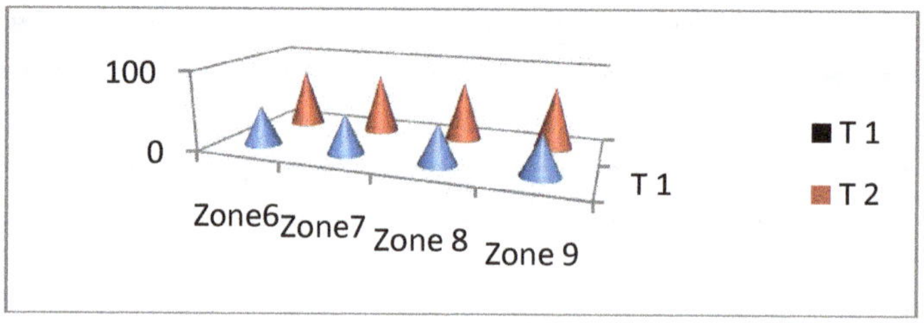

The tables present the initial and final test results that quantified the precision of the players through free throws on deliminated areas of handball gate. The recorded results have shown the following average values.

Zone 3 recorded a percentage of 48.90% successful throws at the initial testing and at the final testing, the accuracy of subjects increased to 81.21%. Differences averages are statistically significant at a threshold of p <0.05. This area (3) is the one that registered the best average of successful throws, actuating means applied to the experiment group especially relating to movements that influenced the throw-up, the players being educated to throw the ball in the moment of maximum acceleration. Also, the coefficient of variation has the lowest amount of throws at the final testing in this area, which means a high homogeneity of this sample group.

Throws in zone 9 first recorded an average of 48.89%, the handball players accuracy increasing to 78.08% at the final testing. Differences averages are statistically significant at a threshold of p <0.05.

Table no. 5

The results of the memory motor test

Statistical indicator	*Value*
Arithmetic average	1.06
Standard deviation	0.79
Min	0
Max	2

The test which aimed assessing the driving memory of the subjects from the experiment group revealed at the end of the research a good memory of the players, so the distribution channels being the following one:

- for the semicircle players, their motor memory was classified as "very good", four of them having no mistake in their execution;

- for the 9m players, their motor memory fall into the category of "good motor memory", 5 of them boasting one mistake and one with 2 mistakes;

-the gool-keepers also exhibit good motor memory, but the mistakes were in number of 2 for the players in this post.

Conclusions

Assessing the level of development of motor skills provide opportunities for effective technical executions, their loyalty being severely limited by the development of motor skills.

At the beginning of our research on technical plan, there have been manifested notable differentiations in the acquisition of handball technique in the experimental group, between the groups of players (9m and semicircle players) the difference between it and the control group evidently decreasing in the reasearch, the differences between the averages being statistically significant at a threshold of $p < 0.05$.

Targeting the preparation process by prioritizing specific executions led to the improvement of content in IV phase of the attack, the attack on the system.

Establishment of the manifestation of quality of mental processes based on tests (attention, memory, thinking), which formed the basis of elaborating working programs with a great degree of objectivity, led to a significant improvement of technology execution and to obtain right motric answers and appropriate game situations.

The driving systems placed in training programs had a custom content, which means they were folded on influencing determinants in acquiring art (fidelity in execution, attention, memory and thinking) and the players gaps were identified in a preliminary investigation .

References

[1]. Dragnea, A., C., Teodorescu-Mate, S., (2002), *Teoria Sportului*, Editura Fest, Bucureşti, pg77.

[2]. Epuran, M., Holdevici, I.,Toniţa, F., (2001), *Psihologia sportului de performanţă.Teorie şi Practică*, Editura Fest, Bucureşti, pg.38.

[3]. Epuran, M., Holdevici, I.,Toniţa, F., (2001), *Psihologia sportului de performanţă.Teorie şi Practică*, Editura Fest, Bucureşti, pg.39.

[4]. Orţănescu, D., Orţănescu, C., (2001), *Învăţarea motrică*, Editura Universitaria, Craiova, pg.58.

36

THE THERAPY WITH KINETIC TAPE APPLICATION IN PEDIATRIC RECOVERY

Andrei DUMITRU
Faculty of Sciences
Department of Kinethic Therapy and Medical Assistance
University of Pitesti
Correspondence address: padrefortete@yahoo.com

Abstract: OBJECTIVES. The purpose of this pilot study is to describe the use of the Kinesio Taping® method for the upper extremity in enhancing functional motor skills in children admitted into an acute rehabilitation program.

METHOD. Fifteen children (10 females and 5 males; 4 to 16 years of age), who were receiving rehabilitation services at the Rehabilitation Institute of Chicago participated in this study. For 13 of the inpatients, this was the initial rehabilitation following an acquired disability, which included encephalitis, brain tumor, cerebral vascular accident, traumatic brain injury, and spinal cord injury. The Melbourne Assessment of Unilateral Upper Limb Function (Melbourne Assessment) was used to measure upper-limb functional change prior to use of Kinesio Tape®, immediately after application of the tape, and 3 days after wearing tape. Children's upper-limb function was compared over the three assessments using analysis of variance.

RESULTS. The improvement from pre- to posttaping was statistically significant, $F(1, 14) = 18.9$; $p < .02$.

CONCLUSION. These results suggest that Kinesio Tape may be associated with improvement in upperextremity control and function in the acute pediatric rehabilitation setting. The use of Kinesio Tape as an adjunct to treatment may assist with the goal-focused occupational therapy treatment during the child's inpatient stay. Further study is recommended to test the effectiveness of this method and to determine the lasting effects on motor skills and functional performance once the tape is removed.

Key words: kineto band; occupational therapy; recovery; evaluation; case study; disabilities

Introduction

Kinesio Tape® is a relatively new technique used in rehabilitation programs to treat upper-arm or hand pain. Although it has been used in the orthopedic and sports settings, it is gaining acceptance as an adjunct in the treatment of other impairments. The use of Kinesio Taping® in conjunction with the child's regular therapy program may favorably influence the cutaneous receptors of the sensorimotor system resulting in subsequent improvement of voluntary control and coordination of the upper limb. Children admitted into an acute rehabilitation program receive intensive daily therapies during their inpatient stay. Important intervention objectives are to strengthen weakened muscles, to improve the quality and active range of motion, and to improve the child's level of independence with activities of daily living [1].

Kinesio Taping®, when applied properly, can theoretically improve the following: strengthen weakened muscles, control joint instability, assist with postural alignment, and relax an over-used muscle. Kinesio Tex™ is the brand name of the tape. The Kinesio Tex tape is more elastic compared to conventional rigid tape. The nonstretch rigid tape is used to limit unwanted joint movement or to protect and support a joint structure. However, data suggest that regular athletic tape does not restrict joint movement. Bragg et al. (2002) found that athletic tape loses its ability to restrict joint motion after 15–20 minutes of exercise. Therefore, the effects of taping may be due to the cutaneous stimulation of the sensorimotor and proprioceptive systems. Taping provides immediate sensorimotor feedback regarding functional abilities.

With the Kinesio Tape applied, patients often report symptom relief, improved comfort level, or stability of the involved joint. The elasticity of Kinesio Tape conforms to the body, allowing for movement. The tape is latex-free, very thin, and stretches in the longitudinal plane. Kinesio Tape has been suggested to provide proprioceptive input in the acute phase of the injury process for lateral ankle sprain. Healthy subjects with good proprioception did not benefit from patellar taping on the knee joint. However, patellar taping for those healthy subjects with poor proprioception appeared to enhance proprioception. The elastic quality and proprioceptive input as well as subtle biomechanical factors may account for the functional changes observed.

When the application procedure is followed correctly, the taped area can be used to facilitate a weakened muscle or to relax an overused muscle. The method for applying the tape varies depending on the specific goals: improve active range of motion, relieve pain, adjust misalignment, or improve lymphatic circulation .Theoretically Kinesio Tex is applied based on treatment goals. The variables in tape application include the amount of prestretch applied to the tape, position of the area to be taped, treatment goals (pain reduction, subcutaneous blood flow, improved muscle function). Unpublished data suggest that applying Kinesio Tex to areas most likely to affect blood circulation, superficial blood flow was increased in all cases where underlying neuromusculoskeletal pathology (pain, tingling, swelling in upper extremity, patella tendonitis, osteoarthritis, hypertension) was present but demonstrated no effect on blood flow in subjects who did not display any pathology. This limited case report suggests that Kinesio Taping may affect superficial blood flow in cases where pathology is present and have no effect on superficial blood flow measures on normal, healthy subjects [2].

Various taping approaches have been adapted to be used clinically in rehabilitation centers for patients who present with shoulder subluxation or shoulder pain. Taping can be used as an adjunct during the rehabilitation program to enhance functional recovery. For the treatment of anterior shoulder impingement, taping was applied to provide proximal scapular stability. The application of the scapular taping used in conjunction with a home exercise program provided relief of shoulder pain and improved overhead reach .

We started using Kinesio Taping at the Rehabilitation Institute of Chicago as an adjunct to therapy in 1998. Typically children who are admitted into an acute pediatric rehabilitation program at the Rehabilitation Institute of Chicago receive 3 hours or more of therapy throughout their inpatient stays. Prior to the intensive rehabilitation program, the Functional Independent Measure (FIM™) is used initially to measure functional outcomes during the length of the inpatient stay . The age range is from 8 years of age to adult and six domains are assessed: self-care, mobility, locomotion, sphincter control, communication, and social cognition. The WeeFIM® measures independent rating and the developmental level of the age of the child from 6 months to 7 years of age (Guide to the Uniform Data Set for Medical Rehabilitation for Children). The WeeFIM and the FIM present uniform data describing the severity of disability and the need for assistance. Both instruments are used as an initial evaluation to measure the basic functional abilities in the six domains prior to the initiation of the therapy program. By considering the child's developmental level and physical ability, intervention can be targeted at the essential skills component necessary for improved independence in self-care function . The therapy program may consist of a daily morning self care program, strengthening exercises through functional activities for the involved upper extremity, improvement of fine motor control, and coordination [3].

The secondary musculoskeletal effects of a neurological assault include muscle weakness or imbalance, pain, limited active and passive range of motion, and poor functional use. The treatment approach of taping is difficult to objectively measure as a viable tool to use to assist with promoting function of the upper extremity. Limited data exist to support the effectiveness of Kinesio Taping as an adjunct to treatment to facilitate attainment of functional motor skills. Therapists often use qualitative assessment tools to measure their results, including subjective clinical observation, anecdotal reporting, or descriptive terminology to assess upper-extremity movement quality. If evidence supports the use of taping this could ultimately justify the rationale for taping children with upper-extremity weakness.

The primary objective of this pilot study was to describe functional hand and arm skills in children admitted into a rehabilitation program subsequent to use of Kinesio Taping.

Method

Subjects

Fifteen children (5 males, 10 females, 4–16 years of age) admitted to the pediatric inpatient program at the Rehabilitation Institute of Chicago participated in this study. Informed consent was obtained from the guardians in accordance with the Institutional Review Board, which approved the study [4]. Study criteria included: decreased muscle strength of the upper extremity as measured by manual muscle testing (poor to fair range) and/or abnormal muscle tone interfering with functional movement as measured by the Modified Ashworth Scale (MAS). This study enrolled children admitted into the pediatric rehabilitation program with varied diagnoses (Table 1). However, all children demonstrated the inclusion criteria of muscle weakness and/or abnormal tone that interfered with upper-extremity functional use. Criteria for selection included children with enough motivation and cognition to follow direction to the Melbourne Assessment of Unilateral Upper Limb Function (Melbourne Assessment), and had no significant behavioral problems. The primary treating therapists recommended those children who were able to follow directions to task, appeared alert and oriented to their surroundings.

Children with dense sensory and motor loss (muscle grade at zero to trace) in the area to be taped were not eligible for the study. Children with significant spasticity on the MAS of 3 or 4 (3 representing considerable increase in tone, passive movement difficult and 4 representing affected parts rigid in flexion or extension) were also not eligible for inclusion as study participants.

Assessing clinical change in the upper extremity in children admitted into a rehabilitation program is a complex measurement task. The results of this study demonstrate that, despite the heterogeneity of the diagnoses in this study, the subjects presented with similar presenting causes for functional losses (muscle weakness and imbalance). The inclusion criteria were established to target children with decreased muscle strength; except for those who presented a muscle grade at zero to trace. The subjects were all evaluated by the same therapist to eliminate the variability found in manual muscle testing. Although this assessment was designed for children with neurological conditions, it was also used in this study for children with muscle weakness from orthopedic condition and/or spinal cord injury (SCI). The subjects in this study were listed by neurological impairments 1–9, and orthopedic and SCI 10–15 (Table 1). The test items of the Melbourne Assessment were taskspecific, which represented the most important components of arm and hand function (Table 2).

Measures

The Melbourne Assessment scores quality of upper-limb function based on 16 criterion-referenced items with 37 subscores, and consisting of 3-, 4-, and 5-point scales to record results. The Melbourne Assessment is an objective standardized measure evaluating the quality of upperextremity function of reach, grasp, release, and manipulation. Each subject's performance is recorded on a videotape for scoring. Each movement test item is subdivided into specific descriptive criteria and assigned a point scale. The raw scores are recorded on the score sheet and later converted to a percentage score (range 0% to 100%). A higher percentage score indicates better quality of arm and hand movements based on the specific test items [5].

The Melbourne Assessment was developed to measure function in children with cerebral palsy. The test–retest reliability of the Melbourne Assessment consisted of a study population of 20 children with cerebral palsy of varying types and severity and indicated that the Melbourne Assessment was highly reliable with the sample population. An initial reliability study resulted in the final 16 items. The development of the clinical test battery quantifies the quality of upper-limb function and demonstrates a strong relationship between the Melbourne Assessment and subjective judgment of the clinicians. Interrater, intrarater, and test–retest reliability were at a high level, indicating the Melbourne Assessment performs very reliably when used for the population it was intended.

Johnson et al. (1994) describes the evaluation of 11 children with cerebral palsy and found agreement with the clinical experts' and the children's score on the objective assessment [6]. By using statistical correlation analysis, the subjective judgment of the clinical experts established the concurrent validity in strong agreement.

Table 1. Physical Characteristic and Taped Areas of the Subjects

Subject Impairments	Sex	Age	Area Taped
1. R hemiplegia/encephalitis	F	4 yrs	forearm supination, triceps, finger extension, thumb extension, palmar stability
2. L hemiplegia/CVA	F	7 yrs	supination, wrist extension, thumb extension
3. L hemiplegia/ seizure	F	7 yrs	scapula stability, supination, encephalomyelitis, palmar stability
4. R hemiplegia/CVA, brain tumor	F	10 yrs	wrist extensor, palmar stability, thumb extension, scapular stability
5. R hemiplegia/brain tumor	F	12 yrs	scapular stability, supination, palmar stability
6. Traumatic brain injury	M	12 yrs	scapular stability, wrist extension, deltoid
7. R hemiplegia/Traumatic brain injury	M	16 yrs	scapula stability, deltoid, supination, palmar stability
8. R hemiplegia/brain stem CVA	M	12 yrs	back extensor, palmar stability thumb extension, postural correction
9. Generalized muscle weakness, cerebral palsy	M	14 yrs	wrist extension, palmar stability, deltoid, thumb extension
10. C2-C6 SCI lesion/brain tumor	F	8 yrs	wrist extension, thumb extension, palmar stability, scapular stability
11. Left shoulder arthritis/sickle cell disease, multifocal osteomyelitis,	F	11 yrs	scapula stability, deltoid
12. SCI C5-6 incomplete/tetraplegia	F	14 yrs	finger extensor, wrist stability
13. SCI C5-6 incomplete/tetraplegia	F	15 yrs	finger flexors, wrist extensors, scapula, deltoid
14. SCI C5-6 incomplete/tetraplegia	F	15 yrs	wrist extension, palmar stability, deltoid
15. SCI C6-7 incomplete/tetraplegia	M	16 yrs	finger flexor, thumb opposition, palmar stability

Note. C2–7 cervical spinal levels 2–7; CVA = cerebral vascular accident; L = left; R = right; SCI = spinal cord injury.

Table 2. Melbourne Assessment Test Items (Randall et al., 1999)

Items	Task
1	Reach forward
2	Reach forward to an elevated position
3	Reach sideways to an elevated position
4	Grasp of crayon
5	Drawing grasp
6	Release of crayon
7	Grasp of pellet
8	Release of pellet
9	Manipulation
10	Pointing
11	Reach to brush from forehead to back of neck
12	Palm to bottom
13	Pronation/supination
14	Hand to hand transfer
15	Reach to opposite shoulder
16	Hand to mouth and down

The evaluation validity of the Melbourne Assessment was used to determine sensitivity to change in the children's upper-limb function. The manual describes the study in detail and concludes that the instrument is significantly sensitive to measure change in function.

Bourke-Taylor (2003) investigated the performance on the Melbourne Assessment as it related to the child's ability to perform functional skills using the Pediatric Evaluation Disability Index (PEDI) [7]. The Melbourne Assessment is a criterion-referenced assessment with items that relate to a child's ability to perform daily living skills. A correlation study comparing the Melbourne Assessment and the PEDI demonstrated concurrent validity between the activities of daily living/self-care domain, the mobility domain, and overall performance on the PEDI. The results confirmed a strong correlation between the Melbourne Assessment as a measure for upper-limb function and functional living skills.

Procedure

Children identified as having upper-extremity movement problems interfering with function were evaluated with the Melbourne Assessment. To prevent bias and to examine inter-tester reliability in administering and scoring the Melbourne Assessment each child's performance was administered and scored by a qualified and experienced occupational therapist familiar with the requirements of each test item and the components of movements scored for each test. A certified occupational therapy assistant was trained to videotape the assessment, which was administered following the guidelines and specific instructions of the assessment.

The Melbourne Assessment was given prior to taping and immediately after application of the Kinesio Tex during the same session to prevent the subject from practicing the skills used in the assessment. The Melbourne Assessment was again administered after the child had worn the tape constantly for three days. The adhesive qualities and elasticity of the Kinesio Tex normally last 3–5 days. Because some children washed their hands frequently, subjecting the tape to excessive wear, the palmar stability tape application was reapplied daily.

An occupational therapist certified in the Kinesio Taping method evaluated the child's ability to use his or her upper extremity for performing functional task. The Kinesio Taping method was applied to assist with a weakened muscle and to improve joint stability and alignment as a means to assist the arm and hand in performing functional task. This therapist was involved only in the taping intervention phase and not the measurement phase of this pilot study [8].

Case Methodology. To illustrate the use of the Melbourne Assessment as a tool to evaluate upper-limb function and the qualitative decision making and processes underlying the application of Kinesio Tex, one subject's clinical case will be described.

A 12-year-old boy in previously good health was admitted to the acute-care hospital with pneumonia. A magnetic resonance image showed extensive areas of acute infarct involving the brain stem, basal ganglia, cerebellum, thalamus, and frontal lobe cortex. A percutaneous gastric tube was placed 1 month after the acute onset of symptoms and he was transferred to the Rehabilitation Institute of Chicago pediatric program. On initial evaluation he presented with spasticity right-sided involvement (lower extremity greater than upper extremity), and dysphagia. He was able to comprehend simple instructions and answered yes or no by a head nod. He was able to use a language board for communication and preferred to use his right hand for pointing.

The boy's right-arm function was evaluated with the Melbourne Assessment. He demonstrated full passive range of motion of both upper extremities. He exhibited mild spasticity of the right upper extremity with a Modified Ashworth Score of 1+ in the biceps and finger flexors slightly increased tone) and 2 in thumb flexors (more marked increase in tone, but affected parts are easily moved). He exhibited flexion of the thoracic-lumbar spine with a posterior pelvic tilt in sitting. He postured his head forward and down with his shoulders protracted. His active range of motion for overhead activities was limited due to decreased trunk stability and poor postural alignment.

During the testing session, he was seen in his wheelchair with the lateral trunk supports removed. He exhibited dystonic movement and overshooting when attempting to reach for items in front and to the side of him. Upon grasping, he was able to maintain the wrist in a neutral position, but he lacked fine finger prehension and used an immature mass grasp and release pattern (Figure 1). Prior to Kinesio Tape application he obtained a 57 out of a maximum possible score of 122 points (47%) on the Melbourne Assessment. The child's greatest difficulties appeared to be: poor trunk control and stability, poor alignment of the shoulder, decreased palmar stability for facilitating finger movements, and decreased thumb stability for thumb-finger prehension. This resulted in difficulty with maintaining a stable base of control for performing functional task such as writing, feeding portions of his meals, moderate assistance for oral and facial hygiene, and dressing [9].

Intervention: Kinesio Tex was applied from distal to proximal attachments of the erector spinae from L5 to T2 spinal level using 2-inch tape on both sides of the trunk to facilitate a functional upright position of the trunk while sitting in the wheelchair. A mechanical correction technique (tape is applied with downward pressure and pulling the elasticity out of portions of the tape as it is applied), was applied to the right protracted shoulder to assist with positioning the shoulder in neutral alignment. Tape was also applied to his right hand from the palm through his web space to provide palmar stability, support the arch, and to facilitate prehension. His thumb was taped to assist with thumb extension (Figure 2). During the initial session, the Melbourne Assessment was repeated immediately after the tape application, with a raw score of 61 (50%). Three days after wearing the Kinesio Tex, a third Melbourne Assessment was completed, resulting in a raw score of 61 out of 122 (50%). His inpatient program consisted of a daily self-care regimen, mat activities to improve trunk control and arm placement, and tabletop activities to improve fine motor skills.

Results

Means and standard deviations for the Melbourne Assessment before taping, immediately after taping, and 3 days of wearing the tape are presented in Table 3. Analysis of variance was used to compare the Melbourne Assessment scores across the 3 time periods. Overall, the Melbourne Scores improved over time, $F(2, 14) = 17.7$, $p < .001$. Further, the improvement from pre- to posttaping was statistically significant, $F(1, 14) = 18.9$, $p < .02$.

Discussion

The primary finding in this study was that the functional status of the upper limb as measured by the Melbourne Assessment improved following the application of Kinesio Tex. The Melbourne Assessment evaluates the ability of unilateral arm and hand function and provides detailed information regarding the child's ability and disability. Through measuring change, it appeared to be adequately sensitive to document the acute change associated with wearing the tape[12]. The items in the Melbourne Assessment were applicable to the population for whom it was developed, but it also appears to be an applicable measurement tool in children with muscle weakness from an orthopedic condition or SCI. Thus, the Melbourne Assessment may have a wider application than to the population with neurological impairment, a hypothesis that will require empirical testing. Potentially it could be used with children with muscle weakness and joint involvement or inflammation regardless of the medical diagnosis. This assessment appears to provide the sensitivity to measure change over time, particularly for children with joint involvement or inflammation and muscle weakness where changes and improvements may be very subtle.

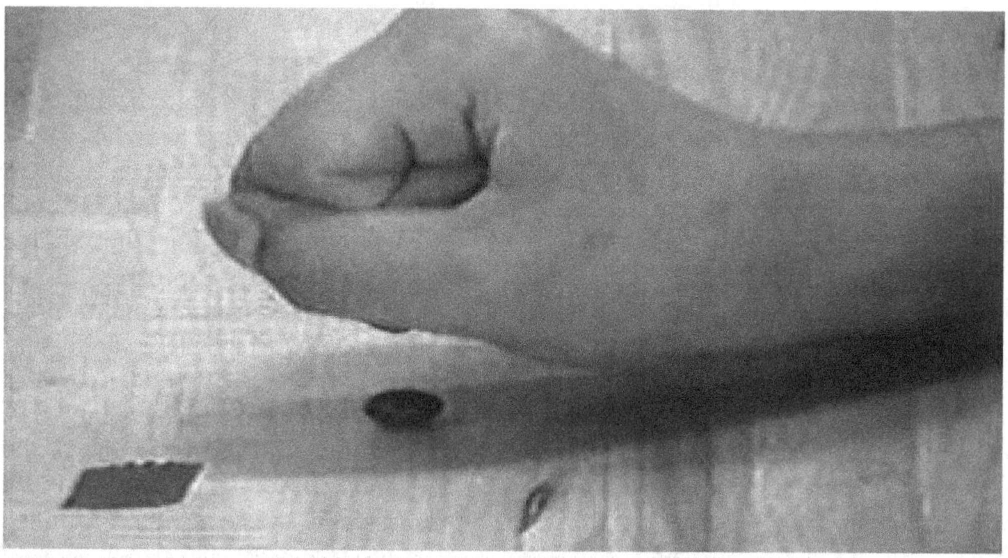

Figure 1. Grasp of pellet-item 7 of Melbourne Assessment.

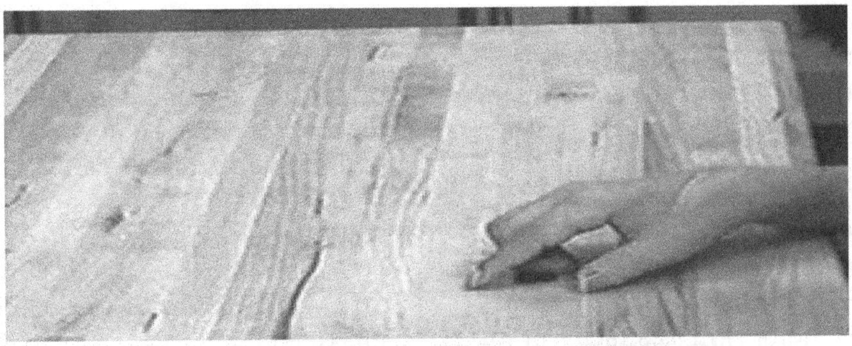

Figure 2. After taping—grasp of pellet-item 7 of Melbourne Assessment.

Table 3. Means and Standard Deviations for the Melbourne Assessment Before, Immediately After Taping, and 3 Days of Wearing the Tape

	Mean	Standard Deviation
Pretape	60.5	23.6
Posttape (immediate)	65.5	23.1
Follow-up (3 days' follow-up)	70.1	23.3

The Melbourne Assessment was able to detect subtle changes in upper-extremity control and movement quality in children that the parents and attending occupational therapist judged to have changed. Other studies have examined the effect of Kinesio Taping in normal subjects and found no difference in maximum leg press or in pain and function following maximal exercise and delayed onset muscle soreness in the taped and untaped conditions. The effects of Kinesio Taping may be so subtle as to be observed only in cases where movement disorders are present. Studies examining effects of the tape on normal subjects may not detect the subtle improvements in movement observed with the Melbourne Assessment. The use of the Kinesio Taping method appeared to have improved purposeful movement, provided needed stability of the shoulder and/or hand, and alignment to perform the task for reach, grasp, release, and manipulation [10].

Although this pilot study demonstrated an association between use of Kinesio Taping and treatment outcome, a number of additional studies are required (1) to determine the sensitivity of using the Melbourne Assessment in detecting small but clinically significant changes for children with SCI or orthopedic conditions, (2) to evaluate the responsiveness to giving the Melbourne Assessment over time to a controlled group, (3) to examine other assessment tools and to determine correlation with results obtained using the Melbourne Assessment, (4) to compare the use of Kinesio Taping application with a control group design to investigate the effectiveness of Kinesio Taping, and (5) to determine the lasting effects on motor skill performance once the tape has been removed.

Limitations

This study was a quasi-experimental design with pre- and postmeasure but no control group. Subject selection was a challenge in the clinical setting as well as the time frame in completing this pilot study. Clinically, this study demonstrated that the Kinesio Taping application may be associated with improvements in upper-extremity function. These improvements were noted as long as the tape was applied;

further studies should examine the duration of the effects once the tape has been removed. The Melbourne Assessment detected a gradient of performance change with Kinesio Taping. After performing the initial assessment the child was then immediately taped and reassessed to prevent any motor learning effects on task familiarization [11]. This eliminates practice of the motor skill as a factor in for the probable change in the quality of arm movement. The natural recovery of children who present with different diagnoses such as SCI posttrauma and a child with brain-based diagnoses may be very different. The immediate change in both diagnostic groups seen after the application of the tape may potentially be attributed to the sensory input provided by the Kinesio Tape, although without a control group no definitive conclusion can be drawn. However, these children are receiving multiple interventions during their inpatient stay, many also likely receiving medications, and one cannot rule out maturation and normal recovery from central nervous system and orthopedic conditions. The continued improvement in upper-limb functional skills observed on day 3 may be the combination of the sensorimotor input of the tape, the continued therapy program, or the natural recovery that is likely occurring at the same time spontaneously.

Conclusion

This change associated with use of Kinesio Taping emerged after 3 days' post-intervention, and is not a long enough assessment of the outcome to support the widespread use of this intervention. However, this pilot study investigated the initial outcome of taping that could ultimately provide the basis for a controlled study to support and document changes in relation to using the Kinesio Taping technique over longer periods. As clinicians we have an obligation to evaluate new treatment techniques with objective measures for assessing change in function. Taping a child's upper extremity can be crucial for participation in activities of daily living, and thus a primary concern to practioners working with children to optimize areas of self-care.

References

[1]. Sbenghe, T. (2002) *Kinesiologie-Ştiinţa mişcării*, Ed. Medicală, Bucureşti, pp. 105-112

[2]. Dragnea, A., Bota Aura, (1999), *Teoria activităţilor motrice*, Editura Didactică şi Pedagogică, Bucureşti, pp. 158-160

[3]. Drăgan, I.,(2002),*Medicina sportivă*. Bucureşti, Ed. Medicala, pp. 152-155

[4]. Grosu, Emilia, (2001) *Învăţarea motorie şi performanţa în sport*, Editura GMI, Cluj-Napoca, pp. 99-102

[5]. Plas, F.,Hangon,E., (2001), *Kinetoterapie activă*. Iaşi, Ed. Polirom, p. 189

[6]. Johnson, L. M., Randall, M. J., Reddihough, D. S., Oke, L. E., Byrt, T. A., & Bach T. M. (1994). Development of a clinical assessment of quality of movement for unilateral upper limb function. *Developmental Medicine & Child Neurology*, vol.36, 965–973.

[7]. Bourke-Taylor, H. (2003). Melbourne assessment of unilateral upper limb function: construct validity and correlation with the pediatric evaluation of disability inventory. *Developmental Medicine & Child Neurology*, vol.45, 92–96.

[8]. Cordun, M., (1995), *Mijloacele kinetoterapeutice în afecţiunile abdomino-ginecologice,* Bucureşti, Ed. Caritas, p. 89

[9]. Cordun, M., (1998), *Kinetologie medicală*. Bucureşti, Ed. Axa, p. 143

[10]. Sbenghe, T., (1999), *Bazele teoretice şi practice ale kinetoterapiei*. Bucureşti, Ed. Medicală, pp. 164-172

[11]. Câmpeanu Melania, (2000), *Gimnastica ritmică sportivă*, Editura Risoprint, Cluj-Napoca pp. 123-125

[12]. Sbenghe T.(1987) „*Kinetoterapia profilactica, terapeutica si de recuperare*", Editura Medicala, Bucuresti, pp. 166-169

PERMISSIONS

 Every chapter published in this book has been scrutinized by our experts. Their significance has been extensively debated. The topics covered herein carry significant findings which will fuel the growth of the discipline. They may even be implemented as practical applications or may be referred to as a beginning point for another development.

The contributors of this book come from diverse backgrounds, making this book a truly international effort. This book will bring forth new frontiers with its revolutionizing research information and detailed analysis of the nascent developments around the world.

We would like to thank all the contributing authors for lending their expertise to make the book truly unique. They have played a crucial role in the development of this book. Without their invaluable contributions this book wouldn't have been possible. They have made vital efforts to compile up to date information on the varied aspects of this subject to make this book a valuable addition to the collection of many professionals and students.

This book was conceptualized with the vision of imparting up-to-date information and advanced data in this field. To ensure the same, a matchless editorial board was set up. Every individual on the board went through rigorous rounds of assessment to prove their worth. After which they invested a large part of their time researching and compiling the most relevant data for our readers.

The editorial board has been involved in producing this book since its inception. They have spent rigorous hours researching and exploring the diverse topics which have resulted in the successful publishing of this book. They have passed on their knowledge of decades through this book. To expedite this challenging task, the publisher supported the team at every step. A small team of assistant editors was also appointed to further simplify the editing procedure and attain best results for the readers.

Apart from the editorial board, the designing team has also invested a significant amount of their time in understanding the subject and creating the most relevant covers. They scrutinized every image to scout for the most suitable representation of the subject and create an appropriate cover for the book.

The publishing team has been an ardent support to the editorial, designing and production team. Their endless efforts to recruit the best for this project, has resulted in the accomplishment of this book. They are a veteran in the field of academics and their pool of knowledge is as vast as their experience in printing. Their expertise and guidance has proved useful at every step. Their uncompromising quality standards have made this book an exceptional effort. Their encouragement from time to time has been an inspiration for everyone.

The publisher and the editorial board hope that this book will prove to be a valuable piece of knowledge for researchers, students, practitioners and scholars across the globe.

LIST OF CONTRIBUTORS

Andrei Dumitru
Faculty of Sciences, Department of Kinethic Therapy and Medical Assistance, University of Pitesti

Anca Jianu
Universitatea Spiru Haret, Sos. Berceni, Nr. 24, Sector 4, Bucureşti

Alina Elena Albină and Constantin Albină
The University of Craiova, the Faculty of Physical Education and Sports, Romania

Sefa Sahan Birol, Elif Ustun and Veysel Temel
Karamanoglu Mehmetbey University, Physical Education and Sports High School, Karaman

H.C. Adrian Dragnea
University of Târgovişte

Cătălin Forţan, Gabriel Mangra, Camelia Vlăsceanu and Cătălin Popescu
University of Craiova

Constantin Albină and Alina Elena Albină
The University of Craiova, Faculty of Physical Education and Sports, Romania

Aurora Ungureanu - Dobre, Doru Stoica and Roxana Dumitru
University of Craiova, Faculty of Physical Education and Sports, Brestei Street, No. 156

Gheorghe Vergu
"Matei Basarab" National College of Informatics, Râmnicu Vâlcea, Henri Coanda Street, No. 21

Claudiu Cristian Teuşdea
Faculty of Physical Education and Sport, Spiru Haret Spiru Haret University

Florentina Popescu
Faculty of Physical Education and Sport Spiru Haret

Porfireanu Maria-Cristiana
Faculty of Physical Education and Academy of Economic Studies

Germina Cosma, Dorina Orţănescu, Ligia RUSU and Roxana Dumitru
University of Craiova, Faculty of Physical Education and Sport

Claudiu Cristian Teuşdea
Faculty of Physical Education and Sport, Spiru Haret Spiru Haret

Ali Gok, Sefa Sahan Birol, Elif Ustun and Mehmet Ali Horozoglu
Karamanoglu Mehmetbey University, Physical Education and Sports High School, Karaman, TURKEY

Mihai Cristian Negoescu and Sanda Toma Urichianu
Ecologic University of Bucharest

Florin Ţurcanu
Universitatea de Medicină şi Farmacie Tîrgu Mureş

Glicheria Dăian
University of Craiova

Razvan Busneag and Carmen Busneag
"Spiru Haret" University - Faculty of Physical Education and Sport, Specialisation: Kinethotherapy and special motricity

Veronica Minoiu
University of Craiova, Faculty of Physical Education and Sports, Romania

Elif Ustun, Veysel Temel and Sefa Sahan Birol
Karamanoglu Mehmetbey University, Physical Education and Sports High School, Karaman

Adin-Marian Cojocaru and Marilena Cojocaru
Spiru Haret University Bucharest, Faculty of Physical Education and Sport

George Cristian Cătună, Butu Ioana Maria and Simona Teodorescu Anemari
Faculty of Physical Education, Sport and Physical Therapy, Spiru Haret University, Berceni Road, nr. 24, sector 4, Bucharest

Diaconescu Dragoş and Dragomir Marian
Universitatea din Craiova, România

Germina-Alina Cosma, Marian Costin Nanu, Mihaela Păunescu and Forţan Cătălin
Faculty of Physical Education and Sport, Brestei Street, no.156, Craiova, România

Daniel Gheorghe and Paula Ivan
Faculty of Physical Education and Sport, Spiru Haret University, Berceni road no 24, Bucharest

Elena Buhociu
Spiru Haret University - Bucharest

Constantin Pehoiu
Valahia University of Târgovişte / Research Centre for Environmental Study, Habitat, Motor Activities and Leisure (Romania)

Dumitru Barbu and Doru Stoica
University of Craiova, Faculty of Physical Education and Sport, Craiova, Romania

Florin Neferu
University C-tin Brâncuşi, Tg.Jiu

Denisa Enescu Bieru, Mihaela Zăvăleanu, Luminiţa Brăbiescu Călinescu and Cătălin Forţan
Faculty of Physical Education and Sport, University of Craiova, Romania

Georgeta Ioana Gheorghe and Dan Gheorghe Păun
Spiru Haret University, Faculty of Physical Education and Sport

Ioan Laurian Păun
Str. Barbu Lăutaru No.10, Brasov School No.1

Mihai Cristian Negoescu
Moldova State University, Faculty of Psychology and Educational Sciences

Ioana Maria Buţu, Simona Anemari Teodorescu and George Cristian Cătună
Faculty of Physical Education, Sport and Physical Therapy, Spiru Haret University, Berceni Road, nr. 24, sector 4, Bucharest

Ilona Ilinca, Eugenia Rosulescu and Mircea Danoiu
University of Craiova, Faculty of Physical Education and Sport, Craiova

Ilona Ilinca and Eugenia Rosulescu
Neuromotor Adults Rehabilitation Center St. Maria, Craiova

Dănut Stoica
University of Physical Education and Sport, Chişinău, Republica Moldova

Valeriu Jurat
University of Physical Education and Sport, Chişinău, Republica Moldova

Dragoş Diaconescu, Eliana Lică, Marian Dragomir and Laurenţiu LICĂ
University of Craiova

Roberta Georgiana Gheţu, Dorina Orţănescu, George Bogdan Burcea and Luminiţa Călinescu Brabiescu
University of Craiova, Faculty of Physical Education and Sport

Index

www.ingramcontent.com/pod-product-compliance
Lightning Source LLC
LaVergne TN
LVHW080654210926
848485LV00003B/374